Breast Pathology: Diagnosis and Insights

Guest Editors

STUART SCHNITT, MD
SANDRA J. SHIN, MD

SURGICAL PATHOLOGY CLINICS

surgpath.theclinics.com

Consulting Editor
JOHN R. GOLDBLUM, MD

September 2012 • Volume 5 • Number 3

SAUNDERS an imprint of ELSEVIER, Inc.

W.B. SAUNDERS COMPANY
A Division of Elsevier Inc.

1600 John F. Kennedy Boulevard • Suite 1800 • Philadelphia, Pennsylvania 19103-2899

http://www.surgpath.theclinics.com

SURGICAL PATHOLOGY CLINICS Volume 5, Number 3
September 2012 ISSN 1875-9181, ISBN-13: 978-1-4557-3942-4

Editor: Joanne Husovski

Surgical Pathology Clinics (ISSN 1875-9181) is published quarterly by Elsevier Inc., 360 Park Avenue South, New York, NY 10010. Months of issue are March, June, September, and December. Business and Editorial Office: Elsevier Inc., 1600 John F. Kennedy Blvd., Ste. 1800, Philadelphia, PA 19103-2899. Accounting and Circulation Offices: Elsevier Inc., 3251 Riverport Lane, Maryland Heights, MO 63043. Periodicals postage paid at New York, NY and at additional mailing offices. Subscription prices are $184.00 per year (US individuals), $212.00 per year (US institutions), $91.00 per year (US students/residents), $230.00 per year (Canadian individuals), $240.00 per year (Canadian Institutions), $230.00 per year (foreign individuals), $240.00 per year (foreign institutions), and $112.00 per year (international & Canadian students/residents). Foreign air speed delivery is included in all *Clinics'* subscription prices. All prices are subject to change without notice. **POSTMASTER:** Send address changes to *Surgical Pathology Clinics*, Elsevier, 3251 Riverport Lane, Maryland Heights, MO 63043. Customer Service: 1-800-654-2452 (US). From outside the United States, call 1-314-447-8871. Fax: 1-314-447-8029. E-mail: JournalsCustomerServiceusa@elsevier.com (for print support) and JournalsOnlineSupport-usa@elsevier.com (for online support).

Reprints. For copies of 100 or more, of articles in this publication, please contact the Commercial Reprints Department, Elsevier Inc., 360 Park Avenue South, New York, NY 10010-1710. Tel. (212) 633-3812; Fax: (212) 462-1935; E-mail: reprints@elsevier.com.

Contributors

CONSULTING EDITOR

JOHN R. GOLDBLUM, MD
Chairman, Professor of Pathology, Department
of Anatomic Pathology, Cleveland Clinics
Lerner College of Medicine, Cleveland Clinic,
Cleveland, Ohio

GUEST EDITORS

STUART J. SCHNITT, MD
Professor, Department of Pathology,
Harvard Medical School, Director,
Anatomic Pathology, Beth Israel Deaconess
Medical Center, Boston, Massachusetts

SANDRA J. SHIN, MD
Chief, Breast Pathology; Director,
Comprehensive Breast Pathology Consultation
Service, Department of Pathology and
Laboratory Medicine, New York-Presbyterian
Hospital—Weill Cornell Medical College,
New York, New York

AUTHORS

ROLA H. ALI, MD, FRCPC
Fellow, Department of Pathology, University
of British Columbia and Consultant Pathologist,
BC Cancer Agency, Vancouver, British
Columbia, Canada

ALESSANDRO BOMBONATI, MD
Assistant Professor, Department of Pathology,
Thomas Jefferson University Hospital,
Philadelphia, Pennsylvania

LAURA C. COLLINS, MD
Associate Professor of Pathology, Associate
Director, Division of Anatomic Pathology, Beth
Israel Deaconess Medical Center, Harvard
Medical School, Boston, Massachusetts

**ANASTASIA CONSTANTINIDOU, MD, MSc,
MRCP**
Research Fellow, Division of Molecular
Pathology, Institute of Cancer Research,
Sutton, United Kingdom

TIMOTHY M. D'ALFONSO, MD
Department of Pathology and Laboratory
Medicine, New York-Presbyterian Hospital—
Weill Cornell Medical College, New York,
New York

DEBORAH DILLON, MD
Assistant Professor of Pathology, Department
of Pathology, Harvard Medical School, Brigham
and Women's Hospital, Boston, Massachusetts

**MALCOLM M. HAYES, MMed Path,
FRCPath, FRCPC**
Clinical Professor of Pathology, Department of
Pathology and Laboratory Medicine, University
of British Columbia and Consultant
Pathologist, BC Cancer Agency, Vancouver,
British Columbia, Canada

BROOKE HOWITT, MD
Department of Pathology, Brigham and
Women's Hospital, Harvard Medical School,
Boston, Massachusetts

NICOLE B. JOHNSON, MD
Staff Pathologist and Instructor in Pathology, Department of Pathology, Beth Israel Deaconess Medical Center, Harvard Medical School, Boston, Massachusetts

ROBIN L. JONES, BSc, MB, MRCP
Associate Professor, Division of Medical Oncology, Fred Hutchinson Cancer Research Center, University of Washington, Seattle, Washington

JENNIFER S. KAPLAN, MD
Department of Pathology, Beth Israel Deaconess Medical Center, Harvard Medical School, Boston, Massachusetts

MELINDA F. LERWILL, MD
Assistant Pathologist, James Homer Wright Pathology Laboratories of the Massachusetts General Hospital; Assistant Professor, Department of Pathology, Harvard Medical School, Boston, Massachusetts

SUSAN C. LESTER, MD, PhD
Assistant Professor, Harvard Medical School; Associate Pathologist, Chief of Breast Pathology Services, Department of Pathology, Brigham and Women's Hospital, Boston, Massachusetts

AMY LY, MD
Instructor of Pathology, Department of Pathology, Harvard Medical School, Brigham and Women's Hospital, Boston, Massachusetts

ALESSANDRA F. NASCIMENTO, MD
Department of Pathology, Baptist Hospital of Miami, Miami, Florida

MARIANNA PHILIPPIDOU, Bsc, MBBS, FRCPath
Consultant Histopathologist, Department of Histopathology, King's College Hospital NHS Foundation Trust, Denmark Hill, London, United Kingdom

SARAH E. PINDER, MB, CHB, FRCPath
Professor of Breast Pathology, Research Oncology, Division of Cancer Studies, King's College London, Guy's and Thomas' Foundation Trust, London, United Kingdom

JORGE S. REIS-FILHO, MD, PhD, FRCPath
Department of Pathology, Memorial Sloan-Kettering Cancer Center, New York, New York

SUNATI SAHOO, MD
Associate Professor, Department of Pathology, UT Southwestern Medical Center, Dallas, Texas

STUART J. SCHNITT, MD
Department of Pathology, Beth Israel Deaconess Medical Center, Harvard Medical School, Boston, Massachusetts

SANDRA J. SHIN, MD
Chief, Breast Pathology; Director, Comprehensive Breast Pathology Consultation Service, Department of Pathology and Laboratory Medicine, New York-Presbyterian Hospital—Weill Cornell Medical College, New York, New York

Contents

> The purpose of this review is to discuss the less common variants and mimics of ductal carcinoma in situ (DCIS). DCIS lesions are heterogeneous in clinical presentation and behavior, morphology, biomarker profile, and identified genetic aberrations. DCIS is most easily recognized when presenting with classical features. The diagnosis is more challenging when a lesion displays less common cytologic features and has architectural patterns that overlap with other benign or malignant entities.

> Invasive lobular carcinoma of the breast is a distinct histologic type with specific clinical, radiologic, and microscopic features, which is increasing in incidence in the Western World. Routine pathologic prognostic factors, including grade, lymph node stage, and size are of significance in predicting outcome in this group of patients who, overall, have survival comparable to those with other subtypes of breast cancer. Variants, however, are seen and these, as well as other standard factors such as histologic grade, have prognostic significance and should be recorded in pathology reports.

> Some inflammatory and reactive lesions of the breast present problems clinically but are treated without resort to biopsy. In others, biopsy is required to make the correct diagnosis and to distinguish the process from malignancy. Still others represent incidental microscopic findings that may create diagnostic problems. This article reviews a number of inflammatory and reactive conditions that are likely to be encountered in routine surgical pathology practice, as well as those that have been recently described.

> This article discusses the most common small glandular proliferations, namely sclerosing lesions (sclerosing adenosis and radial scar), tubular carcinoma, and epithelial displacement after needle core biopsy, as well as less common entities, such as low-grade adenosquamous carcinoma, microglandular adenosis, and syringomatous adenoma. Due to significant morphologic overlap, these entities are easily mistaken for one another. The similarities and differences among these lesions in their clinicopathologic features, radiologic findings, and immunohistochemical profiles are emphasizesd.

> Vascular lesions represent a minority of tumors originating in the breast. The most common entities are benign and include hemangiomas and angiolipomas. Malignant

vascular lesions (angiosarcomas) are rare and may be primary or secondary to radiation. Also appreciated in association to radiotherapy is the development of cutaneous atypical vascular lesion affecting the skin of the breast. The relationship of the latter to radiation-associated angiosarcoma is controversial and remains to be elucidated. This article reviews the most likely encountered vascular lesions in the breast, with emphasis on key pathologic diagnostic features and potential diagnostic pitfalls.

Epithelial-myoepithelial proliferations of the breast are a heterogeneous poorly defined group of lesions characterized morphologically by dual differentiation into ductal (luminal) and myoepithelial cells. They include neoplastic and non-neoplastic entities that have overlapping morphologic features that may give rise to diagnostic difficulty. Many of these entities are low grade or of uncertain malignant potential but the biology of some of these rare lesions remains to be elucidated. This article discusses the differential diagnosis of epithelial-myoepithelial lesions of the breast and highlights the morphologic features of some of these entities.

This article reviews the conceptual and practical implications of the intrinsic subtype classification of breast cancers and the limitations of this approach. It presents the most extensively validated gene expression assays proposed as predictors of clinical outcome and discusses their potential clinical utility and limitations.

Breast cancer is a common source of systemic metastatic disease. Distinguishing metastatic breast cancer from other types of malignancies can be diagnostically challenging but is important for correct treatment and prognosis. Nonmammary tumors can also metastasize to the breast, although this is a rare phenomenon. Differentiating a metastasis to the breast from a primary breast cancer can likewise be difficult. Knowledge of the clinical history and careful morphologic evaluation are the cornerstones of diagnosis. A panel of immunohistochemical stains tailored to the differential diagnosis at hand can provide helpful information in ambiguous cases.

Neoadjuvant therapy (NAT) originally reserved for the treatment of inflammatory and locally advanced breast cancers is currently offered to women with earlier-stage and operable breast carcinoma. NAT allows more women to be eligible for breast conservation surgery and provides an opportunity to assess the response of carcinomas to therapy. This review focuses on the predictors of therapeutic response in pretreatment tumor, evaluation of post-treatment breast and lymph node specimens and classification systems to evaluate degree of response to NAT.

At the time of breast cancer diagnosis, multiple features of the tumor are routinely assessed to evaluate for prognostic and predictive factors. Prognostic factors provide information about the patient's likely clinical course and include tumor stage (composed of lymph node status, tumor size, and presence of chest wall involvement), tumor histologic type and grade, estrogen and progesterone receptor expression, and HER2 status. These traditional prognostic factors are reviewed with particular attention to problematic areas in classification. Several newer prognostic tests may be able to provide information beyond the traditional prognostic factors and are presented.

SURGICAL PATHOLOGY CLINICS

RELATED INTEREST

MRI Clinics, May 2010
Breast MRI
Linda Moy, and Cecilia L. Mercado, *Guest Editors*

DOWNLOAD
Free App!

Review Articles
THE CLINICS

NOW AVAILABLE FOR YOUR iPhone and iPad

Preface
Breast Pathology: Diagnostic Dilemmas

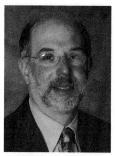
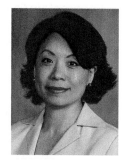

Stuart J. Schnitt, MD   Sandra J. Shin, MD
Guest Editors

We are pleased to serve as guest editors for this issue of *Surgical Pathology Clinics* focusing on breast pathology. This issue should be viewed as a companion to the 2009 issue of *Surgical Pathology Clinics* entitled "Current Concepts in Breast Pathology" and edited by Dr Laura Collins. Given that there are no overlaps in topics between these two issues, together they provide a more comprehensive review of contemporary issues in breast pathology than either alone.

In this issue, you will find reviews written by leading experts in breast pathology that deal with diagnostic and differential diagnostic considerations in less common variants and mimics of DCIS, invasive lobular carcinoma and its variants, inflammatory and reactive lesions, small glandular proliferations, vascular lesions, metastases to and from the breast (including the uses and limitations of adjunctive immunostains to arrive at the correct diagnosis), and combined epithelial-myoepithelial lesions. In addition, there are reviews addressing several timely topics in breast pathology including the evaluation of breast specimens from patients treated with neoadjuvant therapy, the molecular classification of breast cancer, and prognostic factors (including both traditional prognostic factors and newer, molecular-based prognostic tests). The text of the articles is complemented by high-quality photomicrographs as well as tabular summaries of diagnostic features, differential diagnostic issues, and pitfalls, where appropriate.

We hope that you find the articles in this issue of *Surgical Pathology Clinics* both highly informative and useful in the daily practice of breast pathology.

Stuart J. Schnitt, MD
Beth Israel Deaconess Medical Center
and Harvard Medical School
Department of Pathology
330 Brookline Avenue
Boston, MA 02215, USA

Sandra J. Shin, MD
New York Presbyterian Hospital-Weill
Cornell Medical College
Department of Pathology and
Laboratory Medicine
525 East 68th Street
New York, NY 10065, USA

E-mail addresses:
sschnitt@bidmc.harvard.edu (S.J. Schnitt)
sjshin@med.cornell.edu (S.J. Shin)

Surgical Pathology 5 (2012) ix
http://dx.doi.org/10.1016/j.path.2012.06.011
1875-9181/12/$ – see front matter © 2012 Elsevier Inc. All rights reserved.

LESS COMMON VARIANTS AND MIMICS OF DCIS

Nicole B. Johnson, MD*, Laura C. Collins, MD

KEYWORDS

- Ductal carcinoma in situ • Unusual variants • Mimics of DCIS

ABSTRACT

The purpose of this review is to discuss the less common variants and mimics of ductal carcinoma in situ (DCIS). DCIS lesions are heterogeneous in clinical presentation and behavior, morphology, biomarker profile, and identified genetic aberrations. DCIS is most easily recognized when presenting with classical features. The diagnosis is more challenging when a lesion displays less common cytologic features and has architectural patterns that overlap with other benign or malignant entities.

OVERVIEW

DCIS is defined as a proliferation of neoplastic epithelial cells confined to the mammary ducts and lobules by a myoepithelial cell layer and basement membrane. DCIS lesions are heterogeneous in clinical presentation and behavior, morphology, and biomarker profile as well as in the genetic aberrations that have been identified. DCIS is most easily recognized when presenting with classical architectural features, such as cribriforming, and a monotonous cellular proliferation. The diagnosis may be more challenging when the lesion displays less common cytologic features and has architectural patterns that overlap with other benign or malignant entities. The purpose of this article is to review the less common variants of DCIS as well as some of the mimics of this heterogeneous group of lesions.

Key Features

- Ductal carcinoma in situ (DCIS) is most easily recognized when presenting with classical architectural features, such as cribriforming, and a monotonous cellular proliferation.

- The diagnosis of DCIS may be more challenging when a lesion displays less common cytologic features and has architectural patterns that overlap with other benign or malignant entities.

- The importance of recognizing DCIS with clear cell change is not as much in distinguishing the 2 variants, glycogen-rich DCIS and lipid-rich DCIS, from each other as in the knowledge that this cytoplasmic alteration can be seen in DCIS; thus, these lesions are able to be separated from other lesions they may mimic, such as lobular carcinoma in situ (LCIS), or even metastatic clear cell carcinomas, such as renal cell carcinoma or malignant melanoma metastatic to the breast.

GROSS FEATURES

The variants of DCIS that are discussed in this article do not have identifying features on gross examination, except perhaps cystic hypersecretory carcinoma, which may have grossly visible cystically dilated spaces, filled with sticky, colloid-like gelatinous material.[1,2]

The authors have no financial disclosures to report.
Department of Pathology, Beth Israel Deaconess Medical Center, Harvard Medical School, 330 Brookline Avenue, Boston, MA 02215, USA
* Corresponding author.
E-mail address: nbjohnso@bidmc.harvard.edu

Surgical Pathology 5 (2012) 529–544
http://dx.doi.org/10.1016/j.path.2012.06.001
1875-9181/12/$ – see front matter © 2012 Elsevier Inc. All rights reserved.

VARIANTS OF DUCTAL CARCINOMA IN SITU

Clear Cell DCIS

The clear cell DCIS group of lesions consists of DCIS variants that display some degree of cytoplasmic clearing (Fig. 1). Included are glycogen-rich DCIS and lipid-rich DCIS with the distinction between each based on the morphology and the contents of the cytoplasm. The importance of recognizing DCIS with clear cell change is not as much in distinguishing these 2 variants from each other as in the knowledge that this cytoplasmic alteration can be seen in DCIS; thus, these lesions are able to be separated from other lesions they may mimic, such as LCIS, or even metastatic clear cell carcinomas, such as renal cell carcinoma or malignant melanoma metastatic to the breast (Table 1).

The intraductal component of *glycogen-rich carcinoma* consists of neoplastic polygonal or columnar cells with clear cytoplasm and central or basally located nuclei primarily arranged in solid nests. The clear cytoplasm is due to the presence of glycogen, which can be confirmed by periodic acid–Schiff (PAS) staining and sensitivity to PAS with diastase digestion. This entity was originally described as having papillary architecture with tall clear cells, cytologically similar to the fetal breast bud epithelial cells of the 13-week human embryo, and somewhat similar to clear cell carcinomas of the female genital tract.[3,4] Glyocogen-rich DCIS lesions have been reported to have papillary (intracystic), solid, micropapillary, and cribriform growth patterns.[5–8]

Lipid-rich DCIS has neoplastic epithelial cells packed with lipid, imparting a foamy appearance to the cytoplasm conferring positive staining with oil red O.[9–11] The tumor cells of lipid-rich DCIS are arranged in an alveolar pattern with hobnailing of the cells.[12] Lipid-rich DCIS is PAS negative and thus can be distinguished from other clear cell DCIS lesions. Lipid-rich invasive carcinoma tends to be hormone receptor negative and more frequently human epidermal growth factor receptor

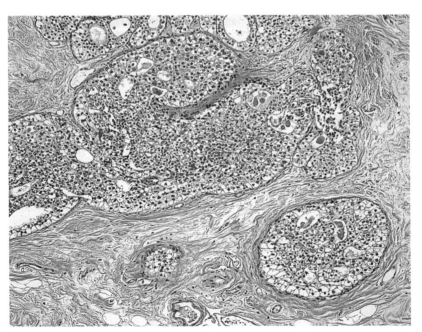

Fig. 1. DCIS with clear cells. Architectural atypia in the form of a cribriforming pattern is present. Nuclear atypia is also readily appreciated. The unusual feature in this example of DCIS is the cytoplasmic clearing. (*Courtesy of* Dr S. Schnitt.)

Table 1
Histochemical stains that may aid in the differentiation of clear cell DCIS

Variant of DCIS	PAS	PAS-d	Alcian Blue	Mucicarmine	Oil Red O	Other
Glycogen rich	+	−	−	−	−	Sudan black−
Signet ring	+	+	+	+	−	
Lipid rich					+	
Secretory	+	+	+	±	−	
Histiocytoid	+		+	+	−	
Apocrine	+	+				
Cystic hypersecretory				Focal+		
Spindle cell/endocrine	+	+	+	+		NSE+ Chromogranin+ Synaptophysin+

Abbreviation: PAS-d, PAS plus diastase.

2 (HER2) positive than invasive carcinoma of no special type.[12,13]

DCIS lesions that should be considered in the differential diagnosis of the aforementioned clear cell DCIS include secretory carcinoma, histiocytoid carcinoma, and signet ring cell carcinoma.

Secretory carcinoma is composed of neoplastic epithelial cells with abundant cytoplasmic secretory material as well as extracellular secretions, which are usually arranged in large cohesive nests. The cytoplasm may appear more eosinophilic and granular than the other clear cell variants.[14,15] In addition to the solid, nested growth pattern, these cells may have a cribriform intraductal growth pattern with rudimentary gland-like spaces.[16] Due to the nested growth pattern, distinction of the in situ from the invasive component can be challenging in secretory carcinomas without the aid of immunohistochemistry for myoepithelial cell markers. These tumors are typically estrogen and progesterone receptor and HER2 negative. Secretory carcinoma is unusual in that it may present in children.

The neoplastic cells of *histiocytoid carcinoma* have abundant foamy or ground glass cytoplasm with small or large vacuoles and eccentric small nuclei with small nucleoli. Rather than the bean-shaped nuclei of histiocytes, the nuclei of histiocytoid carcinoma are round. Most reports of histiocytoid carcinoma are of invasive lesions, which are thought to be a variant of lobular carcinoma or apocrine carcinoma. These cells may, however, be seen in a ductal pattern, supported by strong membranous staining with E-cadherin and the presence of an associated component of DCIS (**Fig. 2**).[17,18] On occasion the bland cytology of histiocytoid DCIS may mimic normal histiocytes contained within a ductal space (**Fig. 3**).

Signet ring cell carcinoma also exhibits clear cytoplasm; however, in contrast to glycogen-rich clear cell carcinomas and lipid-rich clear cell carcinomas, the nuclei of signet ring cell carcinoma are eccentrically located and compressed by the cytoplasm. In addition, the cytoplasm contains a mucin vacuole rather than glycogen or lipid. There has been much debate regarding the classification of signet ring cell carcinoma, in particular the invasive

Differential Diagnosis

Several mimics of DCIS occur and should be considered in the differential diagnosis of DCIS:

- Usual ductal hyperplasia (UDH)
  - Florid
  - Gynecomastoid hyperplasia
- LCIS
  - LCIS involving collagenous spherulosis
  - LCIS involving UDH
  - LCIS with comedo necrosis
  - Pleomorphic LCIS
- Invasive carcinoma
  - Invasive cribriform carcinoma
  - Adenoid cystic carcinoma
  - Invasive carcinoma with a nested growth pattern
  - Extensive lymphovascular space invasion

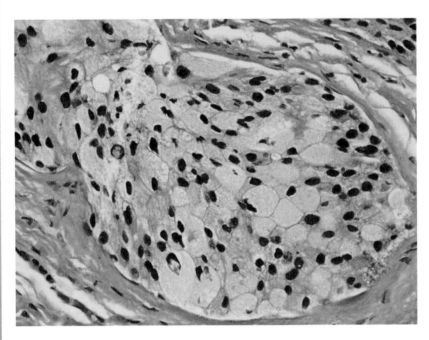

Fig. 2. Histiocytoid DCIS. In this case of DCIS, the neoplastic cells have abundant foamy cytoplasm, with occasional intracytoplasmic vacuoles. The nuclei are enlarged and more rounded than those of benign histiocytes.

component. Investigators have categorized signet ring cells variably as lobular, ductal, or colloid carcinoma. In situ signet ring cell carcinoma most often displays a lobular growth pattern but can occasionally show ductal growth with architectural changes, such as cribriforming, characteristic of DCIS.[19,20] The particular importance of this lesion is in the knowledge that signet ring cell DCIS can be subtle with focal involvement of otherwise benign structures that may easily be overlooked.[20]

Mucinous DCIS

Mucinous DCIS is associated with mucin; however, what differentiates this lesion from the many other variants of DCIS with cytoplasmic

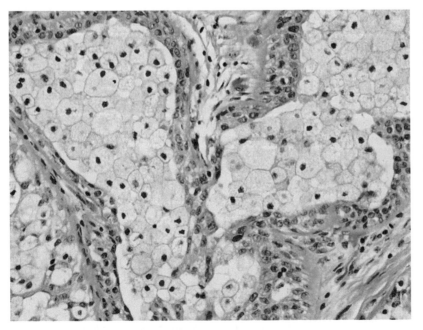

Fig. 3. Benign histiocytes within a duct. The histiocytes in this duct have similar cytoplasmic characteristics to the cells of histiocytoid DCIS (see **Fig. 2**). In contrast to histiocytoid DCIS, however, these cells have a lower nuclear-to-cytoplasmic ratio and lack cytologic atypia. Note also the normal epithelium at the periphery of the space.

mucin is its abundant intraluminal mucin. The neoplastic cells of mucinous DCIS line cystically dilated mucin-filled ducts and may or may not contain appreciable intracytoplasmic mucin (**Fig. 4**). Most mucinous DCIS lesions exhibit micropapillary, cribriform, or solid architectural patterns and often harbor calcifications and foci of necrosis. Intraluminal capillaries are often present within the mucin contents of the ductal spaces.[21] Thus, the presence of neovascularization cannot be used to distinguish in situ from invasive lesions. Difficulty arises when the ducts rupture with extrusion of mucin and possibly tumor cells into the stroma, making the distinction between mucinous DCIS and mucinous carcinoma difficult. Features that favor displaced DCIS cells secondary to duct rupture rather than invasive carcinoma include a limited area of free floating epithelial cells, the detached cells seeming to be lifted off the duct wall (ie, remain as a strip of cells), and the presence of myoepithelial cells within the free floating epithelial cell clusters. The absence of myoepithelial cells, however, does not preclude the diagnosis of DCIS in this situation. DCIS cells may also be displaced by a prior core needle biopsy procedure; adjacent biopsy site changes support this interpretation. As well as differentiating mucinous carcinoma from mucinous DCIS, mucocele-like lesions also enter into the differential diagnosis because of the cystically dilated spaces and abundant mucinous contents. There is a lack, however, of epithelial proliferation and cytologic atypia in mucocele-like lesions enabling ready separation of the 2 entities.

Apocrine DCIS

Apocrine DCIS has the characteristic architectural patterns of DCIS (cribriform, solid, micropapillary, and so forth) but cytologically the cells differ in that they have a lower nuclear-to-cytoplasmic ratio, abundant eosinophilic cytoplasm, and round nuclei with prominent nucleoli. Lesions with low-grade nuclear atypia can be difficult to differentiate from benign apocrine proliferations. Compared with benign apocrine proliferations, low nuclear grade apocrine DCIS is reported to consist of cells with abundant eosinophilic cytoplasm that lack coarse cytoplasmic granularity and that tend not to display the apical cytoplasmic snouts of apocrine metaplasia.[22] More objective evidence can be found in 3-fold to 4-fold nuclear enlargement, which should be present to render a diagnosis of DCIS (**Fig. 5**).[23,24] In contrast to low-grade apocrine DCIS, high-grade nuclear features are more easily recognized with cells that are pleomorphic with large sometimes bizarre nuclei, vesicular chromatin, and single or multiple prominent nucleoli. The mere presence of apocrine type cells often calls to mind benign conditions, which may result in underdiagnosis.[22] Conversely, bear in mind that occasional enlarged nuclei and nucleoli in a background of apocrine change do not suffice for a diagnosis of DCIS. This is important to consider particularly when interpreting atypical apocrine proliferations involving sclerosing adenosis and papillomas. Because assessing the degree of nuclear atypia in apocrine cells can be difficult, identification of diagnostic areas of DCIS with characteristic architectural and cytologic features is

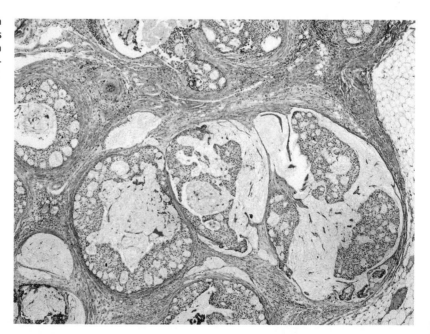

Fig. 4. Mucinous DCIS. In this example of mucinous DCIS, a cribriform pattern predominates. Abundant intraluminal mucin is evident.

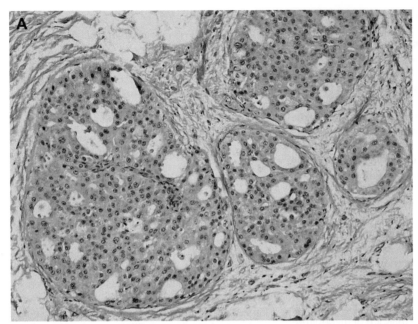

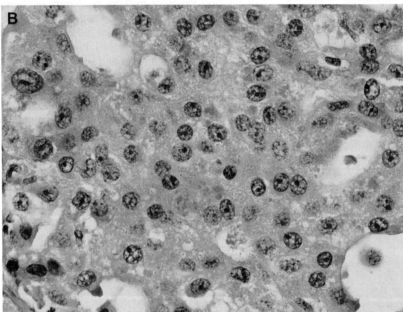

Fig. 5. Apocrine DCIS. (*A*) At low power, the cribriform pattern and apocrine differentiation in this proliferation are readily recognized. Comparison with areas of apocrine metaplasia, when present, facilitate appreciation of the higher nuclear-to-cytoplasmic ratio seen in the DCIS cells. (*B*) Higher power reveals the striking nuclear atypia and variability in nuclear size (*upper left*) characteristic of apocrine DCIS.

helpful in this setting. Unlike their benign counterparts, the cells of apocrine DCIS become more disorganized and crowded, forming cribriform spaces, rigid bars, or micropapillae. As with ADH and DCIS of classical types, some investigators have tried to categorize these proliferations by requiring a minimum span; however, there is no agreement on the size cutoff for the diagnosis of apocrine DCIS.[23,24]

Cystic Hypersecretory Carcinoma

The cystic hypersecretory carcinoma form of DCIS is associated with dense, homogenous, eosinophilic secretions. In contrast to secretory carcinoma, however, the ducts involved by this form of DCIS become cystically dilated by the secretions and have an associated atypical micropapillary proliferation. The lesion is often composed of multiple cystically dilated spaces and the secretions may display artifacts, such as parallel cracks and retraction.[1] The cysts are lined by atypical epithelial cells with enlarged hyperchromatic nuclei (Fig. 6). The cells often have cytoplasmic vacuoles and are arranged in disorderly short, blunt micropapillae. Those cases without micropapillary epithelial projections and which lack recognizable cytologic atypia should be considered cystic hypersecretory hyperplasia rather than carcinoma[1]

and cystic hypersecretory hyperplasia with atypia if nuclear atypia is present without micropapillary projections.[2] Importantly, the cytologic changes are reported to be heterogeneous in their distribution and, therefore, the degree of atypia seen may be affected by sampling. Thus, the entire lesion should be examined microscopically and, if diagnosed on percutaneous needle biopsy, the entire tumor should be excised.[1,25]

Fig. 6. Cystic hypersecretory hyperplasia and carcinoma. (*A*) Intermediate-power image of this lesion reveals cystically dilated spaces containing dense secretions (*upper right*). (*B*) At higher power, an atypical micropapillary proliferation is evident as well as marked cytologic atypia. These latter features are sufficient for a diagnosis of DCIS.

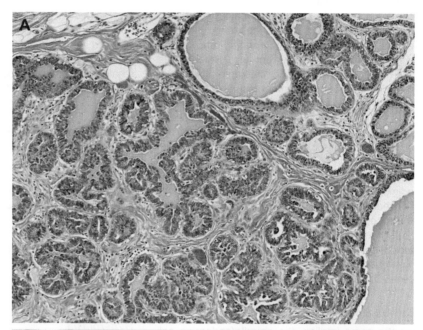

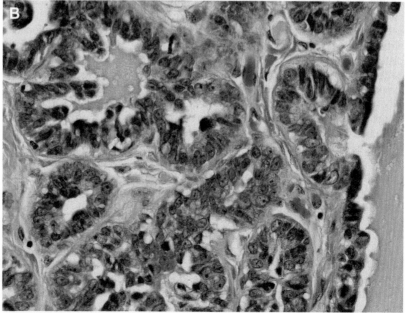

Clinging Carcinoma

The entity, clinging carcinoma, was first described by Azzopardi.[26] In contrast to the better-recognized variants of DCIS, which have cellular proliferations that fill the spaces involved, this variant of intraductal carcinoma was termed, *clinging*, to describe the cells' tendency to cling to the periphery of the structure in which they arise, comprising usually one but occasionally up to a few cell layers. These cells were noted to involve the lobules primarily, with or without concurrent ductal involvement. When originally described, this entity included lesions with both low-grade cytologic atypia (monomorphic, hyperchromatic nuclei) and high-grade cytologic atypia (enlarged, pleomorphic nuclei with vesicular chromatin, and prominent nucleoli). In the current era, lesions with low-grade and high-grade cytologic atypia are now categorized as 2 distinct lesions, namely flat epithelial atypia (or ductal intraepithelial neoplasia 1a) for the former clinging carcinoma of the monomorphic type and clinging carcinoma (or DCIS, clinging pattern) for the latter variant.[27] Azzopardi described the lesion with high-grade nuclear atypia as a subtype of comedo carcinoma, although also acknowledging that luminal necrosis is usually minimal or absent.[26] There is little difficulty with the recognition of clinging carcinoma due to the high-grade cytologic atypia (Fig. 7); however, the lack of cellular proliferation may cause an observer to overlook the dilated acini if there is not concurrent DCIS of other architectural patterns present.

Spindle/Endocrine Cell Carcinoma

As the name implies, the spindle/endocrine cell carcinoma variant of DCIS is composed of spindle cells arranged predominantly in a solid sheet of streaming cells, fascicles, and whorls, which distend the ducts,[28,29] exhibiting a festooning pattern.[28,30] In some cases, intracytoplasmic lumens, focal microglandular formation with mucin production, and fibrovascular cores can also be identified.[28,29,31] The neoplastic cells have been described as enlarged (twice the size of normal ductal cells), monomorphic, elongated, and evenly spaced apart. The cytoplasm is granular and the nuclei have fine chromatin with small nucleoli.[28,29] The morphologic expression of their neuroendocrine phenotype is supported by positive staining of the tumor cells for synaptophysin, chromogranin, and neuron-specific enolase. Rare cells may display signet ring cell morphology and clear cytoplasm.[28] An association with mucinous carcinoma, another tumor that shares the neuroendocrine phenotype, has also been reported.[31] The monotony of the cellular proliferation is usually readily

recognized. The streaming pattern and whorling of the cells, however, may raise the differential diagnostic consideration of UDH. If there is doubt about the distinction of these 2 lesions, use of cytokeratin (CK) 5/6 and estrogen receptor immunostains can aid in the differential diagnosis. In UDH, both immunostains show a heterogeneous pattern of staining. In spindle cell/endocrine DCIS, the CK 5/6 is negative and the estrogen receptor immunostain is strongly and diffusely positive.

Small Cell Carcinoma/Oat Cell Carcinoma of the Breast

The rare lesion, small cell carcinoma/oat cell carcinoma of the breast, shares the same morphologic features as those seen in small cell carcinoma elsewhere in the body. The neoplastic cells are small and hyperchromatic with scant cytoplasm and display the characteristic molding of nuclei and crush artifact. There is evidence of neuroendocrine differentiation by immunohistochemical staining. In those cases described of small cell carcinoma of the breast, an invasive component accompanied the small cell DCIS lesions and displayed aggressive features, including high mitotic activity, necrosis, and lymphovascular space invasion. The presence of an intraductal component supports the primary nature of the lesions,[32] although metastatic disease should always be considered in cases without in situ disease.

MIMICS OF DUCTAL CARCINOMA IN SITU

Usual Ductal Hyperplasia and Gynecomastoid Hyperplasia

The mimic of DCIS most frequently encountered is UDH. Appreciation of criteria for the nuclear and architectural features can usually facilitate distinction of these 2 entities, although morphologic overlap exists particularly in regard to DCIS with intermediate-grade nuclei and spindle cell DCIS. Typically, UDH is diagnosed when a space is filled with a crowded population of epithelial cells with overlapping nuclei and a haphazard arrangement. Rather than polarization around luminal spaces, which are often slit-like in UDH, the nuclei seem to stream in the same axis as the cellular bridge. The nuclei are usually ovoid and show variability in size and shape. Often nuclear grooves and inclusions can be seen. The cells of UDH typically become smaller toward the center of the involved space. Admixed foci of apocrine metaplasia and luminal macrophages favor a benign diagnosis but are by no means exclusively seen in UDH. The aforementioned features contrast with the monotonous population of neoplastic epithelial cells of

Fig. 7. Clinging carcinoma (DCIS, clinging pattern). (*A*) Low-power image shows a dilated space filled with secretion, possibly necrosis, but lacking any significant cellular proliferation. (*B*) Higher power reveals the marked cytologic atypia and necrosis in this example of clinging carcinoma.

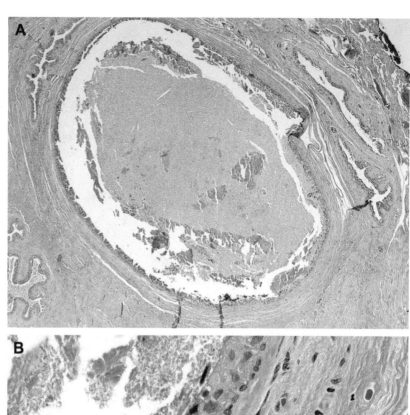

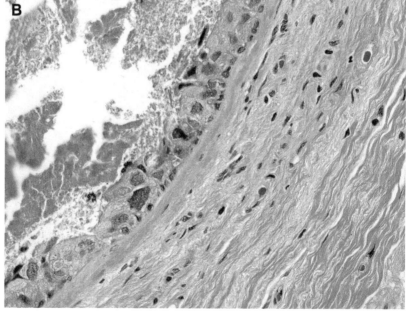

intermediate nuclear grade DCIS and spindle cell DCIS, which on first impression can appear deceptively similar to UDH because of the low-power appearance of swirling. Attention to the monotony of the proliferation and to polarization of cells around any spaces that may be present, even if they are more slit-like in shape, should prevent misdiagnosis. If these features go unnoticed, additional cues to the correct diagnosis include pagetoid involvement of adjacent benign structures as well as areas of classical cribriform DCIS.[28,29]

Immunohistochemistry is particularly helpful in cases proving difficult to distinguish on hematoxylin-eosin staining alone. CK 5/6 and estrogen receptor are the most useful pair of antibodies to use with UDH, showing heterogeneous staining for both CK 5/6 and estrogen receptor (**Fig. 8**), and with DCIS, showing absence of staining for CK 5/6 and strong, diffuse staining for estrogen receptor.

Gynecomastoid hyperplasia may enter the differential diagnosis with micropapillary DCIS. In

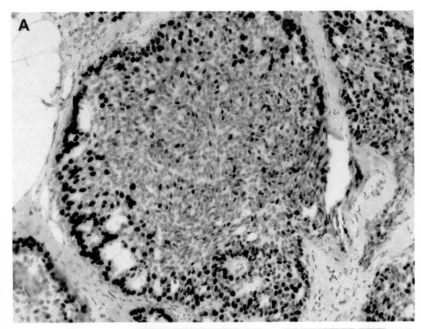

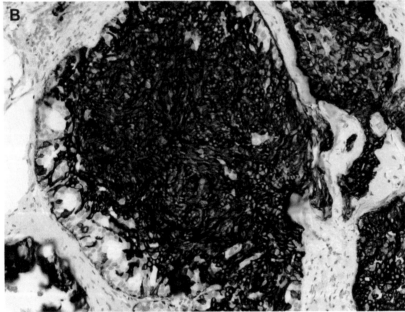

Fig. 8. Immunostains for estrogen receptor and CK 5/6 in UDH. (*A*) An estrogen receptor immunostain in UDH shows a heterogeneous pattern of staining. In contrast, DCIS would show strong diffuse staining for estrogen receptor. (*B*) CK 5/6 immunostain in UDH shows a mosaic pattern of staining. There would be an absence of staining in low and intermediate nuclear grade DCIS lesions.

gynecomastoid hyperplasia, the micropapillations have a broad base with a narrow, pinched tip in which the nuclei of the epithelial cells often appear hyperchromatic and pyknotic (**Fig. 9**). In contrast, the micropapillations of micropapillary DCIS have a narrower base with a bulbous tip and the nuclei are the same size and have the same appearance throughout the micropapillae (see **Fig. 9**).

Lobular Carcinoma In Situ

The solid patterns of DCIS and of LCIS share some morphologic features, including a monomorphic population of cells, spaced evenly apart, with low-grade nuclear atypia. Features that can aid in the distinction of these 2 lesions include the identification of intracytoplasmic vacuoles and cellular dyshesion preferentially in LCIS and the

Fig. 9. (*A*) Gynecomastoid hyperplasia. In gynecomastoid hyperplasia, the micropapillations have a broad base and a narrow pinched tip with hyperchromatic nuclei. (*B*) Micropapillary DCIS, in which the micropapillations have a narrow base and a broad, bulbous tip, with nuclei that are enlarged and the same size throughout the proliferation.

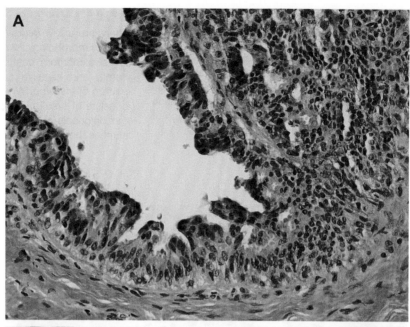

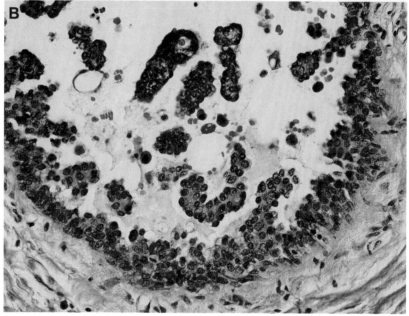

presence of polarization of cells into microacinar structures in DCIS. The neoplastic cells of DCIS retain their cell-cell adhesion whereas the neoplastic cells of LCIS have a defective E-cadherin gene, conferring a loss of cellular cohesion, which can be appreciated histologically. This feature can also be evaluated with the use of E-cadherin and p120 catenin immunohistochemical stains. The cells of DCIS and normal ductal epithelium show membranous staining with E-cadherin and p120 catenin immunohistochemical stains. The defective E-cadherin gene in LCIS is reflected in loss or reduction of membranous staining for E-cadherin and the displacement of p120 catenin protein from the cell membrane into the cytoplasm of the neoplastic cells.

High nuclear grade, calcifications, and necrosis tend to favor a diagnosis of DCIS; however, it is increasingly recognized that these features can be seen in LCIS, in particular pleomorphic LCIS.

These LCIS variants are being seen more frequently due to the widespread use of screening mammography and are often detected because of their association with microcalcifications. Again, cellular cohesion and areas of polarization with hints of microacinar formation are a helpful clue to the ductal rather than lobular nature of these solid proliferations (for an expanded discussion of LCIS variants by Murray and Brogi, see Ref.[33]).

Invasive Carcinoma

There are a few invasive carcinomas that display striking morphologic similarities to DCIS, including invasive cribriform carcinoma, adenoid cystic carcinoma, and invasive carcinomas with a nested pattern of invasion. When the invasive component consists of small or angular nests of tumor cells, the diagnosis is readily recognized. In some instances, however, the invasive tumor is composed

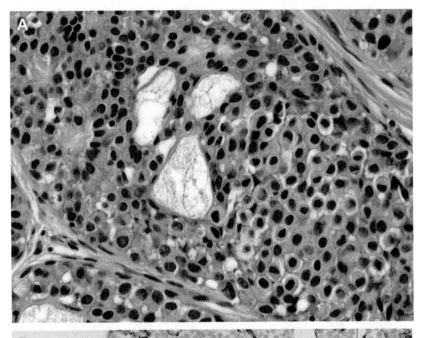

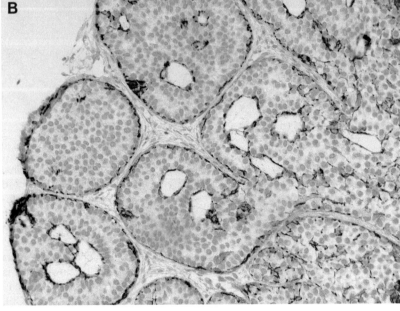

Fig. 10. LCIS in collagenous spherulosis. (A) This image shows a monomorphic, cribriform proliferation that may on first pass resemble DCIS. But the presence of myoepithelial cells surrounding the punched-out spaces as well as the presence of a cuticle of basement membrane material support a diagnosis of collagenous spherulosis. The monomorphic proliferation is due to the involvement by LCIS. Note the cellular dyshesion and occasional cytoplasmic vacuoles. (B) An E-cadherin immunostain highlights the myoepithelial cells while showing an absence of staining in the LCIS cells.

Fig. 11. LCIS and ADH involving the same space. Rigid bridges and bars and cytologic atypia support the diagnosis of ADH in this space. Also present is a dyshesive population of monomorphic cells characteristic of LCIS.

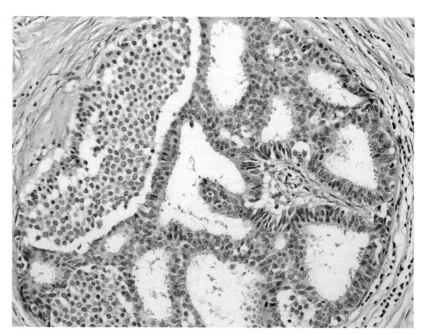

Table 2
Features distinguishing the mimics of DCIS

Mimic	Features of Mimics	Features of DCIS
Usual ductal hyperplasia	• Overlapping nuclei • Polymorphous • Loose peripheral spaces • Nuclei streaming parallel to cellular bridges • Cytokeratin 5/6+ • Heterogeneous staining with estrogen receptor	• Evenly spaced nuclei • Monomorphic • Rigid spaces • Polarization, nuclei perpendicular to axis of cellular bridges • Cytokeratin 5/6 absent • Estrogen receptor strongly, diffusely +
LCIS	• Dyshesive • Rarely pleomorphic nuclei • Occasional calcifications and/or comedo necrosis • E-cadherin − • Cytoplasmic staining with p120 catenin	• Cohesive • Polarization around spaces • More frequent pleomorphism, calcifications and necrosis • E-cadherin membrane + • Membranous staining with p120 catenin
Invasive carcinoma	Involved spaces disrupting existing benign ducts Absent myoepithelial cell markers on immunohistochemistry	Involved spaces conform to ductal/ lobular pattern Presence of myoepithelial cells (highlighted by immunohistochemistry)
Collagenous spherulosis	• Spaces filled with eosinophilic or amphophilic, often fibrillary material • No polarization of cells around spaces • Presence of myoepithelial cells around cribriform spaces • Dyshesive nature of cell population if LCIS involving collagenous spherulosis	• Spaces may be filled with homogenous eosinophilic secretions, calcifications or necrosis • Polarization of tumor cells around spaces

of large rounded nests of tumor cells mimicking solid pattern DCIS, and the invasive nature of these lesions may only be appreciated when identified as a metastatic focus in a lymph node. Features that may alert to the diagnosis are perineural invasion or the irregular arrangement of large nests of tumor cells that seem to bluntly permeate through the framework of the existing normal ducts and lobules. Other clues to the correct diagnosis include the identification of areas of more classical patterns of invasive carcinoma, which may be present. Even if an invasive component is recognized, determining the extent of invasive versus in situ disease can be challenging if both lesions have a similar pattern of large rounded nests or a cribriform architecture. In this situation, use of immunohistochemical stains for myoepithelial cells (such as p63, smooth muscle myosin heavy chain, and calponin) aid in the confirmation and determination of extent of an invasive component as well as highlighting the presence of any DCIS with positive staining of the myoepithelial cell layer.

Extensive lymphovascular space invasion may also be misinterpreted as DCIS. In this instance, the lymphatic spaces are vastly and extensively distended by tumor emboli conforming to the rounded spaces. Cribriforming and comedo necrosis may also be present compounding the impression of DCIS. Clues to the correct diagnosis, in the absence of an associated invasive component in the material available for review, include the arrangement of the putative nests of DCIS around normal ducts and lobules and proximity to the vascular bundle. Use of immunohistochemistry for antibodies against lymphatic endothelial cells, such as D2-40, may be helpful. This antibody may also stain myoepithelial cells, however, so care should be taken in the interpretation of this immunostain in this particular differential diagnosis.[34]

Dimorphic Populations

Some confusion can be caused when 2 different cellular proliferations occupy the same ductal space. For instance, when LCIS involves collagenous spherulosis, the resulting morphologic features may mimic cribriform pattern DCIS (Fig. 10). The spherules appear as punched-out spaces, but the spaces are usually filled with eosinophilic or amphophilic basement membrane material that may have a fibrillary quality. The concurrent proliferation of atypical, monomorphic epithelial cells may lend credence to the misinterpretation of the lesion as DCIS; however, the atypical cells are not cohesive and do not polarize

Pitfalls

! Spindle cell/endocrine DCIS may closely resemble UDH.
- Appreciation of the evenly spaced, monomorphic cells with areas of polarization, and luminal mucin point to a diagnosis of DCIS.

! DCIS, intermediate nuclear grade, solid pattern may mimic UDH.
- Calcifications and necrosis favor DCIS.
- Nuclear grooves and inclusions, associated macrophages, and apocrine metaplasia favor UDH.

! Invasive carcinoma with large rounded nests may mimic solid pattern DCIS.
- Haphazard arrangement between existing ducts and lobules and presence of perineural invasion, as well as the absence of a myoepithelial cell layer indicate invasive carcinoma rather than DCIS.

around the spaces. The spindled nuclei of myoepithelial cells can be seen at the periphery of the cribriform spaces. Pleomorphic LCIS can also involve collagenous spherulosis, conferring even greater cytologic atypia on the cribriform proliferation, thereby mimicking a high-grade DCIS. Again, appreciation of the cytologic dyshesion and the presence of myoepithelial cells surrounding the cribriform spaces is an alert to the correct diagnosis in this situation.

Additionally, DCIS (or atypical ductal hyperplasia [ADH]) and LCIS can populate the same ductal space (Fig. 11); LCIS can involve areas of usual ductal hyperplasia; and, rarely, 2 morphologically distinct populations of DCIS may coexist within a duct or involve a papilloma. Use of adjunctive immunohistochemical stains as discussed previously, may be helpful in separating out these different entities. Features distinguishing the mimics from DCIS are summarized in Table 2.

SUMMARY

There is tremendous heterogeneity to DCIS, including variable morphologic features as well as biomarker profiles and genetic alterations. Although it may not be necessary to distinguish each variant using a barrage of stains, it is important to be aware of the different variants of DCIS to recognize these lesions, especially when evaluating core needle biopsy specimens. Furthermore, appreciation of the mimics of DCIS leads to greater accuracy in distinguishing these proliferative lesions.

REFERENCES

1. Rosen PP, Scott M. Cystic hypersecretory duct carcinoma of the breast. Am J Surg Pathol 1984; 8(1):31–41.

2. Guerry P, Erlandson RA, Rosen PP. Cystic hypersecretory hyperplasia and cystic hypersecretory duct carcinoma of the breast. Pathology, therapy, and follow-up of 39 patients. Cancer 1988;61(8): 1611–20.

3. Hull MT, Priest JB, Broadie TA, et al. Glycogen-rich clear cell carcinoma of the breast: a light and electron microscopic study. Cancer 1981;48(9): 2003–9.

4. Hull MT, Warfel KA. Glycogen-rich clear cell carcinomas of the breast. A clinicopathologic and ultrastructural study. Am J Surg Pathol 1986;10(8):553–9.

5. Hayes MM, Seidman JD, Ashton MA. Glycogen-rich clear cell carcinoma of the breast. A clinicopathologic study of 21 cases. Am J Surg Pathol 1995; 19(8):904–11.

6. Gurbuz Y, Ozkara SK. Clear cell carcinoma of the breast with solid papillary pattern: a case report with immunohistochemical profile. J Clin Pathol 2003;56(7):552–4.

7. Kuroda H, Sakamoto G, Ohnisi K, et al. Clinical and pathological features of glycogen-rich clear cell carcinoma of the breast. Breast Cancer 2005; 12(3):189–95.

8. Markopoulos C, Mantas D, Philipidis T, et al. Glycogen-rich clear cell carcinoma of the breast. World J Surg Oncol 2008;6:44.

9. Aboumrad MH, Horn RC, Fine G. Lipid-secreting mammary carcinoma: report of a case associated with Paget's disease of the nipple. Cancer 1963; 16:521.

10. Ramos CV, Taylor HB. Lipid-rich carcinoma of the breast. A clinicopathologic analysis of 13 examples. Cancer 1974;33(3):812–9.

11. Guan B, Wang H, Cao S, et al. Lipid-rich carcinoma of the breast clinicopathologic analysis of 17 cases. Ann Diagn Pathol 2011;15(4):225–32.

12. Kimura A, Miki H, Yuri T, et al. A case report of lipid-rich carcinoma of the breast including histological characteristics and intrinsic subtype profile. Case Rep Oncol 2011;4(2):275–80.

13. Shi P, Wang M, Zhang Q, et al. Lipid-rich carcinoma of the breast. A clinicopathological study of 49 cases. Tumori 2008;94(3):342–6.

14. McDivitt RW, Stewart FW. Breast carcinoma in children. JAMA 1966;195(5):388–90.

15. Tavassoli FA, Norris HJ. Secretory carcinoma of the breast. Cancer 1980;45(9):2404–13.

16. Botta G, Fessia L, Ghiringhello B. Juvenile milk protein secreting carcinoma. Virchows Arch A Pathol Anat Histol 1982;395(2):145–52.

17. Gupta D, Croitoru CM, Ayala AG, et al. E-cadherin immunohistochemical analysis of histiocytoid carcinoma of the breast. Ann Diagn Pathol 2002;6(3): 141–7.

18. Jager J, Bassler R. Intraductal, lipid forming histiocytoid breast cancer. Contribution to the differential diagnosis of intraductal lipophage proliferations. Pathologe 1991;12(1):44–7 [in German].

19. Hull MT, Seo IS, Battersby JS, et al. Signet-ring cell carcinoma of the breast: a clinicopathologic study of 24 cases. Am J Clin Pathol 1980;73(1):31–5.

20. Fisher ER, Tavares J, Bulatao IS, et al. Glycogen-rich, clear cell breast cancer: with comments concerning other clear cell variants. Hum Pathol 1985; 16(11):1085–90.

21. Gadre SA, Perkins GH, Sahin AA, et al. Neovascularization in mucinous ductal carcinoma in situ suggests an alternative pathway for invasion. Histopathology 2008;53(5):545–53.

22. Raju U, Zarbo RJ, Kubus J, et al. The histologic spectrum of apocrine breast proliferations: a comparative study of morphology and DNA content by image analysis. Hum Pathol 1993;24(2):173–81.

23. O'Malley FP. Non-invasive apocrine lesions of the breast. Curr Diagn Pathol 2004;10:211–9.

24. O'Malley FP, Bane AL. The spectrum of apocrine lesions of the breast. Adv Anat Pathol 2004;11(1): 1–9.

25. Shin SJ, Rosen PP. Carcinoma arising from preexisting pregnancy-like and cystic hypersecretory hyperplasia lesions of the breast: a clinicopathologic study of 9 patients. Am J Surg Pathol 2004;28(6): 789–93.

26. Azzopardi JG. Problems in breast pathology. Philadelphia: WB Saunders; 1979.

27. Tavassoli FA, Devilee P, editors. Tumours of the breast and female genital organs. Lyon (France): IARC Press; 2003.

28. Tsang WY, Chan JK. Endocrine ductal carcinoma in situ (E-DCIS) of the breast: a form of low-grade DCIS with distinctive clinicopathologic and biologic characteristics. Am J Surg Pathol 1996;20(8):921–43.

29. Farshid G, Moinfar F, Meredith DJ, et al. Spindle cell ductal carcinoma in situ. An unusual variant of ductal intra-epithelial neoplasia that simulates ductal hyperplasia or a myoepithelial proliferation. Virchows Arch 2001;439(1):70–7.

30. Cross AS, Azzopardi JG, Krausz T, et al. A morphological and immunocytochemical study of a distinctive variant of ductal carcinoma in-situ of the breast. Histopathology 1985;9(1):21–37.

31. Maluf HM, Koerner FC. Carcinomas of the breast with endocrine differentiation: a review. Virchows Arch 1994;425(5):449–57.

32. Papotti M, Gherardi G, Eusebi V, et al. Primary oat cell (neuroendocrine) carcinoma of the breast. Report of four cases. Virchows Arch A Pathol Anat Histopathol 1992;420(1):103–8.

33. Collins L, editor. Current concepts in breast pathology. 1st edition. Philadelphia: Elsevier Inc; 2009.

34. Rabban JT, Chen YY. D2-40 expression by breast myoepithelium: potential pitfalls in distinguishing intralymphatic carcinoma from in situ carcinoma. Hum Pathol 2008;39(2):175–83.

INVASIVE LOBULAR CARCINOMA OF THE BREAST

Marianna Philippidou, Bsc, MBBS, FRCPath[a],*,
Sarah E. Pinder, MB, CHB, FRCPath[b]

KEYWORDS

- Breast cancer • Invasive lobular carcinoma • Histopathology

ABSTRACT

Invasive lobular carcinoma of the breast is a distinct histologic type with specific clinical, radiologic, and microscopic features, which is increasing in incidence in the Western World. Routine pathologic prognostic factors, including grade, lymph node stage, and size are of significance in predicting outcome in this group of patients who, overall, have survival comparable to those with other subtypes of breast cancer. Variants, however, are seen and these, as well as other standard factors such as histologic grade, have prognostic significance and should be recorded in pathology reports.

OVERVIEW

Features of lobular carcinoma, described in the seminal article in which lobular carcinoma in situ (LCIS) was first recorded by Foote and Stewart,[1] include tumor cells arranged in a linear fashion and a tendency to grow in a circumferential fashion around ducts and lobules. Foote and Stewart also observed that, although an in situ component did not always accompany the tumor, the histologic pattern of LCIS was sufficiently distinctive to be considered a specific form.

Invasive lobular carcinoma (ILC) comprises 3% to 15% of breast carcinomas.[2–4] It occurs in a wide age range (28 through 86 years) with a mean age at diagnosis of 63 years. It is more common in older women,

those older than age 75 years of age compared with 35 years or younger.[5] ILC seems to be increasing in incidence at a greater rate than carcinoma of ductal/ no special type (14.4% per year vs 1.2% per year, respectively), at least in the Western world.[6] This increase, at a population level, seems, at least in part, related to the use of hormone replacement therapy; the increase in ILC in women on hormone replacement therapy is more marked than the increase in ductal/no special type lesions and is seen across all ages[7] and across disease stages, sizes, and nodal status.[8]

Bilaterality of disease is considered more common in patients with ILC compared with other types of carcinoma, with the reported relative risk ranging from 1.6 (95% CI, 0.7–3.6) to 2.0 (95% CI, 0.8–8.4) in 3 studies.[9–11] Other series, however, have not demonstrated an increased incidence of multicentricity and/or bilaterality with ILC beyond that of ductal/no special type cancers,[12,13] despite that this is reported widely in textbooks and the medical literature.

DIAGNOSIS OF INVASIVE LOBULAR CARCINOMA

Patients with ILC most commonly present with a mass or vague diffuse nodularity, although they may be detected by mammographic breast screening. In general, the clinical and gross pathologic features are not distinct from other forms of invasive breast cancer.

Disclosure: The authors have no interests or conflicts to declare.
[a] Department of Histopathology, King's College Hospital NHS Foundation Trust, Denmark Hill, London, United Kingdom
[b] Research Oncology, Division of Cancer Studies, King's College London, Guy's and Thomas' Foundation Trust, 3rd Floor, Bermondsey Wing, Great Maze Pond, London SE1 9RT, United Kingdom
* Corresponding author.
E-mail address: marianna.philippidou@nhs.net

Surgical Pathology 5 (2012) 545–566
http://dx.doi.org/10.1016/j.path.2012.06.006
1875-9181/12/$ – see front matter © 2012 Published by Elsevier Inc.

surgpath.theclinics.com

Radiologically, ILC may be occult and is less often associated with microcalcification than other types of invasive carcinoma, although it is often suspected if a low-density mass is seen on mammography. ILC is also often associated with, and not isolated from, the main glandular density of the breast on mammograms. Intriguingly, ILC, more often than ductal/no special type breast cancer, varies in appearances between the craniocaudal and mediolateral oblique mammogram views; approximately 40% of spiculate masses related to ILC on craniocaudal views appear as distortions or asymmetric densities on mediolateral oblique mammograms.[14]

MRI may be especially helpful in the radiologic assessment of ILC, with increased sensitivity in detection and evaluation of these lesions,[15] particularly if the index lesion is difficult to assess on standard mammography. The current UK National Institute for Health and Clinical Excellence guidelines recommend that if on needle core biopsy there is proved ILC, MRI of that breast should

be considered for assessment of tumor size if breast-conserving surgery is to be undertaken. The authors have assessed the reliability of diagnosis of ILC on core biopsy and find that, without E-cadherin immunohistochemical evaluation (discussed later), 86 of 93 cases of ILC were correctly categorized on core biopsy (including 13 of 17 of the pleomorphic variant; 92.5%), whereas 4 of 7 mixed ductal/no special type and lobular mixed lesions were also correctly identified as bearing an ILC component (Philippidou and Pinder, personal communication, 2012).

MICROSCOPIC FEATURES OF INVASIVE LOBULAR CARCINOMA

ILC can be of classical type or variant forms, including alveolar, solid, tubulolobular, pleomorphic lobular, or mixed appearance. To be classified as ILC, 90% of the tumor should be of the appropriate cytomorphology, and to be regarded as a "pure" variant, more than 90% of the tumor should be composed of this type. The mixed-type of lobular carcinoma includes those lesions with an admixture of the different lobular subtypes. ILC can also be seen in association with other histologic types, such as ductal/no special type (Fig. 1) or, less commonly, with other special-type lesions, when less than 90% of the lesion is ILC, and the other special type makes up the remainder. In tumors of mixed subtypes, such as mixed ILC and ductal/no special type, the component parts are typically seen in distinct areas, with foci of typical ILC but discrete areas of the other subtype of carcinoma. The term, *mixed*, should not be used for lesions that show incomplete features of either type, such as a ductal/no special type carcinoma that shows some, but not convincing, infiltrating lobular features.

DIFFERENTIAL DIAGNOSIS

On cytology, diagnosis of ILC presents diagnostic challenges and problems, mainly due to the sparse cellularity resulting in false-negative reports.[16] As in histologic sections, the tumor cells are uniform, usually small to medium-sized, with

---

Pathologic Key Features
OF INVASIVE LOBULAR CARCINOMA OF THE BREAST

Gross features
- No specific gross features: typically a pale tumor, poorly defined, and sometimes difficult to assess and measure on macroscopic examination

- Average size 2.4 mm

Microscopic findings
- Cells show discohesive pattern of infiltration with little stromal reaction

- Nuclei typically moderately pleomorphic (other than pleomorphic variant)

- Intracytoplasmic lumina/vacuoles are common

- Subtypes include classical, tubulolobular, alveolar, solid, pleomorphic, and mixed variants

- Usually histologic grade 2, except tubulolobular (grade 1) and pleomorphic (grade 3) variants

- LCIS present in 66% of cases

Immunohistochemistry
- Negative or reduced staining for E-cadherin is typical

- Usually positive for estrogen and progesterone receptors

- Usually negative for HER2 (approximately 99% cases) (except pleomorphic variant)

Differential Diagnosis
OF INVASIVE LOBULAR CARCINOMA OF THE BREAST

- Other non-lobular invasive breast cancer types
- Lymphoid population, either benign or lymphomatous.

Fig. 1. A mixed tumor composed of separate areas of ductal/no special type and classical invasive lobular components, with high-grade solid architecture ductal carcinoma in situ. (*A*) At medium power, the no special type areas (*left*) can be seen as small, cohesive clusters of large, pleomorphic epithelial cells whereas the invasive lobular portion forms typical single files of infiltrative cells (*right*). (*B*) At high power, the difference in the cytologic features is seen, with the small, regular cells of the invasive lobular component (*top*) approximately twice the size of mature lymphoid cells (*bottom left*). The invasive no special type cells are much larger with prominent nucleoli (*bottom right*).

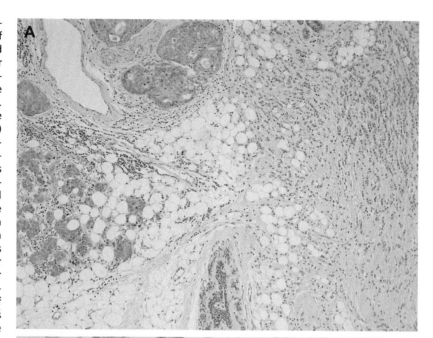

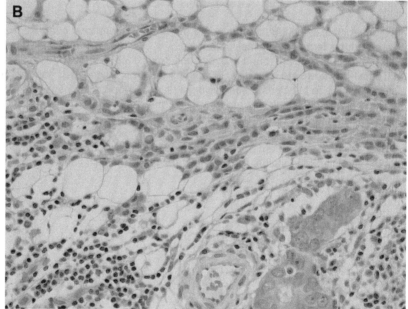

a uniform staining pattern. Occasionally central mucoid globules resulting in intracytoplasmic lumina are helpful diagnostically. The same features are helpful in needle core biopsy as in excision specimens, although the appearances may be subtle and the diagnosis may be missed, or mistaken for a lymphoid infiltrate.

CLASSICAL INVASIVE LOBULAR CARCINOMA

Classical ILC typically infiltrates in single strands (**Figs. 2** and **3**), although small clusters and islands can be admixed. The carcinoma cells show lack of cohesion and often appear dispersed within the stroma or adipose tissue. There is commonly little, or no, stromal reaction to the infiltrate, which may subtly invade more widely than anticipated grossly or clinically. Another characteristic of ILC is the tendency of the tumor cells to arrange themselves around ducts and lobules in a concentric fashion resulting in a targetoid appearance (**Fig. 4**). In cases where there is a prominent lymphocytic reaction around the tumor, it may be subclassified as

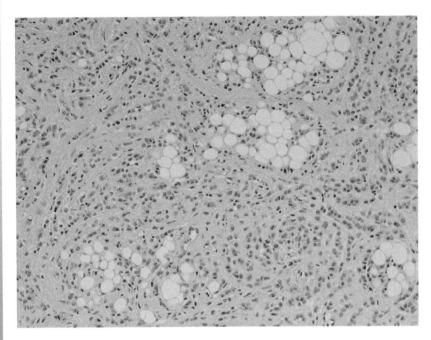

Fig. 2. Classical variant of ILC infiltrating through stroma and fat without a significant host reaction. Tumor cells invade as single files.

a lymphoepithelial-like lobular carcinoma but this is rare and the term is not widely used.

The carcinoma cells are round to ovoid, uniform, and small to moderate in size. Sometimes an eccentrically placed nucleus is seen giving a plasmacytoid appearance. Nucleoli are usually inconspicuous. The cells may contain intracytoplasmic lumina (**Fig. 5**) containing sialomucins, often seen on H&E stains but also demonstrable with mucicarmine or alcian blue stains. Occasionally these secretions overtake the cytoplasm, pushing the nucleus to one side and resulting in a signet ring configuration.

Associated lobular in situ neoplasia (atypical lobular hyperplasia or LCIS) is often present (**Fig. 6**). The cytology of the cells in the in situ process is essentially similar to those of the invasive component with expansion of the lobules by moderately sized, discohesive cells with intracytoplasmic vacuoles.

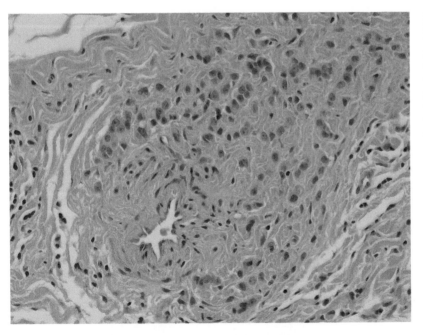

Fig. 3. Classical variant of ILC infiltrating through fibrous stroma close to a small blood vessel. Single files of moderately sized tumor cells show discohesion. Slightly unusually for the classical variant, single prominent nucleoli are evident.

Fig. 4. A signet ring cell variant of classical ILC surrounding a normal small ducts in a targetoid fashion. Tumor cells are moderate in size but the cytoplasm is markedly distended by intracytoplasmic vacuoles of mucin.

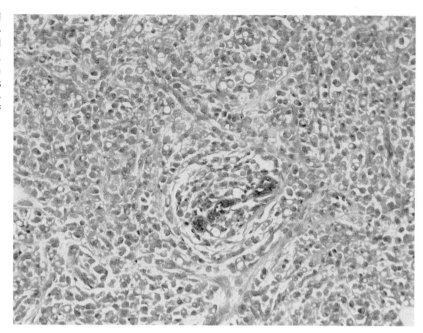

VARIANT FORMS OF LOBULAR CARCINOMA

Variant forms constitute approximately 23% of lobular carcinomas diagnosed. These include ILCs in which a substantial proportion of the tumor growth pattern is nonlinear and thus the cytology of the cells is that of ILC, but the architecture is not that of the classical variant. These include solid subtypes and tubulolobular and pleomorphic forms as well as an alveolar variant, where the tumor is composed of small clusters or aggregates of 20 cells or more (Fig. 7) but which has the same cytologic features as in classical ILC. In the solid variant, the tumor grows as a solid sheet (Figs. 8 and Fig. 9). In the latter case, E-cadherin immunohistochemistry may be helpful (see Fig. 8C and discussed later) if there is doubt of the lobular nature of the invasive tumor, for example in core biopsy.

TUBULOLOBULAR CARCINOMA

The tubulolobular variant of ILC has some morphologic features intermediate between classical ILC and tubular carcinoma but the tubules in this form of ILC are small and round and formed from cells of typical lobular morphology, admixed with the linear cords of single cells of classical ILC (Fig. 10). The tubules of tubular carcinoma are classically angulated and the cells lack the discohesion, regularity, and cytologic features of ILC. Specifically, the infiltrating single files of classical ILC are not seen in tubular carcinoma. Both tubulolobular and tubular carcinomas, however, are of histologic grade 1 and both have an excellent prognosis.[17,18] Elastosis is commonly present in tubulolobular carcinomas, with some reports that an intraduct papillary or cribriform element may also be seen.[18]

PLEOMORPHIC LOBULAR CARCINOMA

Pleomorphic lobular carcinoma shows the same infiltrative pattern as classical lobular (Fig. 11A), including the typical single files and small clusters, but the tumor cells exhibit cellular atypia, nuclear pleomorphism, and, often, prominent nucleoli (see Fig. 11B, C; Fig. 12). The cells are large with more abundant eosinophilic cytoplasm and show high cytonuclear grade features (score 3 for the pleomorphism/atypia component of histologic grade). Some have emphasized the apocrine features seen in some forms of this variant[19–21] and some cases are immunoreactive to gross cystic disease fluid protein 15 (GCDFP-15). There are limited data, however, on the reproducibility of diagnosis of this uncommon form and improved guidelines on the criteria that should be applied are required.

DIFFERENTIAL DIAGNOSIS - E-CADHERIN

Historically, investigators have described "formidable" problems in distinguishing ductal and lobular varieties of infiltrating breast carcinoma.[22]

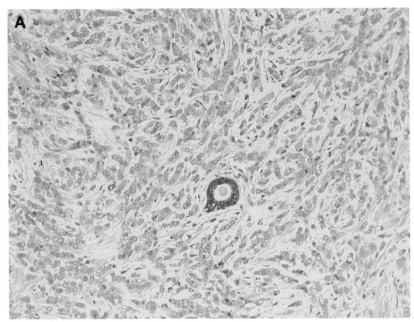

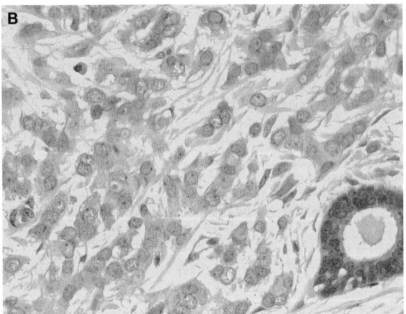

Fig. 5. (*A*) ILC of classical variant surrounding a benign small ductule. Tumor cells are forming single files and small clusters and trabeculae (more than 1 cell thick). (*B*) High power of same tumor shows intracytoplasmic vacuoles in the tumor cells.

More recently, however, the recognition of aberrations in E-cadherin in these lesions has proved helpful in diagnosis, at least in some cases; E-cadherin is a cell-to-cell adhesion molecule, connecting the E-cadherin membrane complex to the intercellular actin cytoskeleton and acting as a tumor invasion suppressor gene. ILC typically shows reduced (dot-like or beaded membrane staining) or absent E-cadherin expression[23–25] as well as low expression of α-catenin, β-catenin, and γ-catenin (see **Figs.** **8C** and **10C**).[25]

The aberrations in immunohistochemical pattern of E-cadherin are associated with mutation (or other functional silencing) of the E-cadherin

Fig. 6. Classical ILC with adjacent LCIS. Infiltrating single files of invasive carcinoma are seen within fibrous stroma, whereas expanded lobules bear a solid proliferation of discohesive cells of similar appearance.

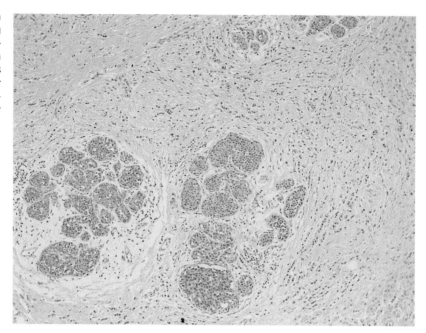

gene (*CDH1*), which maps at chromosome 16q22.1, in ILC. That mutations of this gene are involved in the etiology of sporadic breast cancers of lobular type is supported by studies of the introduction of conditional E-cadherin mutations into a mouse model based on epithelium-specific knockout of p53,[26] which induces tumors histologically akin to human ILC.

Absence of membrane E-cadherin expression immunohistochemically is typical of lobular carcinoma (both in situ and invasive) but some positivity in approximately 15% of lobular lesions has been reported.[27,28] For example, Choi and colleagues[27] found that weak, partial, or incomplete E-cadherin positivity was seen in 14% of lobular cases (11.5% weak/partial fragmented and 2.1% focal/dot-like cytoplasmic). Conversely, most ductal/no special type carcinomas show continuous membranous positivity; for example, Qureshi and colleagues[29] found E-cadherin reactivity in 203 (99.5%) of 204 of invasive ductal/no special type carcinomas but other series have shown reduced/weak staining in up to 29% of ductal lesions.[28] Morphologically pure ductal/no special type carcinomas (in particular, grade 3 lesions) can also lose E-cadherin

membrane reactivity but this is not usually a significant diagnostic dilemma.

Also, variation in E-cadherin immunoreactivity with different antibodies is reported[28] and there is a lack of reproducibility of assessment of E-cadherin immunostaining. Thus, even with E-cadherin added to morphologic examination, the categorization of a lesion as ILC remains problematic in some cases. In one study of 161 lesions previously classified as lobular (in situ or invasive), 3 pathologists agreed with the previous morphologic diagnoses of lobular neoplasia or infiltrating lobular carcinoma in 100 (71.4%), 2 pathologists agreed in 26 (18.6%), and only 1 pathologist diagnosed the lesion as lobular in 14 (10%) of lesions. All 3 pathologists disagreed with the previous diagnoses of lobular neoplasia/ ILC but agreed that the lesion was of ductal type (DCIS or invasive) in 21 cases (13.0%).

An occasional difficulty which may be faced is that of subclassification of an invasive breast cancer with classical ILC morphology that is E-cadherin immunopositive, or conversely, a tumor without significant lobular features that shows an absence of E-cadherin expression. There is little agreement in how to categorize these lesions;

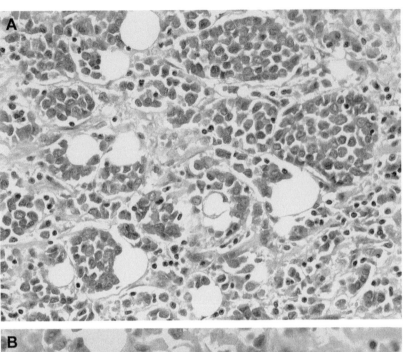

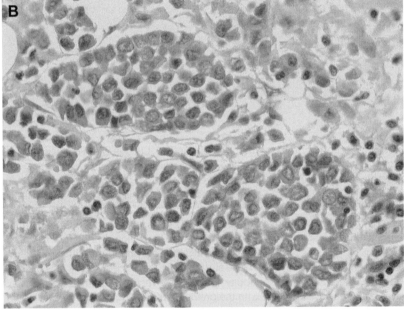

Fig. 7. Alveolar lobular carcinoma (A) Clusters of discohesive cells are seen at medium power. These formed the entire tumor, without single files of infiltration or other architectural patterns. (B) High power shows the discohesion of the tumor cells, which have moderately atypical nuclei and abundant eosinophilic cytoplasm.

some experts report such cases based on the histologic morphology (arguing that the behavior and outcome data from the literature is based on such analysis) whereas others suggest that the molecular features (namely E-cadherin loss) should take precedence as reflecting the molecular changes. There are limited data on the outcome of patients with ILC that shows E-cadherin positivity, but this indicates that the behavior of these ILCs is not different from those that are E-cadherin

Fig. 8. Solid lobular carcinoma (A) Medium-power H&E of a core biopsy bearing solid sheets of tumor cells showing discohesion. (B) Higher power shows some cytologic features of ILC, including moderate cell size, lack of marked pleomorphism, abundant cytoplasm, and discohesion.

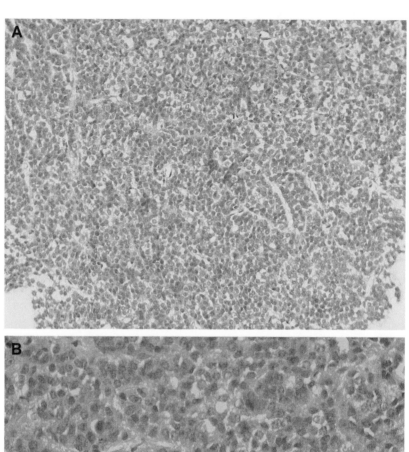

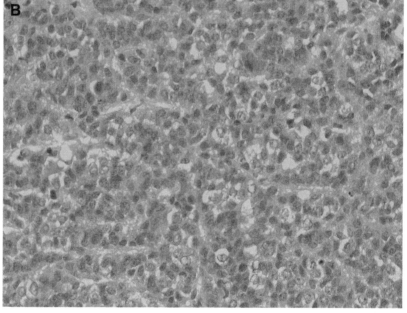

negative.[28] Such cases tend to show evidence of impairment of the overall E-cadherin/catenin membrane complex, despite immunoreactivity for E-cadherin immunohistochemically, for example,

diffuse cytoplasmic expression of catenins, such as p120 catenin, which is similar to E-cadherin negative ILCs. At present, therefore, an approach that includes description of both morphologic

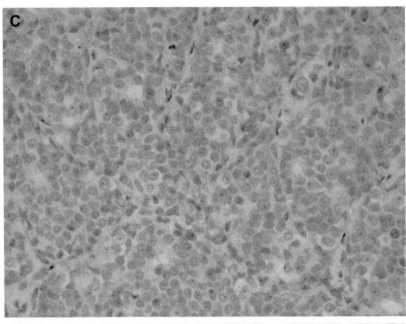

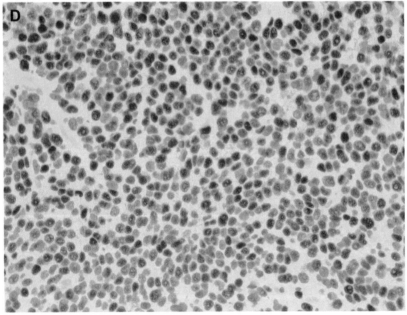

Fig. 8. (*C*) E-cadherin immunostaining on the tumor in this core biopsy showed no membrane immunoreactivity. (*D*) Estrogen receptor staining showed moderate intensity reactivity in 100% of tumor cell nuclei.

features and the immunophenotype seems sensible; thus, categorization of a lesion as having ILC histologic features but which is E-cadherin positive or, conversely, which seems of ductal/no special type but shows E-cadherin negativity will allow accrual of data on the clinical significance of these uncommon forms of lesion and is our present recommendation.

Fig. 9. Solid lobular carcinoma. Invasive breast carcinoma, solid lobular variant. Sheets of tumor cells, without clearly evident cell boundaries and moderate size are seen without a infiltrating single file or trabecular pattern.

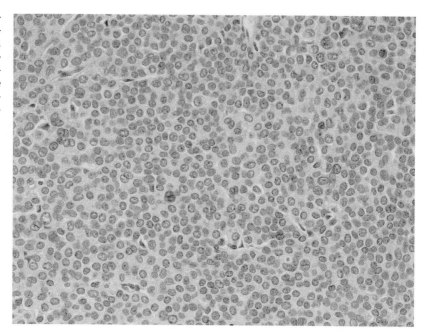

DIFFERENTIAL DIAGNOSIS—OTHER PITFALLS

Apart from other histologic invasive tumor types, differential diagnosis of ILC includes lymphoid infiltrates, both benign and malignant (**Fig. 13**). Unfortunately, lymphomas can be difficult to distinguish from ILC and the only way to avoid the potential pitfall is to consider the diagnosis. In uncertain or problematic cases, immunohistochemical evaluation should be undertaken. Once the diagnosis is considered, immunohistochemistry enables diagnosis with relative ease: ILC expresses cytokeratin markers but not lymphoid markers and conversely, although rarely lymphomas can express cytokeratins, other specific markers (such as lymphocyte common antigen), and relevant B, or, less commonly, T-cell markers are positive in a primary breast lymphoma.

ILC can, however, also be missed in the background of increase cellularity seen with a coexisting chronic inflammatory reaction (**Fig. 14**) and care should be taken to assess adjacent tissue thoroughly. Even when not associated with chronic inflammation, ILC can be subtle (**Fig. 15**A) and, because it typically does not have a significant host reaction, may be missed. This is particularly the case with very small foci in a needle core biopsy or at the margins of an excision specimen. Care should be taken in assessment and a low threshold for assessment of cytokeratin markers highlights the epithelial nature of the cells, which may also mimic plasma cells (see **Fig. 15**B).

The diagnosis of metastatic ILC may be more problematic than other invasive breast cancer types, both in lymph nodes and other distant sites (discussed later). As in the primary lesion, cytologic examination (either preoperative fine-needle aspiration cytology or intraoperative touch imprint cytology) of sentinel lymph node specimens may be especially difficult, as may be frozen section assessment. It is useful to check the histologic type of the primary lesion as reported on the core or excision biopsy, if available, when examining such intraoperative samples, so that there is awareness of a potential pitfall before examining the lymph node cytology or histology (**Fig. 16**). The infiltrate in the lymph nodes may be more diffuse and discohesive (as in the primary lesion) (**Fig. 17**) and may occasionally mimic sinus histiocytosis. Epithelial markers assist in reaching the correct diagnosis in tricky cases and highlight the tumor cells of the ILC.

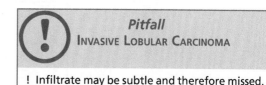

> **(!)** ***Pitfall***
> **INVASIVE LOBULAR CARCINOMA**
>
> ! Infiltrate may be subtle and therefore missed.

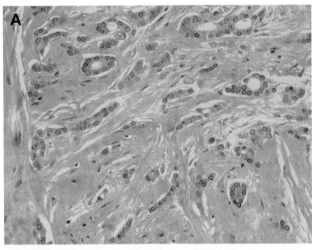

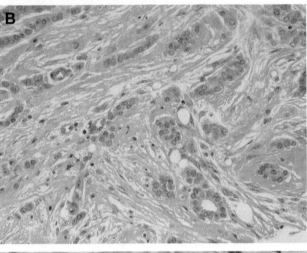

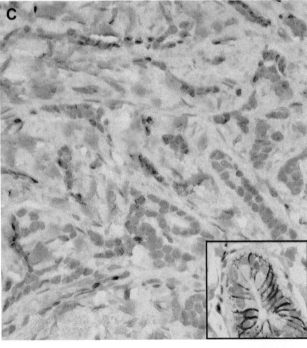

Fig. 10. (*A* and *B*) Tubulolobular variant. H&E. An admixture of small round tubular structures and single files of infiltrating carcinoma cells is seen in this variant along with, in this case, small clusters of cancer cells without lumina but of the same cytologic appearance (*C*) E-cadherin immunostaining in this case, confirmed that faint, incomplete, focal membrane reactivity only was seen (inset shows internal control membrane reactivity of a normal duct in the adjacent tissue).

Fig. 11. Pleomorphic lobular carcinoma (*A*) This invasive carcinoma has an architectural infiltrative pattern typical of classical ILC with single cells and infiltrating files of cells extending through fibrous tissue (*B*) Higher power confirms that the tumor cells are large and pleomorphic with abundant cytoplasm. Some cells bear intracytoplasmic vacuoles.

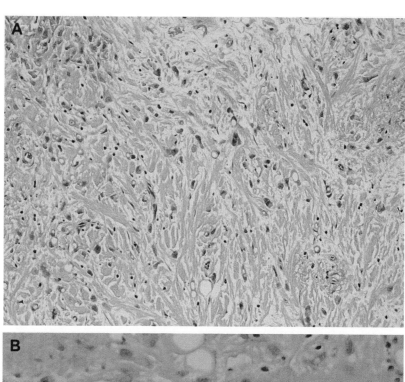

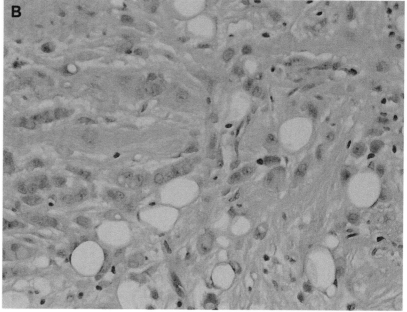

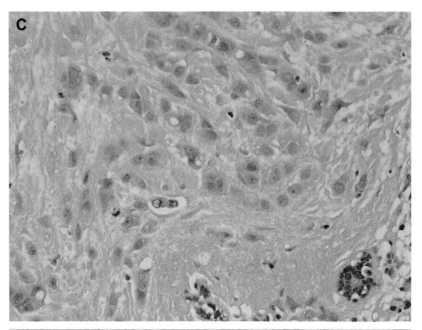

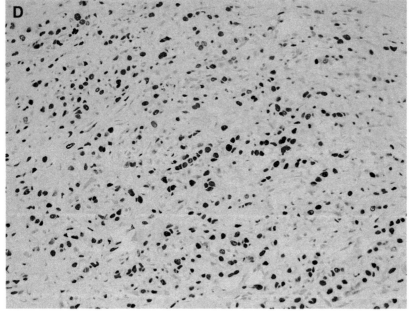

Fig. 11. (*C*) The size of the tumor cells can be appreciated by comparison with adjacent normal epithelial cells (*bottom right*) or lymphoid cells or erythrocytes if there is no normal epithelium present, such as in a core biopsy. (*D*) The pleomorphic ILC cells nevertheless uniformly, express estrogen receptor of moderate to strong intensity. This tumor was also HER2 negative (not shown).

OTHER BIOMARKERS

The majority (87.5%) of ILCs are positive for estrogen receptor (see **Figs.** 8D and 11D) and 75% are positive for progesterone receptor (PR).[30] Some are also positive for GCDFP-15, predominantly those with pleomorphic or signet ring cytology, as well as cyclin D1 (80% of cases).[31–33] HER2 positivity is rarely detected and can be seen in less than 1% of ILCs overall.[34]

Fig. 12. Pleomorphic lobular carcinoma. High-power H&E of a pleomorphic ILC showing the large, discohesive tumor cells with abundant eosinophilic cytoplasm, pleomorphic nuclei with prominent nucleoli and mitotic figure.

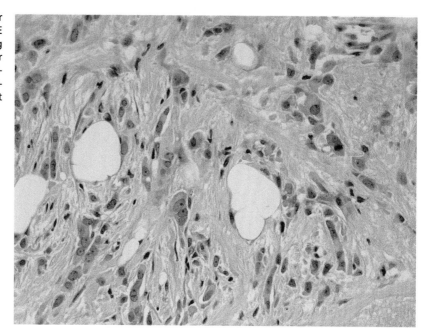

Fig. 13. High-grade B-cell lymphoma. H&E. A discohesive infiltrate of large atypical cells with pleomorphic nuclei, clumped chromatin and multiple prominent nucleoli is seen (*left*) with adjacent small mature lymphoid forms (*right*). The nuclear features would be unusual, but this could be mistaken for ILC. A low threshold for immunohistochemistry is such cases is advised; confirmation of the absence of cytokeratin marker positivity and expression of lymphocyte common antigen and B-cell markers enables the diagnosis of high grade B-cell lymphoma.

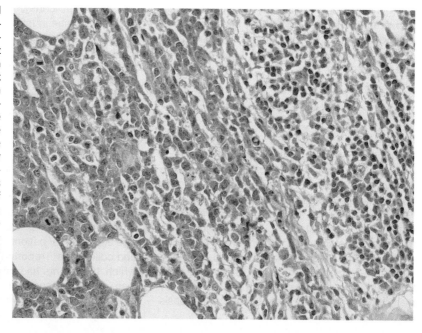

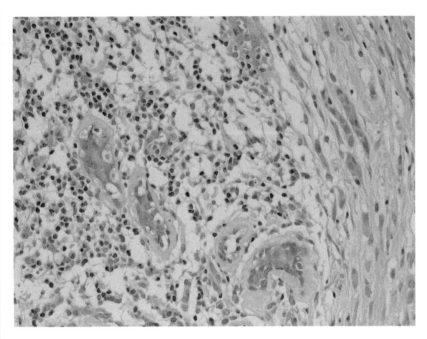

Fig. 14. In the presence of associated chronic inflammation, a scanty infiltrate of ILC can be missed. Although this case shows a perilobular chronic inflammatory cell infiltrate, the nature of the classical ILC (*right*) is seen to be distinct, formed of single files of cells with more abundant cytoplasm, which are more overtly epithelial in nature.

The pleomorphic variant has been reported as positive or shows equivocal HER2 immunostaining in up to 81% of lesions, but this includes those with either 2+ or 3+ reactivity.[35] Similarly, basal cytokeratins, such as CK5/6, have been described in up to 17% of ILCs,[36] predominantly those cases of histologic grade 3 and lesions that are estrogen receptor negative.

STAGING AND PROGNOSIS

Patients with ILC have the same prognosis as those with invasive ductal/no special type carcinoma when other prognostic factors are taken into consideration. Several studies have reported on the prognosis of patients with ILC; Newman[2] found that 14% of patients with stage I and 46% with stage II disease died, with follow-up averaging approximately 8 years. Ashikari and colleagues[37] reported 5-year and 10-year survival rates of 86% and 74%, respectively, for stage I patients with ILC treated by mastectomy not further stratified on the basis of tumor size.[37]

In multivariate analysis, histologic grade, tumor stage, size, and nodal status remain prognostically significant in ILC,[38] as in other invasive breast cancers. Significantly, histologic grading of ILC remains of value in this tumor type and should be undertaken. Although most (76%) patients with ILC have tumors of histologic grade 2 (scoring 3 for tubules, 2 for pleomorphism, and 1 for mitoses), tubulolobular forms are of histologic grade 1 and pleomorphic variants typically of histologic grade 3. Thus, 12% of ILCs are grade 1 and 12% grade 3 in some large series.[38] Conversely, lymphovascular invasion is less commonly seen in ILC than other types and is not of independent significance for prognosis in multivariate analysis, presumably because of the infrequency with which it is identified.[38]

Limited series suggest that pleomorphic ILC is an aggressive tumor with a frequent recurrence rate and death of patients from disease. Middleton and colleagues[35] reported a series of 38 cases, of which 19 patients had follow-up data available; 9 were dead of disease between 2 months to 9 years later and 3 were alive with disease with 2 months to 14 years follow-up. Although patients with

Fig. 15. Subtle classical ILC. H&E. (*A*) Scanty small cords or single cells of invasive carcinoma in a core biopsy or close to an excision margin can easily be missed. On this moderate-power view, the increase in cellularity of the field of view is apparent and closer inspection allows the correct diagnosis to be reached. (*B*) In the same case, high-power view shows short rows of cells, somewhat resembling plasma cells, with small regular nuclei, close to the margin of this wide local excision specimen. In such situations, or in needle core biopsy from a mass lesion, a low threshold for cytokeratin immunohistochemistry allows a correct diagnosis of classical ILC to be reached, because these tumor cells express epithelial markers.

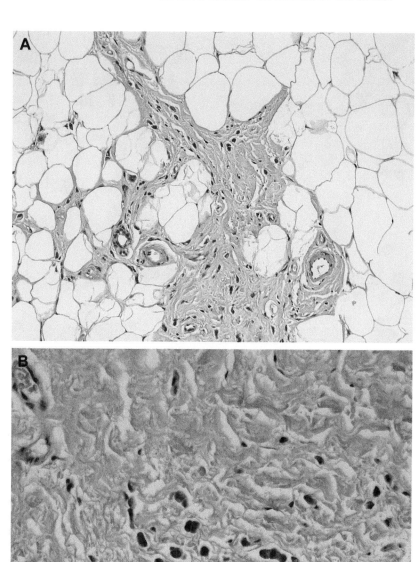

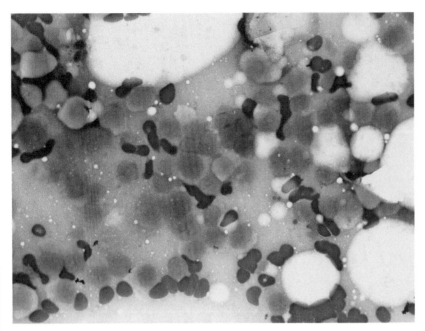

Fig. 16. Ultrasound-guided fine-needle aspiration cytology (FNAC) specimen (Giemsa-stained) of axillary lymph node. Although FNACs from ILCs are recognized as more difficult to diagnose on occasions, this FNAC from enlarged axillary lymph node in a patient with known ILC (same case as see **Fig. 8**) shows moderately sized cells with clearly evident cytoplasm, some with conspicuous nucleoli. The appearances are those of metastatic carcinoma.

classical ILC have a better prognosis than those with variant forms as a group,[39] including solid and pleomorphic variants, those with tubulolobular carcinoma have an excellent prognosis.[17] Thus, histologic variant is a predictor of prognosis within the broader group of ILCs; the tubulolobular variant has a significantly lower risk of regional (17%) and distant (13%) recurrence relative to the other subtypes, whereas the solid variant has significantly higher risk of recurrence (82% and 54%, respectively).

Among patients with ILC, 32% to 43% have associated axillary nodal metastases at diagnosis and 8% have distant metastases. ILC typically has a distinct pattern of metastasis, including spread to the bone marrow, orbit, peritoneum and retroperitoneum, leptomeninges, gastrointestinal tract (**Fig. 18**), and gynecologic organs, in the latter, for example, causing ovarian enlargement and resulting in a Krukenberg tumor; it forms pulmonary or pleural metastases less frequently than ductal/no special type.[40,41]

TREATMENT OF INVASIVE LOBULAR CARCINOMA

Breast-conserving surgery (wide local excision) with radiotherapy or mastectomy, depending on the site and size of the tumor and patient choice, is an appropriate treatment modality for ILCs as for other invasive breast cancers. Nonrandomized studies indicate that patient survival and local recurrence rates are similar to those of ductal/no special type carcinoma at 5 years[42,43] when managed by breast-conserving surgery therapy. A tendency, however, for later recurrence in patients who are followed up for 10 years has been reported.[44]

Conversion from wide local excision to mastectomy because of positive margins after re-excision has been reported as being required more frequently in patients treated for ILC by initial breast-conserving surgery.[45] This is particularly the case for those who have been treated with neoadjuvant (primary) chemotherapy[46]; approximately half of patients with ILC in some series are described as requiring completion mastectomy to obtain complete excision of disease, because of incomplete resection margins after neoadjuvant therapy. There is also evidence that ILC may intrinsically be less responsive to neoadjuvant chemotherapy than invasive carcinoma of ductal/no special type.[47,48] Conversely, a better response to adjuvant endocrine therapy is described,[49] with a greater improvement in survival in patients with ILC receiving hormone therapy compared with those matched patients with ductal/no special type breast cancers.

Fig. 17. Lymph node metastasis of ILC. (*A*) On medium-power H&E, a diffuse infiltrate of discohesive cells is seen in the sinus (*bottom left*) and the parenchyma of the lymph node. (*B*) Higher power shows that these are moderate in size, with abundant cytoplasm, but with a high nuclear-to-cytoplasmic ratio, prominent nucleoli, and relatively uniform cytology, indicating that these are not histiocytic in origin but are metastasis from primary ILC of the breast.

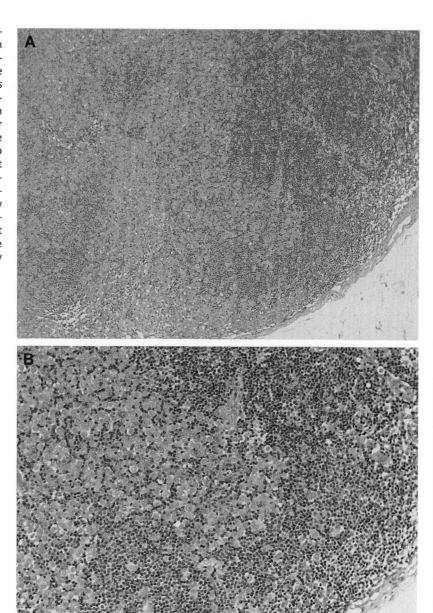

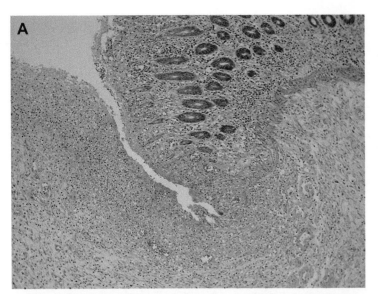

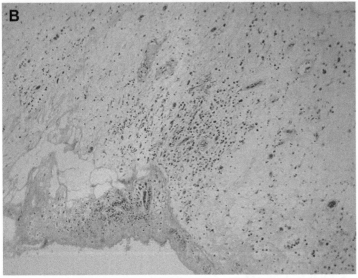

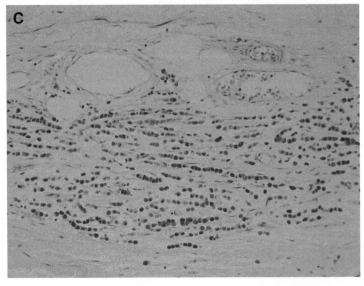

Fig. 18. Colonic resection for large bowel obstruction due to metastatic classical ILC. H&E. (*A*) Ulceration of the luminal surface of the large bowel is seen on low-power H&E; (*B*) the serosal surface is edematous with congestion of small blood vessel and shows increased cellularity, which on higher-power view H&E (*C*) shows single files of discohesive cells of metastatic ILC.

SUMMARY

ILC of the breast is a distinct histologic type with specific clinical, radiologic, and microscopic features, which is increasing in incidence in the Western world. *CDH1* is typically mutated and E-cadherin immunohistochemistry usually negative in ILC. The aberrant expression of this cell adhesion molecule is associated with the histologic features of diffuse, single-file infiltration. Routine pathologic prognostic factors, including grade, lymph node stage, and size, are of significance in predicting outcome in this group of patients who, overall, have survival comparable to those with other subtypes of breast cancer. Variants of the classical type, however, are seen and these have prognostic significance and should be recorded in pathology reports.

REFERENCES

1. Foote FW Jr, Stewart FW. Lobular carcinoma in situ: a rare form of mammary cancer. Am J Pathol 1941; 17:491–6.
2. Newman W. Lobular carcinoma of the female breast. Report of 73 cases. Ann Surg 1966;164:305–14.
3. Richter GO, Dockerty MB, Clagett OT. Diffuse infiltrating scirrhous carcinoma of the breast. Special consideration of the single filing phenomenon. Cancer 1967;20:363–70.
4. Henson D, Tarone R. A study of lobular carcinoma of the breast based on the Third National Cancer Survey in the United States of America. Tumori 1979;65:133–42.
5. Singh R, Hellman S, Heimann R. The natural history of breast carcinoma in the elderly: implications for screening and treatment. Cancer 2004;100(9):1807–13.
6. Verkooijen HM, Fioretta G, Vlastos G, et al. Important increase of invasive lobular breast cancer incidence in Geneva, Switzerland. Int J Cancer 2003;104:778–81.
7. Biglia N, Mariani L, Sgro L, et al. Increased incidence of lobular breast cancer in women treated with hormone replacement therapy: implications for diagnosis, surgical and medical treatment. Endocr Relat Cancer 2007;14:549–67.
8. Li CI, Malone K, Porter PL, et al. Relationship between menopausal hormone therapy and risk of ductal, lobular and ductal-lobular breast carcinomas. Cancer Epidemiol Biomarkers Prev 2008;17(1):43–50.
9. Schaapveld M, Visser O, Louwman WJ, et al. The impact of adjuvant therapy on contralateral breast cancer risk and the prognostic significance of contralateral breast cancer: a population based study in the Netherlands. Breast Cancer Res Treat 2008;110(1):189–97.
10. Malone KE, Begg CB, Haile RW, et al. Population-based study of the risk of second primary contralateral breast cancer associated with carrying a mutation in BRCA1 or BRCA2. J Clin Oncol 2010; 28(14):2404–10.
11. Kurian AW, McClure LA, John EM, et al. Second primary breast cancer occurrence according to hormone receptor status. J Natl Cancer Inst 2009; 101(15):1058–65.
12. Sastre-Garau X, Jouve M, Asselain B, et al. Infiltrating lobular carcinoma of the breast. Clinicopathologic analysis of 975 cases with reference to data on conservative therapy and metastatic patterns. Cancer 1996;77(1):113–20.
13. Dawson LA, Chow E, Goss PE. Evolving perspectives in contralateral breast cancer. Eur J Cancer 1998;34:2000–9.
14. Garnett S, Wallis M, Morgan G. Do screen-detected lobular and ductal carcinoma present with different mammographic features? Br J Radiol 2009;82:20–7.
15. Mann RM, Hoogeveen YL, Blickman JG, et al. MRI compared to conventional diagnostic work-up in the detection and evaluation of invasive lobular carcinoma of the breast: a review of existing literature. Breast cancer Res Treat 2008;107:1–14.
16. Tsuchiya S. Cytological characteristics of invasive lobular carcinoma of the human breast. Med Mol Morphol 2008;41(3):121–5.
17. Pereira H, Pinder SE, Sibbering DM, et al. Pathological prognostic factors in breast cancer. IV: should you be a typer or a grader? A comparative study of two histological prognostic features in operable breast carcinoma. Histopathology 1995;27(3):219–26.
18. Ellis IO, Galea M, Broughton N, et al. Pathological prognostic factors in breast cancer. II. Histological type. Relationship with survival in a large study with long-term follow-up. Histopathology 1992;20(6):479–89.
19. Tan PH, Harada O, Thike AA, et al. Histiocytoid breast carcinoma: an enigmatic lobular entity. J Clin Pathol 2011;64(8):654–9 [Epub 2011 Mar 12].
20. Gupta D, Croitoru CM, Ayala AG, et al. E-cadherin immunohistochemical analysis of histiocytoid carcinoma of the breast. Ann Diagn Pathol 2002;6(3): 141–7.
21. Frolik D, Caduff R, Varga Z. Pleomorphic lobular carcinoma of the breast: its cell kinetics, expression of oncogenes and tumour suppressor genes compared with invasive ductal carcinomas and classical infiltrating lobular carcinomas. Histopathology 2001;39(5): 503–13.
22. Martinez V, Azzopardi JG. Invasive lobular carcinoma of the breast: incidence of variants. Histopathology 1979;3:467–88.
23. Mastracci TL, Tjan S, Bane AL, et al. E-cadherin alterations in atypical lobular hyperplasia and lobular carcinoma in situ of the breast. Mod Pathol 2005;18(6):741–51.
24. Loffe O, Silverberg SG, Simsir A. Lobular lesions of the breast: immunohistochemical profile and

comparison with ductal proliferations. Mod Pathol 2000;13:23A.

25. Moriya T, Kozuka Y, Kanomata N, et al. The role of immunohistochemistry in the differential diagnosis of breast lesions. Pathology 2009;41(1):68–76.

26. Derksen PW, Liu X, Saridin F, et al. Somatic inactivation of E-cadherin and p53 in mice leads to metastatic lobular mammary carcinoma through induction of anoikis resistance and angiogenesis. Cancer Cell 2006;10(5):437–49.

27. Choi YJ, Pinto MM, Hao L, et al. Interobserver variability and aberrant E-cadherin immunostaining of lobular neoplasia and infiltrating lobular carcinoma. Mod Pathol 2008;21(10):1224–37.

28. Rakha EA, Patel A, Powe DG, et al. Clinical and biological significance of E-cadherin protein expression in invasive lobular carcinoma of the breast. Am J Surg Pathol 2010;34(10):1472–9.

29. Qureshi HS, Linden MD, Divine G, et al. E-cadherin status in breast cancer correlates with histologic type but does not correlate with established prognostic parameters. Am J Clin Pathol 2006;125:377–85.

30. Riva C, Dainese E, Caprara C, et al. Immunohistochemical study of androgen receptors in breast carcinoma. Evidence of their frequent expression in lobular carcinoma. Virchows Arch 2005;447:695–700.

31. Radhi JM. Immunohistochemical analysis of pleomorphic lobular carcinoma: higher expression of p53 and chromogranin and lower expression of ER and PgR. Histopathology 2000;36:156–60.

32. Wells CA, El-Ayat GA. Non-operative breast pathology: apocrine lesions. J Clin Pathol 2007;60(12):1313–20.

33. Mazoujian G, Bodian C, Haagensen DE Jr, et al. Expression of GCDFP-15 in breast carcinomas. Relationship to pathologic and clinical factors. Cancer 1989;63:2156–61.

34. Bilous M, Ades C, Armes J, et al. Predicting the HER2 status of breast cancer from basic histopathology data: an analysis of 1500 breast cancers as part of the HER2000 International Study. Breast 2003;12:92–8.

35. Middleton LP, Palacios DM, Bryant BR, et al. Pleomorphic lobular carcinoma: morphology, immunohistochemistry, and molecular analysis. Am J Surg Pathol 2000;24(12):1650–6.

36. Fadare O, Wan SA, Hileeto D. The expression of cytokeratin 5/6 in invasive lobular carcinoma of the breast: evidence of a basal-like subset? Hum Pathol 2008;39:331–6.

37. Ashikari R, Huvos AG, Urban JA, et al. Infiltrating lobular carcinoma of the breast. Cancer 1973;31:110–6.

38. Rakha EA, El-Sayed ME, Menon S, et al. Histologic grading is an independent prognostic factor in invasive lobular carcinoma of the breast. Breast Cancer Res Treat 2008;111(1):121–7.

39. du Toit RS, Locker AP, Ellis IO, et al. Invasive lobular carcinomas of the breast—the prognosis of histopathological subtypes. Br J Cancer 1989;60:605–9.

40. Harake MD, Maxwell AJ, Sukumar SA. Primary and metastatic lobular carcinoma of the breast. Clin Radiol 2001;56(8):621–30.

41. Bhat-Nakshatri P, Appaiah H, Ballas C, et al. SLUG/SNAI2 and tumour necrosis factor generate breast cells with CD44+/CD24- phenotype. BMC Cancer 2010;10:411.

42. Stolier AJ, Barre G, Bolton JS, et al. Breast conservation therapy for invasive lobular carcinoma: the impact of lobular carcinoma in situ in the surgical specimen on local recurrence and axillary node status. Am Surg 2004;70(9):818–21.

43. Hannoun-Levi JM, Ferré M, Raoust I, et al. [Accelerated partial breast irradiation using interstitial high dose rate brachytherapy: preliminary clinical and dosimetric results after 61 patients]. Cancer Radiother 2008;12(6–7):532–40 [in French].

44. Stucky CC, Gray RJ, Wasif N, et al. Increase in contralateral prophylactic mastectomy: echoes of a bygone era? Surgical trends for unilateral breast cancer. Ann Surg Oncol 2010;17(Suppl 3):330–7.

45. Yeatman TJ, Cantor AB, Smith TJ, et al. Tumour biology of infiltrating lobular carcinoma. Implications for management. Ann Surg 1995;222:549–61.

46. Straver ME, Rutgers EJ, Rodenhuis S, et al. The relevance of breast cancer subtypes in the outcome of neoadjuvant chemotherapy. Ann Surg Oncol 2010;17(9):2411–8.

47. Cristofanilli M, Gonzalez-Angulo A, Sneige N, et al. Invasive lobular carcinoma classic type: response to primary chemotherapy and survival outcomes. J Clin Oncol 2005;23:41–8.

48. Katz A, Saad ED, Porter P, et al. Primary systemic chemotherapy of invasive lobular carcinoma of the breast. Lancet Oncol 2007;8(1):55–62.

49. Rakha EA, El-Sayed ME, Powe DG, et al. Invasive lobular carcinoma of the breast: response to hormonal therapy and outcomes. Eur J Cancer 2008;44(1):73–83.

IMPORTANT INFLAMMATORY AND REACTIVE LESIONS OF THE BREAST

Jennifer S. Kaplan, MD, Stuart J. Schnitt, MD*

KEYWORDS

- Mammary duct ectasia • Lymphocytic mastopathy/diabetic mastopathy
- Idiopathic granulomatous mastitis/lobular granulomatous mastitis • Sarcoidosis
- Squamous metaplasia of lactiferous ducts • Nodular fasciitis • IgG4-related sclerosing mastitis
- Eosinophilic mastitis • Reactive spindle cell nodules • Inflammatory myofibroblastic tumors
- Reactions to foreign materials • Treatment effects

ABSTRACT

Some inflammatory and reactive lesions of the breast present problems clinically but are treated without resort to biopsy. In others, biopsy is required to make the correct diagnosis and to distinguish the process from malignancy. Still others represent incidental microscopic findings that may create diagnostic problems. This article reviews a number of inflammatory and reactive conditions that are likely to be encountered in routine surgical pathology practice, as well as those that have been recently described.

MAMMARY DUCT ECTASIA (PERIDUCTAL MASTITIS)

OVERVIEW

Mammary duct ectasia occurs primarily in perimenopausal and postmenopausal women, and is characterized by varying amounts of periductal inflammation, periductal fibrosis, and duct dilatation.[1] Patients may present with pain, nipple discharge, nipple retraction, and/or a mass. The clinical findings may mimic those of carcinoma. Mammography may demonstrate a ductal pattern of calcification that simulates the pattern of mammographic calcifications seen in association with ductal carcinoma in situ (DCIS).

GROSS FEATURES

In the early stages, the lesion is confined to the large subareolar ducts, but later an entire mammary segment may be involved. Cut section of the gross specimen often reveals dilated ducts with thick walls. The ducts may contain pasty, yellow-brown, intraluminal secretions, an appearance that may be mistaken for DCIS with comedo necrosis. The intervening stroma may be fibrotic.

MICROSCOPIC FEATURES

A wide spectrum of histologic changes is observed in this condition. Some cases are characterized by inspissation of lipid-rich material within ducts with

Key Features
OF MAMMARY DUCT ECTASIA

- Clinically may present with pain, nipple discharge, nipple retraction, and/or mass
- Disorder of extralobular ducts; may involve entire breast segment
- Early lesions: periductal inflammation with prominent plasma cells
- Later lesions: duct dilatation with periductal fibrosis and inspissated secretions

Department of Pathology, Beth Israel Deaconess Medical Center, Harvard Medical School, 330 Brookline Avenue, Boston, MA 02215, USA
* Corresponding author.
E-mail address: sschnitt@bidmc.harvard.edu

Surgical Pathology 5 (2012) 567–590
http://dx.doi.org/10.1016/j.path.2012.06.009

surgpath.theclinics.com

568

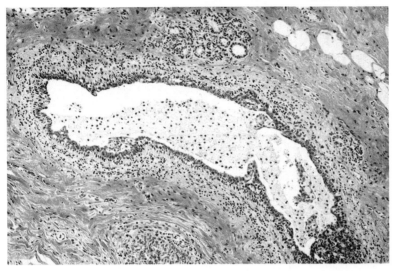

Fig. 1. Duct ectasia. This ectatic duct contains intraluminal foamy histiocytes and there is periductal chronic inflammation composed of lymphocytes and plasma cells.

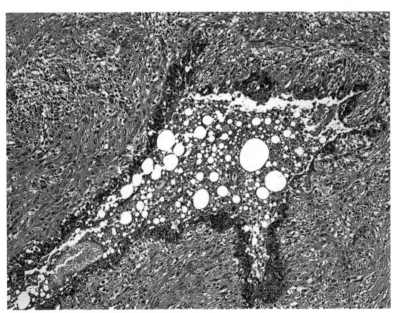

Fig. 2. Duct ectasia. Duct with inspissated secretions and periductal chronic inflammation.

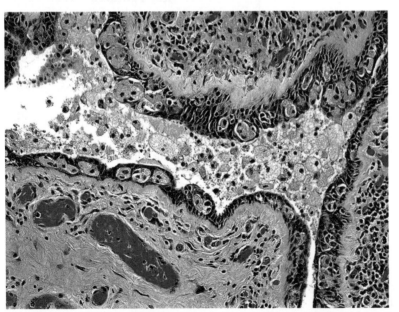

Fig. 3. Duct ectasia. Foamy histiocytes are present in the duct lumen and in the duct epithelium. There is periductal chronic inflammation with lymphocytes and plasma cells.

Fig. 4. Duct ectasia. The duct epithelium is attenuated and the lumen is filled with foamy histiocytes. There is periductal chronic inflammation including a poorly formed granuloma to the right side of the duct.

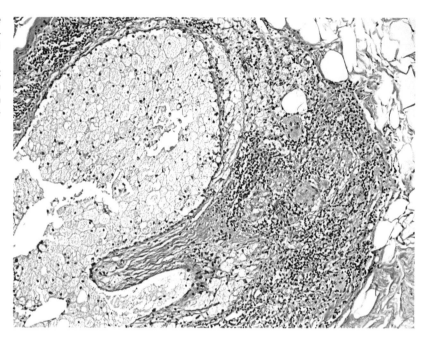

evidence of duct leakage or rupture and prominent periductal inflammation. Plasma cells may be a prominent component of the periductal inflammatory infiltrate. Foamy histiocytes are typically present within the inspissated intraductal secretions and may infiltrate the wall and the epithelium of involved ducts (**Figs. 1–3**). In some cases, histiocytes containing lipofuscin pigment ("ochrocytes")

are present. Less frequently, the periductal inflammatory infiltrate may be granulomatous or xanthogranulomatous (**Fig. 4**). Occasionally, there is an acute inflammatory component, and this can result in abscess or fistula formation.

In other cases, periductal fibrosis predominates (**Fig. 5**). This is often accompanied by ectasia of the ducts and/or obliteration of duct lumens. The

Fig. 5. Duct ectasia. In this example of later stage duct ectasia, there is prominent periductal fibrosis.

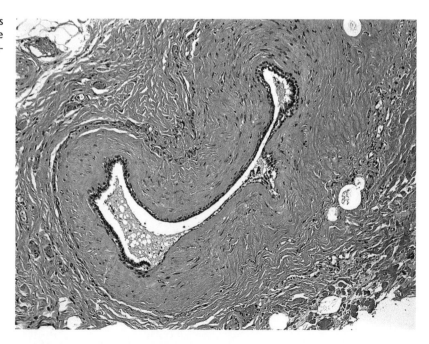

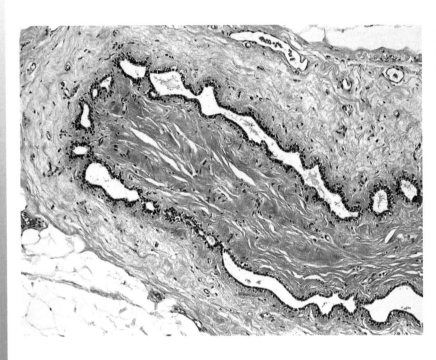

Fig. 6. Duct ectasia. The duct lumen is obliterated by fibrous tissue, which is surrounded by a "garland" of epithelial-lined spaces.

obliterated lumens may be surrounded by a ring of epithelial-lined tubular structures, sometimes referred to as "the garland pattern" (**Fig. 6**), or 1 or 2 epithelial-lined spaces may be seen to one side of an obliterated duct.

Variable degrees of ectasia of extralobular ducts is commonly identified in breast tissue obtained at autopsy and in surgically excised material; this has been observed in 30% to 40% of women older than 50 years. Clinically evident mammary duct ectasia, as described previously, however, occurs much less frequently,[2] and simply observing ectatic ducts in breast tissue sections is insufficient for a diagnosis of mammary duct ectasia (**Fig. 7**).

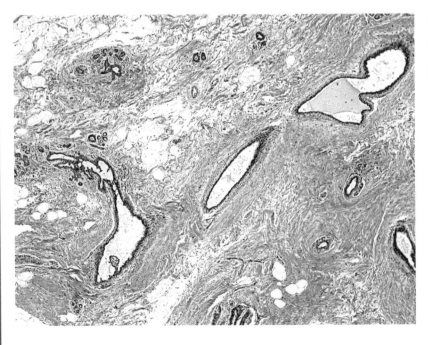

Fig. 7. Ectatic ducts in breast tissue from a postmenopausal woman. This should not be misinterpreted as the entity of mammary duct ectasia.

DIFFERENTIAL DIAGNOSIS

Duct ectasia may be difficult to distinguish from cysts in cases in which there is prominent ductal dilatation with little or no inflammatory component; however, duct ectasia is a disorder of extralobular ducts, whereas cysts arise in the terminal duct lobular units (TDLUs). If necessary, elastic tissue stains can be used to help make this distinction, as ducts contain elastic tissue in their walls whereas cysts do not.

Changes similar or identical to those seen in mammary duct ectasia (ductal dilatation, inspissation of secretions, periductal inflammation, and periductal fibrosis) may result when there is more proximal duct luminal obstruction by an intraductal lesion, such as an intraductal papilloma. A diagnosis of "duct ectasia" should not be made in such cases; the diagnosis of mammary duct ectasia should be reserved for cases in which no mechanical cause for duct obstruction is identified.

PATHOGENESIS

The pathogenesis of this condition has not been fully established. It has been postulated that periductal inflammation leads to periductal fibrosis, which subsequently results in ductal dilatation.[2] It has also been suggested, however, that periductal mastitis and duct ectasia represent 2 separate entities, based on differences between women with these 2 disorders with regard to age, clinical history, and smoking history.[3] In particular, smoking has been reported to be associated with periductal inflammation but not with duct dilatation. Mammary duct ectasia is an uncommon finding in children; the occurrence in this age group suggests a possible anomalous developmental etiology.[4]

LYMPHOCYTIC MASTOPATHY/DIABETIC MASTOPATHY

OVERVIEW

Lymphocytic mastopathy/diabetic mastopathy, which primarily affects young to middle-aged women, is most commonly seen in association with type 1 (insulin-dependent) diabetes, but similar histologic changes have been described in association with other autoimmune diseases, such as Hashimoto thyroiditis, in patients with

various types of autoantibodies in their serum, in patients without diabetes or other autoimmune diseases, in patients with type 2 diabetes, and in men.[5–7] Patients present with palpable or mammographically detected breast masses, predominantly located in the subareolar region, which may be multiple and have been reported to be bilateral in up to one-fifth of patients.[7]

MICROSCOPIC FEATURES

Histologic examination shows a characteristic constellation of features.[7] These include dense, keloidlike fibrosis; periductal, perilobular, and perivascular lymphocytic infiltrates (primarily composed of B-lymphocytes); and epithelioid myofibroblasts in the stroma (**Figs. 8–12**). The appearance of these latter cells may be alarming and, particularly when numerous, may lead to an erroneous diagnosis of an invasive carcinoma or a granular cell tumor.[8]

PROGNOSIS

Although the pathogenesis of this condition is unknown, it may represent an autoimmune reaction. Recurrences have been reported in up to one-third of patients.[7]

Key Features
OF LYMPHOCYTIC MASTOPATHY

- Patients present with palpable or radiographically detectable breast mass(es); may be bilateral

- Associated with autoimmune disorders, particularly type 1 (insulin-dependent) diabetes

- Histologic constellation of periductal, perilobular, and perivascular lymphocytic infiltrates, dense, keloidlike fibrosis, and epithelioid myofibroblasts

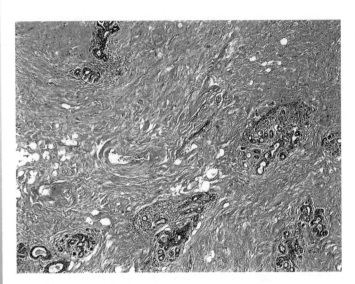

Fig. 8. Lymphocytic mastopathy (diabetic mastopathy). Stromal fibrosis and peril-obular chronic inflammatory infiltrates are evident.

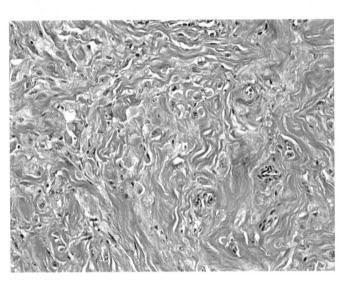

Fig. 9. Lymphocytic mastopathy (diabetic mastopathy). The fibrotic stroma contains epithelioid myofibroblasts.

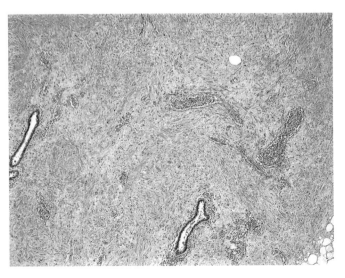

Fig. 10. Lymphocytic mastopathy (diabetic mastopathy). In this low-power image, peri-ductal and perivascular lymphocytic infil-trates and stromal fibrosis are evident.

Fig. 11. Lymphocytic mastopathy (diabetic mastop-
athy). Higher-power view
of the same case shown in
Fig. 10, illustrating periductal and perivascular lym-
phocytic infiltrates and
fibrotic stroma containing
epithelioid myofibroblasts.

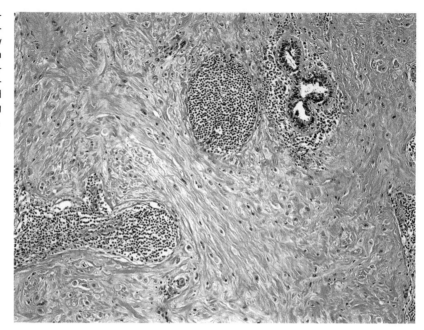

Fig. 12. Lymphocytic mastopathy (diabetic mastop-
athy). In this case, the
epithelioid myofibroblasts
are particularly promi-
nent, and could be miscon-
strued as epithelial cells in
the stroma.

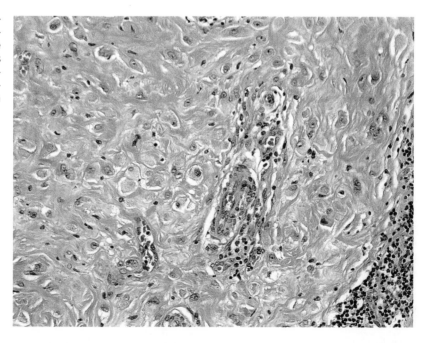

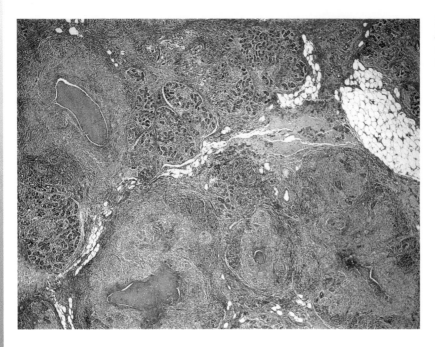

Fig. 13. Tuberculous mastitis. At scanning magnification, numerous necrotizing granulomas are evident.

GRANULOMATOUS LESIONS

Some infections, including those caused by mycobacteria, fungi, and parasites, are typically associated with granulomatous inflammation but are rare in Western countries. The histologic appearance of the granulomas in these disorders resembles those seen in other sites and will not be described further here (**Figs. 13** and **14**). In addition, non-necrotizing, sarcoid-type granulomas may be seen in the stroma of some breast carcinomas.[9] Finally, as noted and illustrated earlier (see **Fig. 4**), granulomatous inflammation may be seen in association with duct ectasia.

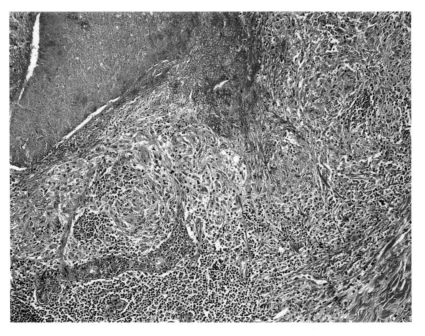

Fig. 14. Tuberculous mastitis. Higher-power view of the case shown in **Fig. 13**, showing the edge of one of the necrotizing granulomas. Acid-fast bacilli were demonstrated in this case.

Fig. 15. Sarcoidosis. At scanning magnification, numerous non-necrotizing granulomas are seen in the breast tissue.

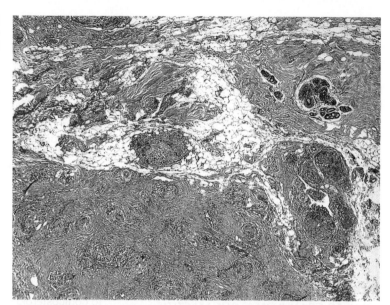

Fig. 16. Sarcoidosis. Confluent granulomas are present at the top of the field. A periductal granuloma is also evident.

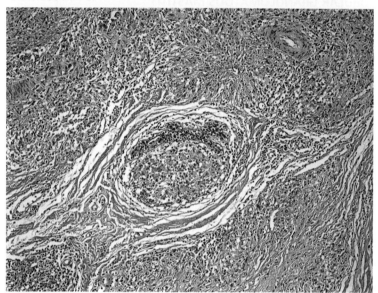

Fig. 17. Sarcoidosis. High-power view of the same case shown in *Fig. 16*, illustrating the non-necrotizing, periductal granuloma.

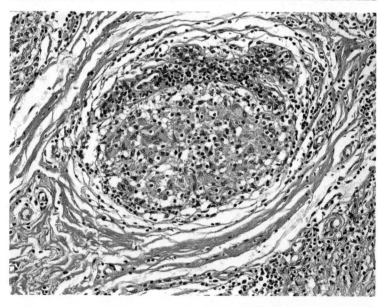

SARCOIDOSIS

Involvement of the breast by sarcoidosis is rare, but when present, may clinically simulate a neoplasm.[10] Histologically, the lesions consist of non-necrotizing granulomas with varying numbers of giant cells in the interlobular and intralobular stroma (**Figs. 15–17**). As in other organs, sarcoidosis is a diagnosis of exclusion, and other causes of granulomatous inflammation, such as infections and reactions to foreign materials, must be ruled out. Sarcoidosis must also be distinguished from idiopathic granulomatous mastitis (see the following section).

IDIOPATHIC GRANULOMATOUS MASTITIS/ LOBULAR GRANULOMATOUS MASTITIS

Overview

The cause of idiopathic granulomatous mastitis/ lobular granulomatous mastitis, an uncommon lesion, is obscure.[11,12] It usually presents as a mass, nearly always in young parous women, and is often related to recent pregnancy. Clinically, the lesion can simulate carcinoma. Bilateral disease sometimes occurs.

Microscopic Features

This lesion is characterized histologically by primarily lobulocentric granulomas that often contain neutrophils. The neutrophils may be numerous enough to create microabscesses (**Figs.** 18 and 19). Foci of necrosis may be present within the granulomas, but true caseous necrosis is not seen.

Differential Diagnosis

Although the lobulocentricity of the granulomas and the presence of neutrophils should raise the possibility of idiopathic granulomatous mastitis, other causes of granulomatous inflammation (such as infections, sarcoidosis, and reaction to foreign materials) should always be excluded.

Prognosis

The pathogenesis of idiopathic granulomatous mastitis is uncertain. Although these lesions may persist or recur, there is some evidence to suggest that patients with this condition respond favorably to corticosteroid therapy.

SQUAMOUS METAPLASIA OF LACTIFEROUS DUCTS

Overview

The keratinizing squamous epithelium of the skin normally extends into the nipple duct orifices for approximately 1 to 2 mm; however, if this epithelium extends more deeply into a nipple duct, keratin may accumulate, filling and obstructing the duct and creating a lesion analogous to an epidermal inclusion cyst. Rupture of the duct will result in the extrusion of keratinaceous debris into the stroma, eliciting a foreign body giant cell inflammatory reaction. Secondary bacterial colonization

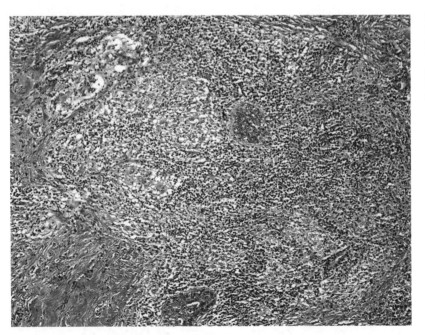

Fig. 18. Idiopathic granulomatous mastitis/lobular granulomatous mastitis. There are lobulocentric granulomas accompanied by a chronic inflammatory cell infiltrate.

Fig. 19. Idiopathic granu-lomatous mastitis/lobular granulomatous mastitis. High-power view of a gran-uloma showing scattered neutrophils.

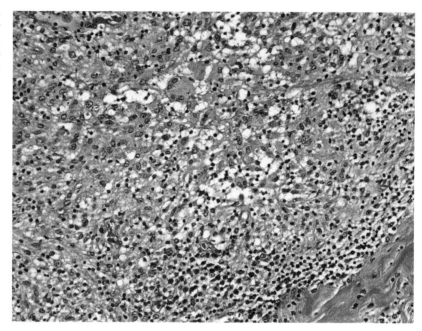

and infection may occur. This condition, known as squamous metaplasia of lactiferous ducts (SMOLD) (also known as Zuska disease and recur-rent subareolar abscess), presents as a red and painful mass near the nipple that may be inter-preted clinically to be an abscess.[13] It may occur at any age and is highly associated with a history of smoking.

Microscopic Features

The initial surgical procedure in patients with SMOLD is often incision and drainage of a presump-tive abscess. Specimens from this type of proce-dure typically consist of fragments of subareolar breast tissue, with or without subcutaneous tissue

Key Features
OF SQUAMOUS METAPLASIA OF
LACTIFEROUS DUCTS

- Clinically, red painful mass near the nipple suggesting abscess

- Highly associated with history of smoking

- Large ducts with squamous metaplasia of epithelium with or without intraluminal keratin; mixed periductal/stromal inflamma-tory infiltrate, including neutrophils and foreign body giant cell reaction

- Treatment requires complete excision of duct(s) involved

and/or skin, and show a mixed inflammatory infil-trate and foreign body giant cell reaction. Areas of abscess formation may be present. The findings of inflammation and foreign body giant cell reaction are not specific; however, in the appropriate clinical context, these findings should raise the suspicion of SMOLD and should prompt careful histologic eval-uation for the presence of keratinaceous debris within the inflammatory infiltrate and for ducts with squamous metaplasia and/or intraluminal keratin, the defining features of this disorder (**Figs. 20–23**). Of note, diagnostic features of SMOLD are more often seen in subsequent excision speci-mens, rather than in specimens from incision and drainage procedures, as more tissue is available for histologic examination.

Prognosis

Antibiotic therapy and/or incision and drainage procedures are generally ineffective. Treatment requires complete excision of the affected duct or ducts with wedge resection of the nipple. Failure to adequately excise the area may result in multiple recurrences or formation of a fistulous tract.[13,14]

NODULAR FASCIITIS

Overview

Nodular fasciitis is uncommonly seen in the breast, but is particularly important to recognize because it may clinically, radiographically, and histologi-cally mimic a malignant tumor.[2] Lesions of nodular

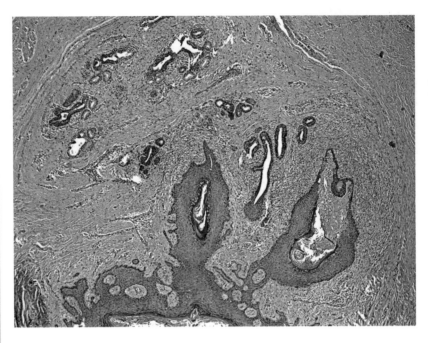

Fig. 20. SMOLD. Squamous metaplasia is seen completely or partially involving several nipple ducts, some of which contain intraluminal keratin. There is an associated stromal inflammatory infiltrate.

fasciitis may occur either in the subcutaneous tissue of the breast or in the mammary parenchyma. As in other sites, nodular fasciitis in the breast presents as a rapidly growing mass that may be painful or tender and disappears spontaneously within a few months.

Histologic Features

The histologic features are identical to those of nodular fasciitis elsewhere. The lesion is generally well circumscribed, but not encapsulated. Plump spindle cells (fibroblasts and myofibroblasts) with a "tissue culture" appearance are present in a stroma

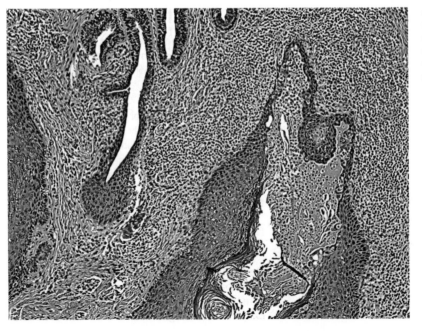

Fig. 21. SMOLD. Higher-power view of the same case shown in Fig. 20, demonstrating duct linings composed of keratinizing squamous epithelium. The periductal inflammation in this case is primarily composed of lymphocytes.

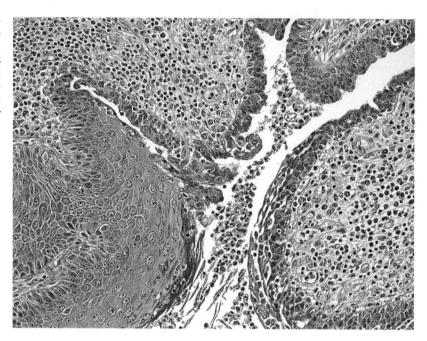

Fig. 22. SMOLD. Squamous metaplasia of the duct epithelium is evident. The duct lumen contains flakes of keratin and neutrophils. The periductal stroma shows chronic inflammation. (*Courtesy of* Dr Susan Lester.)

that ranges from loose and myxoid to collagenized. The spindle cells are arranged in short fascicles and whorls. The nuclei have prominent nucleoli, but are relatively uniform in appearance. Mitotic figures are readily identifiable and may be numerous. Extravasated erythrocytes and patchy lymphoid infiltrates are commonly seen in the stroma. The cellularity of the lesions varies; early lesions are highly cellular, whereas regressing lesions show less cellularity and more stromal collagen deposition (**Figs. 24–26**). Mammary ducts and lobules are usually not present within the lesion. The spindle cells typically express actin, but this may be focal. Desmin expression is also occasionally seen.

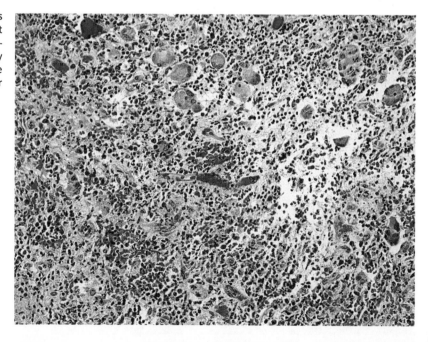

Fig. 23. SMOLD. In this case, there is prominent acute and chronic inflammation and foreign body giant cell reaction in the stroma. (*Courtesy of* Dr Susan Lester.)

580

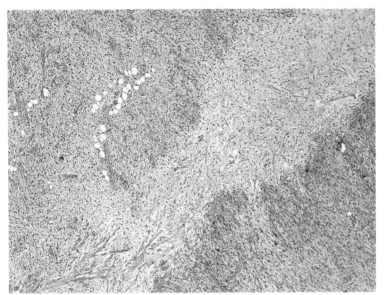

Fig. 24. Nodular fasciitis. This lesion is characterized by a variably cellular proliferation of spindle cells. The stroma shows focally prominent myxoid change. No mammary ducts or lobules are present in the lesion.

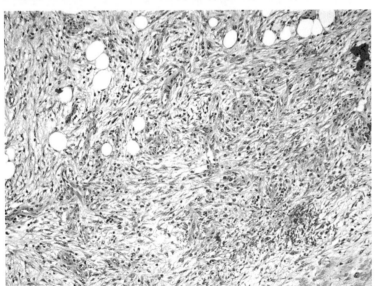

Fig. 25. Nodular fasciitis. Spindle cells, myxoid stroma, and extravasated erythrocytes are evident.

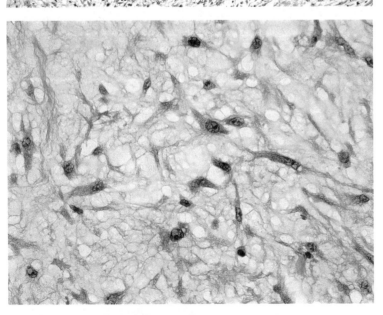

Fig. 26. Nodular fasciitis. The spindle cells exhibit a "tissue culture" appearance.

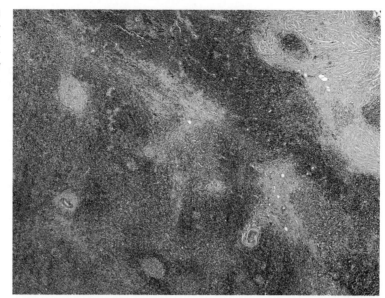

Fig. 27. IgG4-related sclerosing mastitis. Low-power view demonstrating diffuse and nodular chronic inflammatory cell infiltrates and stromal fibrosis. A few germinal centers are present. (*Courtesy of* Dr John K.C. Chan.)

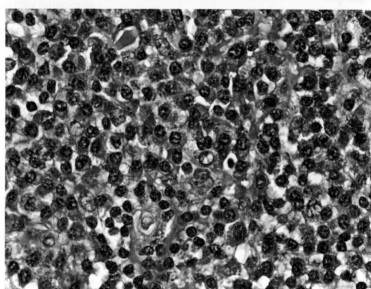

Fig. 28. IgG4-related sclerosing mastitis. High-power view demonstrating numerous plasma cells. (*Courtesy of* Dr John K.C. Chan.)

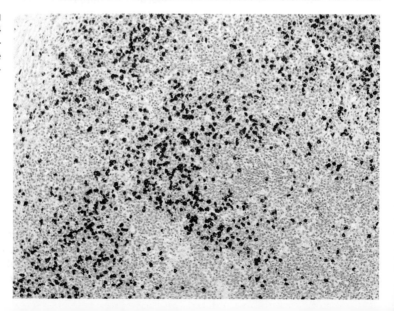

Fig. 29. IgG4-related sclerosing mastitis. Immunostain for IgG4 demonstrates numerous IgG4-positive plasma cells within the inflammatory infiltrate. (*Courtesy of* Dr John K.C. Chan.)

Differential Diagnosis

The major differential diagnostic considerations are malignant spindle cell tumors (including spindle cell carcinomas and sarcomas) and fibromatosis. Nodular fasciitis lacks the nuclear atypia of sarcomas and most spindle cell carcinomas and does not have the long, sweeping fascicles and infiltrative edge of fibromatosis. Furthermore, in contrast to spindle cell carcinomas, the cells of nodular fasciitis lack cytokeratin expression.

Prognosis

Although nodular fasciitis will spontaneously regress, the clinical presentation of a growing mass in the breast virtually always prompts a biopsy or excision. Local excision is adequate treatment.

IGG4-RELATED SCLEROSING MASTITIS

This recently described lesion is part of a growing family of IgG4-related sclerosing diseases and is characterized by discrete, painless breast masses that may be unilateral or bilateral. The masses consist of dense, diffuse, or nodular lymphoplasmacytic infiltrates with lymphoid follicles and a large component of IgG4+ plasma cells along with stromal sclerosis with lobular atrophy (Figs. 27–29). Patients may also have elevated serum levels of IgG4. In some patients, lesions are limited to the breast but in others, extramammary sites may be involved as well. The clinical course appears to be benign.[15]

EOSINOPHILIC MASTITIS

Breast manifestations of systemic diseases and noninfectious inflammatory diseases are rare. However, eosinophilic mastitis, which presents as a palpable breast mass, has been reported in association with peripheral eosinophilia, hypereosinophilic syndrome, Churg-Strauss syndrome, and allergic conditions. Histologically, there is extensive eosinophilic infiltration around ducts and lobules. Lymphocytes and plasma cells may be admixed within the infiltrate (Figs. 30 and 31). The epithelium of the involved ducts and lobules often appears reactive with enlarged nuclei and prominent nucleoli. These rare lesions may be locally aggressive and can recur following excision without control of the underlying disorder.[16]

REACTIVE SPINDLE CELL NODULES

Reactive spindle cell nodules (RSCNs), similar in appearance to the postoperative spindle cell nodules reported in the genitourinary tract and thyroid, may also occur in the breast.[17] These are most often seen following needle biopsy of lesions with a prominent stromal component, such as papillary lesions and complex sclerosing lesions. RSCNs consist of intersecting fascicles of plump spindle cells with admixed blood vessels, collagen fibers, and a mixed inflammatory infiltrate, including lymphocytes, plasma cells, and macrophages, some of which are hemosiderin-laden. The spindle cells, which have an immunophenotype consistent with myofibroblasts, show mild to moderate pleomorphism and rare mitotic figures (Figs. 32 and 33). Distinguishing RSCNs from other spindle cell lesions of the breast may be challenging; a history of a previous needling procedure and the presence of other changes associated with biopsy sites, such as hemosiderin and foamy histiocytes, help lead to the diagnosis of RSCN.

INFLAMMATORY MYOFIBROBLASTIC TUMOR

Inflammatory myofibroblastic tumors of the breast are rare and, like those of other sites, are characterized by a proliferation of bland myofibroblasts with an admixed polymorphous inflammatory cell infiltrate composed of prominent plasma cells, lymphocytes, and eosinophils. Fibrosis and collagen deposition may be present, and varying amounts of myxoid and/or vascular areas may be seen. Clinically, these lesions often present as palpable and discrete masses that may mimic carcinoma. Recurrences have been reported and rare cases may metastasize. Some studies have demonstrated clonality in inflammatory myofibroblastic tumors, suggesting a neoplastic rather than reactive etiology.[18,19]

REACTIONS TO FOREIGN MATERIAL

BIOPSY SITE MARKING DEVICES

Overview

Marking devices are now commonly placed in the breast following core needle biopsy so that the location of the biopsy site can be identified on subsequent radiologic examination. Those most commonly used are composed of bovine collagen plugs and pellets of a resorbable copolymer, similar to Vicryl suture material.

Microscopic Features

The histologic changes associated with these marking devices differ. The collagen plugs appear as broad bands of eosinophilic, acellular material. There is an accompanying inflammatory infiltrate

Fig. 30. Eosinophilic mastitis. In this breast core-needle biopsy specimen, there is a stromal inflammatory infiltrate with a prominent component of eosinophils.

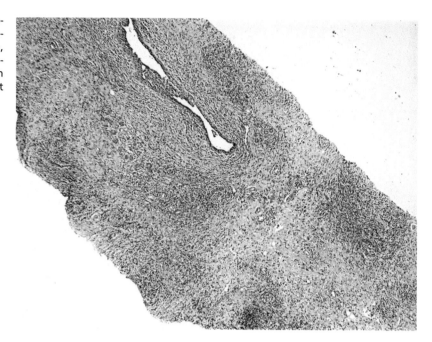

composed of lymphocytes, plasma cells, eosinophils, and occasionally neutrophils, initially at the periphery of the plug, but later within the plug, admixed with the collagen fibers. Foreign body–type giant cells are uncommon. With time, the plug is infiltrated by granulation tissue and there is deposition of native collagen. The copolymer pellets, which may dissolve during tissue processing, are initially associated with a fibrotic rim, with sparse lymphocytes and eosinophils, around empty spaces. Later biopsies show a histiocytic and foreign body–type giant cell reaction around the empty spaces and infiltration of the spaces by fibrinous material.[20]

Fig. 31. Eosinophilic mastitis. High-power view of the same case shown in **Fig. 30,** showing numerous eosinophils and scattered lymphocytes and plasma cells.

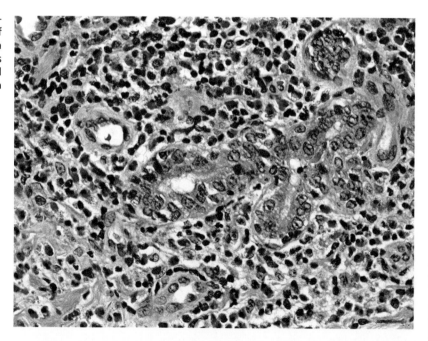

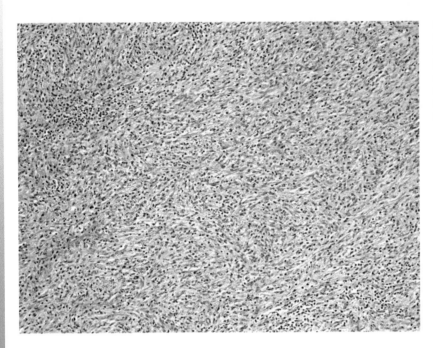

Fig. 32. Reactive spindle cell nodule. The lesion is composed of fascicles of spindle cells in a collagenous stroma with admixed blood vessels, chronic inflammatory cells, and hemosiderin.

REACTIONS TO MAMMARY IMPLANTS

Overview

A variety of tissue reactions have been reported in association with mammary implants.[21] The most common is the formation of a fibrous capsule in the surrounding tissue. In 10% to 40% of patients there is contracture of this capsule, which results in breast tightness or firmness and deformation of the implant, necessitating either capsulotomy or removal of the implant and the surrounding capsule.

Microscopic Features

Histologic examination of the capsular tissue shows varying degrees of fibrosis, chronic inflammation,

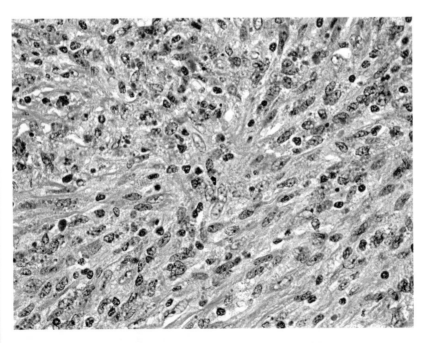

Fig. 33. Reactive spindle cell nodule. The spindle cells are mildly atypical and have plump nuclei. There is prominent hemosiderin deposition.

Fig. 34. Breast implant capsule with synovial metaplasia.

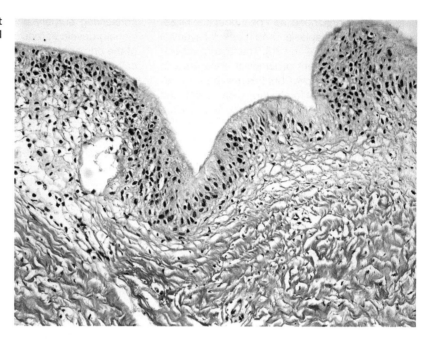

fat necrosis, granulation tissue, fibrin deposition, histiocytes, foreign body giant cells, and calcifications. Additionally, in the case of silicone gel implants, silicone (and where it has been used as part of the implant shell, polyurethane) may be present within the capsule. Silicone gel leakage may be seen even in the absence of implant rupture, and characteristically produces oval, cystic spaces that appear empty or contain amorphous, pale material, which is not birefringent with polarized light.[22] Silicone can diffuse to a variety of sites around the body, and silicone lymphadenopathy has been reported in axillary lymph nodes; hematogenous dissemination can also occur. Some capsules surrounding breast implants develop a cellular lining that histologically, immunohistochemically, and ultrastructurally resembles either normal synovium or synovium with papillary hyperplasia (proliferative synovitis) and has physiologic properties similar to synovium.[21] This change has

Fig. 35. Breast implant capsule with synovial metaplasia. In this case, the lining of the implant capsule resembles proliferative synovitis.

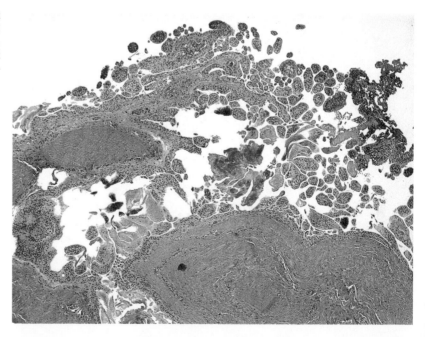

been variably described as "pseudoepithelialization," "synovial metaplasia," and "capsular synovial hyperplasia" (**Figs. 34** and **35**). The factors associated with development of synovial metaplasia in this setting are not known, but this may be a consequence of mechanical forces (eg, micromotion and friction) between the implant and the surrounding tissue.

Mesenchymal tumors, such as fibromatosis and sarcomas, have been reported in association with both silicone and saline mammary implants. This phenomenon appears to be rare, however, with only 24 cases reported to date. Whether there is a cause-and-effect relationship between the implants and these mesenchymal lesions remains to be determined.[23] Most recently, examples of anaplastic large-cell lymphoma have been reported to occur in association with implant capsules.[24]

TREATMENT EFFECTS

RADIATION

Overview

Radiation-induced changes in the skin of the breast are identical to those described in irradiated skin from other sites and include epidermal atrophy and telangiectasia.[25] The nature of these changes is, in part, dependent on the interval between irradiation and histologic examination. Patients with invasive cancer and DCIS treated by breast-conserving surgery and radiation therapy occasionally develop areas of fat necrosis in the vicinity of the primary tumor site. These lesions may clinically, mammographically, and macroscopically resemble carcinoma.[26] Although the diagnosis of fat necrosis can be readily made on core needle biopsy, whether the changes in the needle biopsy samples are fully representative of the lesion in the breast may be a matter of concern. In such cases, careful clinical-radiologic-pathologic correlation is essential to avoid the underdiagnosis of breast cancer recurrence. If there is doubt about whether or not the core biopsy samples are representative, a surgical excision should be performed.

Microscopic Features

A characteristic constellation of histologic changes is observed in non-neoplastic breast tissue in patients treated by breast-conserving surgery and radiation therapy.[27] The most frequent finding is that of scattered atypical epithelial cells in the TDLU, usually associated with variable degrees of lobular sclerosis and atrophy (**Figs 36** and **37**). These atypical cells are large, with enlarged, diffusely hyperchromatic nuclei, generally small or inconspicuous nucleoli, and finely vacuolated eosinophilic cytoplasm. The cells often protrude into the lumen of the involved duct or acinus but do not show evidence of proliferation, such as cellular stratification, loss of polarity, or mitotic activity.

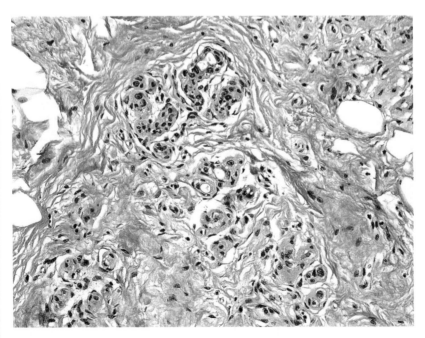

Fig. 36. Radiation effect. Several terminal duct lobular units are present in this image and show variable sclerosis. Scattered enlarged epithelial cells with atypical nuclei are evident.

Fig. 37. Radiation effect. The acini in the terminal duct lobular units shown in this image show sclerosis and scattered atypical epithelial cells.

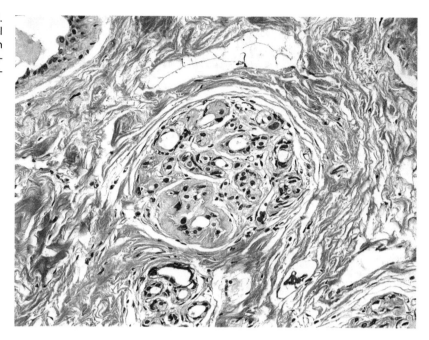

Additional pathologic changes that may be observed in non-neoplastic irradiated breast tissue include epithelial atypia in large (extralobular) ducts, atypical fibroblasts in the stroma, and vascular changes, such as myointimal hyperplasia in small arteries and prominent capillary endothelial cells.[27] These changes tend to be most pronounced in cases in which the alterations in the TDLU are marked, however. It is important to note that stromal fibrosis, a well-recognized feature of radiation effect in other organs, is so variable in both irradiated and nonirradiated breasts that it cannot by itself be considered a constant and reliable histologic indicator of prior irradiation in the breast.

Differential Diagnosis

The most important differential diagnosis is distinguishing radiation effects from carcinoma to prevent an incorrect diagnosis of tumor recurrence. The distinction between radiation change and lobular carcinoma in situ is not difficult because of the characteristic histologic appearance of the latter, ie, a monotonous population of relatively small cells that fill and distend small ducts and acini. The differentiation of radiation-induced changes from DCIS involving the TDLU (cancerization of lobules) may be more difficult; however, when DCIS involves the TDLU, there is generally evidence of cellular proliferation, as characterized by cellular stratification, loss of polarity, and distension of the involved ducts and acini. In addition, the nuclei in carcinoma cells tend to show irregularly dispersed chromatin and variably prominent nucleoli. Finally, necrosis of varying degrees may be seen with DCIS, and mitoses may be apparent. Conversely, the epithelial cells in areas of radiation change generally show maintenance of cellular polarity and cohesion, lack of stratification, a diffuse homogeneous increase in chromatin, usually small or inconspicuous nucleoli, and no evidence of necrosis or mitotic activity. In some instances of radiation change, there may be extensive lobular fibrosis and atrophy with distortion of the lobular architecture. Entrapment of acini containing atypical epithelial cells may result in a pseudoinfiltrative pattern, thereby simulating invasive carcinoma; however, the lobulocentric configuration of such areas is usually apparent on low-power examination.

CHEMOTHERAPY

In patients treated with neoadjuvant chemotherapy, non-neoplastic breast tissue shows atrophic changes and a considerable reduction in the volume of lobular tissue compared with untreated women of similar age. Lobular sclerosis is often present, as well as attenuation of the epithelium lining the ducts and lobules; this results in the appearance of a prominent myoepithelial cell layer.[28–30] Nuclear atypia in the non-neoplastic epithelium, similar to that described previously, after radiation treatment is seen in some patients treated with chemotherapy.[29–31]

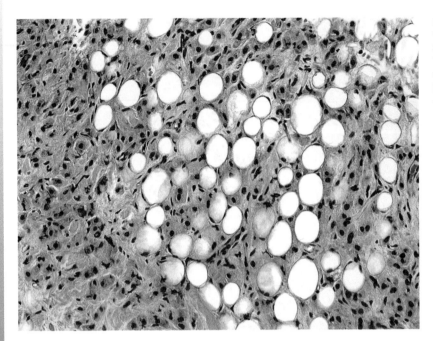

Fig. 38. Histiocytoid variant of invasive lobular carcinoma. The presence within fat of tumor cells with abundant, foamy cytoplasm mimics the appearance of fat necrosis.

MIMICS OF INFLAMMATORY AND REACTIVE LESIONS

A variety of lesions may mimic inflammatory and reactive processes. Desmoid-type fibromatosis may mimic a scar in the breast. The presence of fat necrosis, foreign body giant cell reaction, and hemosiderin deposition favors a diagnosis of scar, whereas nuclear expression of β-catenin favors fibromatosis.[32] Similarly, low-grade fibromatosislike metaplastic carcinoma can be misinterpreted as a scar. Immunostains for cytokeratin or p63 may be required to make this distinction. Spindle cell metaplastic carcinomas with a fasciitis-type pattern may be difficult to distinguish from nodular fasciitis. Again, immunostains for cytokeratin or p63 may be of value in distinguishing between these lesions. Lymphoproliferative and hematopoietic lesions, including chronic lymphocytic leukemia, low-grade B-cell lymphomas, and extramedullary hematopoiesis, among others, may mimic inflammatory infiltrates in the breast. Careful attention to the pattern and cytologic features of the infiltrates and appropriate

---

Pitfalls
DIAGNOSIS OF INFLAMMATORY AND REACTIVE LESIONS OF THE BREAST

! Inflammatory and reactive lesions may mimic neoplasms
  - Epithelioid myofibroblasts in lymphocytic mastitis may mimic invasive carcinoma
  - Spindle cells in reactive spindle cell nodule and nodular faciitis may mimic benign and malignant spindle cell neoplasms
  - Atypical epithelial cells in radiation changes may mimic DCIS or even invasive carcinoma
  - Scars may mimic fibromatosis

! Neoplasms may mimic reactive and inflammatory lesions
  - Fibromatosis and low-grade fibromatosislike metaplastic carcinoma may mimic scars
  - Lymphoma and classic invasive lobular carcinoma may mimic chronic inflammatory cell infiltrates
  - Histiocytoid variant of invasive lobular carcinoma may mimic histiocytic infiltrates of fat necrosis

immunostains may be required to arrive at the correct diagnosis. Some invasive lobular carcinomas with only patchy involvement of the breast and/or widely dispersed cells may be mistaken for inflammatory infiltrates, particularly on low-power examination. Examination of the cells at higher power may be necessary to make this distinction. The histiocytoid variant of invasive lobular carcinoma may in some areas closely mimic fat necrosis (Fig. 38); cytokeratin immunostains may be required to make the correct diagnosis.

REFERENCES

1. Haagensen CD. Diseases of the breast. 3rd edition. Philadelphia: W. B. Saunders; 1986.
2. Dixon JM, Anderson TJ, Lumsden AB, et al. Mammary duct ectasia. Br J Surg 1983;70(10): 601–3.
3. Dixon JM, Ravisekar O, Chetty U, et al. Periductal mastitis and duct ectasia: different conditions with different aetiologies. Br J Surg 1996;83(6):820–2.
4. McHoney M, Munro F, Mackinlay G. Mammary duct ectasia in children: report of a short series and review of the literature. Early Hum Dev 2011;87(8): 527–30.
5. Schwartz IS, Strauchen JA. Lymphocytic mastopathy. An autoimmune disease of the breast? Am J Clin Pathol 1990;93(6):725–30.
6. Lammie GA, Bobrow LG, Staunton MD, et al. Sclerosing lymphocytic lobulitis of the breast—evidence for an autoimmune pathogenesis. Histopathology 1991;19(1):13–20.
7. Ely KA, Tse G, Simpson JF, et al. Diabetic mastopathy. A clinicopathologic review. Am J Clin Pathol 2000;113(4):541–5.
8. Ashton MA, Lefkowitz M, Tavassoli FA. Epithelioid stromal cells in lymphocytic mastitis—a source of confusion with invasive carcinoma. Mod Pathol 1994;7(1):49–54.
9. Bassler R, Birke F. Histopathology of tumour associated sarcoid-like stromal reaction in breast cancer. An analysis of 5 cases with immunohistochemical investigations. Virchows Arch A Pathol Anat Histopathol 1988;412(3):231–9.
10. Gansler TS, Wheeler JE. Mammary sarcoidosis. Two cases and literature review. Arch Pathol Lab Med 1984;108(8):673–5.
11. Kessler E, Wolloch Y. Granulomatous mastitis: a lesion clinically simulating carcinoma. Am J Clin Pathol 1972;58(6):642–6.
12. Donn W, Rebbeck P, Wilson C, et al. Idiopathic granulomatous mastitis. A report of three cases and review of the literature. Arch Pathol Lab Med 1994; 118(8):822–5.
13. Lester S. Subareolar abscess (Zuska's Disease): a specific disease entity with specific treatment
and prevention strategies. Pathol Case Rev 1999; 4(5):189–93.
14. Meguid MM, Oler A, Numann PJ, et al. Pathogenesis-based treatment of recurring subareolar breast abscesses. Surgery 1995;118(4):775–82.
15. Cheuk W, Chan AC, Lam WL, et al. IgG4-related sclerosing mastitis: description of a new member of the IgG4-related sclerosing diseases. Am J Surg Pathol 2009;33(7):1058–64.
16. Komenaka IK, Schnabel FR, Cohen JA, et al. Recurrent eosinophilic mastitis. Am Surg 2003;69(7):620–3.
17. Gobbi H, Tse G, Page DL, et al. Reactive spindle cell nodules of the breast after core biopsy or fine-needle aspiration. Am J Clin Pathol 2000;113(2):288–94.
18. Khanafshar E, Phillipson J, Schammel DP, et al. Inflammatory myofibroblastic tumor of the breast. Ann Diagn Pathol 2005;9(3):123–9.
19. Hill PA. Inflammatory pseudotumor of the breast: a mimic of breast carcinoma. Breast J 2010;16(5): 549–50.
20. Guarda LA, Tran TA. The pathology of breast biopsy site marking devices. Am J Surg Pathol 2005;29(6): 814–9.
21. Schnitt SJ. Tissue reactions to mammary implants: a capsule summary. Adv Anat Pathol 1995;2(1): 24–7.
22. Kossovsky N, Freiman CJ. Silicone breast implant pathology. Clinical data and immunologic consequences. Arch Pathol Lab Med 1994;118(7):686–93.
23. Balzer BL, Weiss SW. Do biomaterials cause implant-associated mesenchymal tumors of the breast? Analysis of 8 new cases and review of the literature. Hum Pathol 2009;40(11):1564–70.
24. de Jong D, Vasmel WL, de Boer JP, et al. Anaplastic large-cell lymphoma in women with breast implants. JAMA 2008;300(17):2030–5.
25. Fajardo LJ. Pathology of radiation injury. New York: Masson Publishing; 1982.
26. Clarke D, Curtis JL, Martinez A, et al. Fat necrosis of the breast simulating recurrent carcinoma after primary radiotherapy in the management of early stage breast carcinoma. Cancer 1983;52(3):442–5.
27. Schnitt SJ, Connolly JL, Harris JR, et al. Radiation-induced changes in the breast. Hum Pathol 1984; 15(6):545–50.
28. Sharkey FE, Addington SL, Fowler LJ, et al. Effects of preoperative chemotherapy on the morphology of resectable breast carcinoma [see comments]. Mod Pathol 1996;9(9):893–900.
29. Kennedy S, Merino MJ, Swain SM, et al. The effects of hormonal and chemotherapy on tumoral and non-neoplastic breast tissue. Hum Pathol 1990;21(2): 192–8.
30. Fisher ER, Wang J, Bryant J, et al. Pathobiology of preoperative chemotherapy: findings from the National Surgical Adjuvant Breast and Bowel (NSABP) protocol B-18. Cancer 2002;95(4):681–95.

31. Pinder SE, Provenzano E, Earl H, et al. Laboratory handling and histology reporting of breast specimens from patients who have received neoadjuvant chemotherapy. Histopathology 2007;50(4):409–17.

32. Abraham SC, Reynolds C, Lee JH, et al. Fibromatosis of the breast and mutations involving the APC/beta-catenin pathway. Hum Pathol 2002;33(1): 39–46.

SMALL GLANDULAR PROLIFERATIONS OF THE BREAST

Timothy M. D'Alfonso, MD, Sandra J. Shin, MD*

KEYWORDS

- Glandular proliferations • Sclerosing lesions • Tubular carcinoma • Epithelial displacement

ABSTRACT

This article discusses the most common small glandular proliferations, namely sclerosing lesions (sclerosing adenosis and radial scar), tubular carcinoma, and epithelial displacement after needle core biopsy, as well as less common entities, such as low-grade adenosquamous carcinoma, microglandular adenosis, and syringomatous adenoma. Due to significant morphologic overlap, these entities are easily mistaken for one another. The similarities and differences among these lesions in their clinicopathologic features, radiologic findings, and immunohistochemical profiles are emphasizesd.

OVERVIEW

In the breast, small glandular proliferations comprise a spectrum of benign, atypical, and malignant lesions. In most cases, the cytologic and architectural features are diagnostic and the entity can be appropriately classified. In some cases, however, particularly those with cytologically bland or uniform cells, the architectural features alone are insufficient to warrant a definitive diagnosis. This is particularly true in limited material, such as needle core biopsies, where tissue fragmentation and inadequate sampling of the lesion compound an already problematic issue. Important clinical, radiologic and pathologic features across the spectrum of small glandular proliferations of the breast will be discussed in the following text. Hopefully this discussion will be useful in guiding pathologists who may encounter a small glandular proliferation of the breast in routine practice (**Tables 1** and **2**).

SCLEROSING ADENOSIS

OVERVIEW

Adenosis refers to a benign lobulocentric glandular proliferation, composed of epithelial and myoepithelial cells, that arises from terminal duct lobular units. The most common form of adenosis is sclerosing adenosis, which denotes adenosis with associated stromal proliferation that frequently compresses the involved glands. Sclerosing adenosis is commonly seen as part of the spectrum of fibrocystic changes in the breast. When foci of sclerosing adenosis become coalescent and mass forming, the terms, *adenosis tumor* and *nodular adenosis*, are used to describe these lesions.

Most cases of sclerosing adenosis are discovered incidentally in surgical specimens or on screening imaging. Less frequently, sclerosing adenosis presents as a palpable abnormality. There is a slight increase in the risk of developing breast cancer in patients with sclerosing adenosis, which is similar to that of other proliferative fibrocystic changes.[1–4] Histologically, sclerosing adenosis is a small glandular proliferation that can mimic invasive carcinoma, particularly in needle core biopsy samples, in which the lesion's lobulocentric growth pattern may be difficult to recognize.

Department of Pathology and Laboratory Medicine, New York-Presbyterian Hospital – Weill Cornell Medical College, New York, NY, USA

* Corresponding author. Department of Pathology and Laboratory Medicine, Surgical Pathology-Starr 1002, 525 East 68th Street, New York, NY 10065.

E-mail address: sjshin@med.cornell.edu

Surgical Pathology 5 (2012) 591–643

http://dx.doi.org/10.1016/j.path.2012.06.007

1875-9181/12/$ – see front matter © 2012 Elsevier Inc. All rights reserved.

Table 1
Pathologic features of small glandular proliferations

Feature	Tubular Carcinoma	Radial Scar	Sclerosing Adenosis	MGA	LGASC	Syringomatous Adenoma	Displaced Epithelium
Growth pattern	Haphazard, infiltrative	Stellate, infiltrative	Lobulocentric, nodular	Haphazard, infiltrative	Infiltrative, sometimes stellate	Infiltrative	Clustered
Gland shape	Open, teardrop-shaped, angulated	Angulated, tubular, distorted	Round, tubular, elongated	Uniform, round	Angulated, branching	Tadpole-shaped with comma-like tails, teardrop, branching	Variable, micropapillary with underlying papillary lesion
Luminal secretion	Occasionally present, basophilic	Not present	Occasionally present	Dense, eosinophilic, PAS positive, diastase resistant	Occasionally present; eosinophilic, condensed	Occasionally present; pink, retracted, PAS positive	Not present
Luminal cytoplasmic snouts	Present	Not present	Not present	Not present	Not present	Not present	Not present
Myoepithelial layer	Not present	Present, may be attenuated or focally absent	Present	Not present	Variably present	Variably present	Variable, may be attenuated or absent
Basement membrane	Not present	Present	Present	Present	Present by electron microscopy in 1 study[92]	Not well studied	Not well studied
Stroma	Desmoplastic, elastotic	Elastotic	Fibrous	Hypocellular fibrous tissue, no stromal reaction	Fibrous or cellular around glands	Fibrous or mildly cellular around glands	Reactive, granulation tissue-like or scar, lacks desmoplasia
Squamous differentiation	Not present	Infrequent	Not present	Not present	Present, variable in degree	Present, keratin cysts	Occasional (reactive) metaplasia
Chronic inflammation; lymphoid aggregates	Not present	Not present	Not present	Not present	Present	Not present (unless with ruptured keratin cyst with associated chronic inflammation and foreign body giant cell reaction)	Occasional, associated with acute and chronic inflammation

Table 2
Immunohistochemical profiles of small glandular proliferations

Immunohistochemical Marker	Tubular Carcinoma	Radial Scar	Sclerosing Adenosis	MGA	LGASC	Syringomatous Adenoma	Epithelial Displacement
ER/PR	+ (Diffuse, strong)	+ (Focal)	+	−	−	−	Variable
Circumferential p63	−	Variable, may be attenuated or focally absent	+	−	Variable or absent	Variable or absent	Variable, may be attenuated or absent
Basement membrane—laminin, collagen IV	−	+	+	+	Not well studied	Not well studied	Not well studied
Circumferential smooth muscle myosin heavy chain	−	Variable, may be attenuated	+	−	Variable in glands and spindle cell metaplasia (stromal)	Variable	Variable, may be attenuated or absent
S-100 protein	−	−	+, Myoepithelium	+	−	−	−

CLINICAL FEATURES

Sclerosing adenosis is most often encountered in premenopausal women in their 30s and 40s.[5–8] Frequently, sclerosing adenosis is found as an incidental microscopic finding associated with other fibrocystic changes. Sclerosing adenosis may be detected on screening imaging and may be biopsied because of the presence of microcalcifications or a mammographic density. Some cases of sclerosing adenosis come to attention as a palpable mass, which can clinically simulate invasive carcinoma.[8,9] Some patients may present with breast pain.[6,8]

IMAGING

Sclerosing adenosis has a variable radiographic appearance and may manifest as microcalcifications, architectural distortion, a mass lesion, or an asymmetric opacity.[6] Calcifications are frequently present and can be amorphous, punctate, pleomorphic and are often clustered.[6,7,10] When a mass is identified, it may be circumscribed or stellate and irregular in appearance.[7] In some patients, especially younger patients with dense breast tissue, a mass may not be identified on mammography but may be discovered on ultrasound examination.[6,7] On sonography, sclerosing adenosis may present as a solid lesion with well-defined borders or may appear ill-defined.[8]

Some cases manifest as acoustic shadowing or heterogeneity, without an identifiable mass.[6]

GROSS FEATURES

Non–mass-forming sclerosing adenosis has the gross appearance of firm nodular breast tissue. Calcifications in sclerosing adenosis may give the tissue a gritty texture on cut section.[5] Often, a discrete gross lesion is not identifiable.

MORPHOLOGIC FEATURES

Sclerosing adenosis is characterized by a proliferation of small glands with a swirling lobulocentric growth pattern accompanied by a fibrous stromal proliferation that compresses and distorts the glands (**Fig. 1**). The glands comprising the lesion are of variable sizes and shapes and consist of epithelial and myoepithelial cell layers. Some glands are open, and in others the lumina are obliterated by the intralobular stroma. Some glands may take on a tubular appearance with angulated contours, which can mimic tubular carcinoma (**Fig. 2**).

The epithelial cells of sclerosing adenosis are cuboidal to low columnar without atypia or mitotic activity. Atypical cytologic features and mitotic figures may be encountered in cases diagnosed during pregnancy or lactation.[5] In some lesions of sclerosing adenosis, the myoepithelial cell layer is prominent, whereas in other lesions, it may be

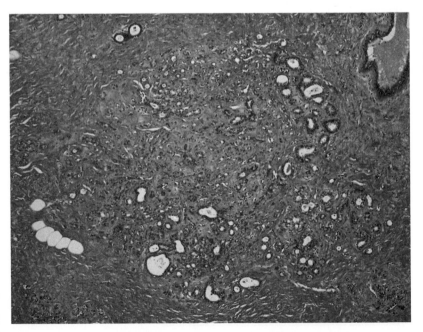

Fig. 1. Sclerosing adenosis is characterized by a lobulocentric proliferation of glands of variable sizes and shapes embedded in a fibrous stroma.

Fig. 2. (*A*) Sclerosing adenosis with angulated and tubular glands. Such cases can mimic invasive ductal carcinoma, in particular, tubular carcinoma. (*B*) A p63 immunostain highlights the nuclei of myoepithelial cells.

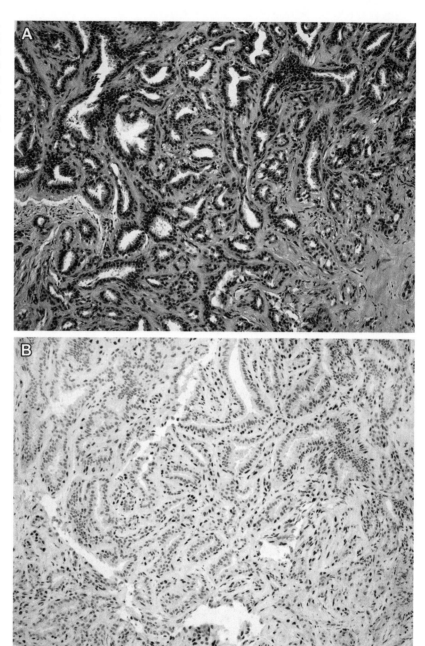

inconspicuous. Myoepithelial cells may undergo myoid metaplasia and take on a spindle-shaped appearance. An eosinophilic, periodic acid–Schiff (PAS)-positive secretion may be present in the lumina of glands. Calcifications are frequently present and can be extensive (**Fig. 3**). Collagenous spherulosis is present in some cases (**Fig. 4**).[11,12] Sclerosing adenosis may secondarily involve radial scars, intraductal papillomas, and fibroadenomas.

Invasion of peripheral nerves may be seen in sclerosing adenosis, and carcinoma should not be diagnosed based on this finding (**Fig. 5**).[13,14] Foci of sclerosing adenosis and, in some cases, even histologically unremarkable ducts may show pseudoinfiltrative growth into adipose tissue, giving the glands an appearance that resembles invasive carcinoma (**Fig. 6**A, B). Identifying myoepithelial cells with immunohistochemical stains, such as

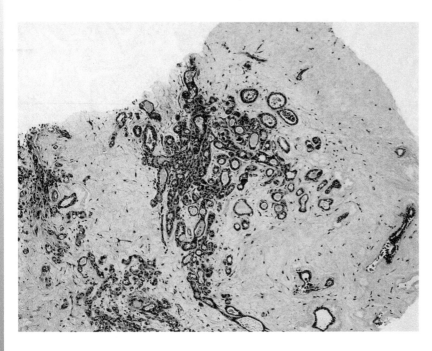

Fig. 3. Sclerosing adenosis in a needle core biopsy sample with epithelial calcifications.

p63, smooth muscle myosin heavy chain, and calponin, is helpful in establishing a benign diagnosis in these scenarios.

In situ carcinoma and atypical hyperplasia may secondarily involve sclerosing adenosis and mimic the appearance of invasive carcinoma. In cases involved by in situ carcinoma, the architectural framework of underlying sclerosing adenosis is maintained and is helpful in making the distinction from invasive carcinoma.[15] Diffuse or partial involvement of duct lobular units by in situ carcinoma may be seen.[16–18] Lobular carcinoma in situ (LCIS) is the most frequent form of in situ carcinoma arising within sclerosing adenosis.[5,15,19] LCIS in

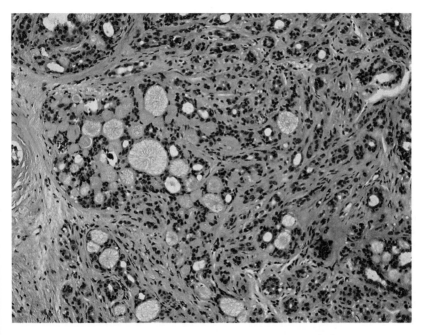

Fig. 4. Sclerosing adenosis with collagenous spherulosis.

Fig. 5. (*A*) Sclerosing adenosis showing invasion of peripheral nerves. (*B*) A calponin immunostain highlights myoepithelial cells in the lesion.

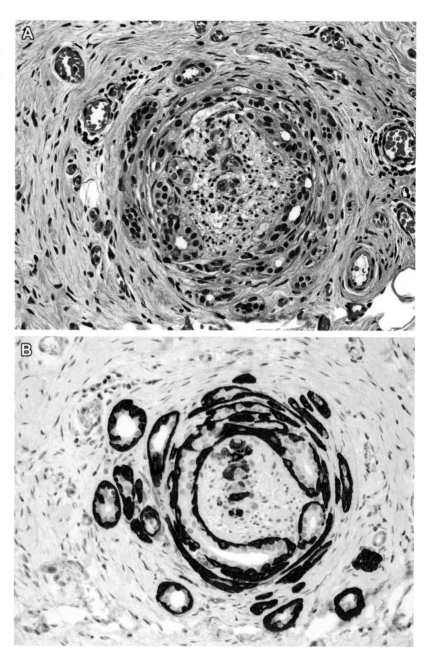

sclerosing adenosis is characterized by nests of uniform cells with small round nuclei, expanding ducts and lobules growing in a lobulocentric pattern and associated with intralobular fibrous stroma.[15,17] Ductal carcinoma in situ (DCIS) involving sclerosing adenosis shows solid, cribriform, and papillary architectural features.[5,16]

DCIS can be associated with necrosis, which may aid in characterizing the lesion as in situ carcinoma.[5] The identification of foci of sclerosing adenosis uninvolved by DCIS may also be helpful in recognizing the presence of underlying adenosis.[18]

Apocrine adenosis is the term given to adenosis or sclerosing adenosis that undergoes apocrine

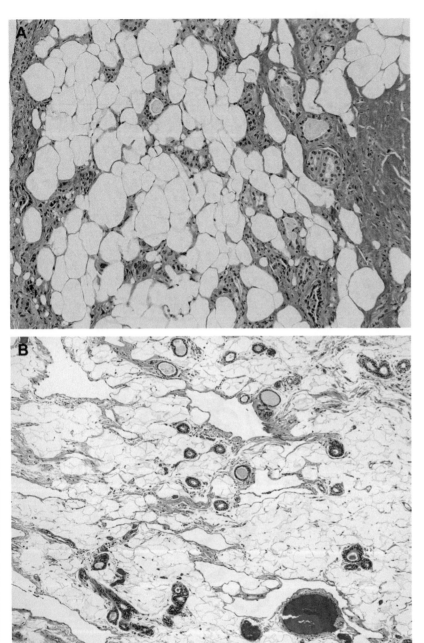

Fig. 6. (*A*) Sclerosing adenosis and (*B*) benign unremarkable glands showing an infiltrative appearance in adipose tissue, which can mimic well-differentiated invasive ductal carcinoma.

metaplasia. Apocrine metaplastic changes can focally or diffusely involve terminal duct lobular units with sclerosing adenosis. The cytoplasm in cells of apocrine adenosis may be granular, eosinophilic, or clear. In some cases, the apocrine epithelial cells exhibit cytologic atypia, which can mimic in situ or invasive carcinoma.[20] These cases are referred to as *atypical apocrine adenosis*. Atypical apocrine adenosis is characterized by cells with apocrine cytoplasmic features that show nuclear hyperchromasia and pleomorphism, prominent nucleoli, and multiple nucleoli (**Fig. 7**).[20–22] Some investigators have suggested that to characterize apocrine adenosis as atypical,

Fig. 7. (*A*) Atypical apocrine adenosis maintains the lobulocentric growth pattern of sclerosing adenosis. (*B*) Apocrine cytoplasmic features and nuclear atypia are present in atypical apocrine adenosis.

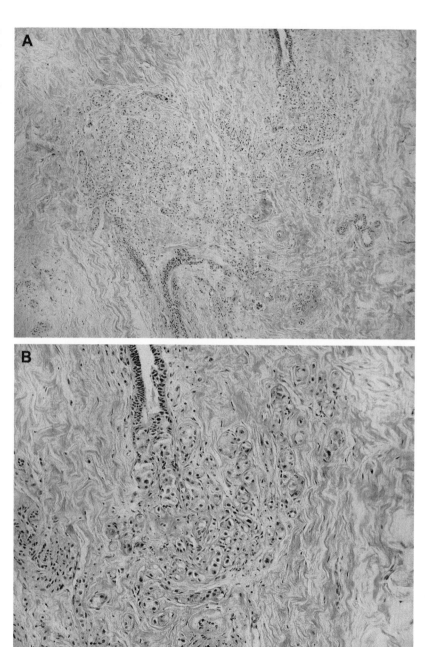

a 3-fold variation in nuclear size should be present.[20,22,23] Mitotic figures are infrequent in atypical apocrine adenosis and are observed more readily in apocrine DCIS.[5] In some cases, atypical apocrine adenosis identified in a needle core biopsy sample represents apocrine DCIS involving sclerosing adenosis, and excisional biopsy is needed to accurately characterize the lesion. As with other apocrine lesions, androgen receptor expression can be seen in atypical apocrine adenosis and can be detected by immunohistochemistry (**Fig. 8**).

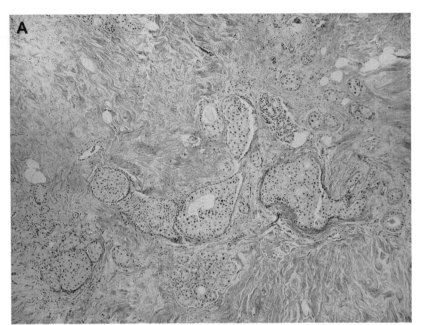

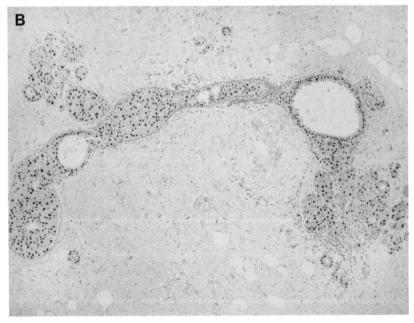

Fig. 8. (*A*) This case of atypical apocrine adenosis diagnosed on a prior needle core biopsy represents apocrine DCIS involving sclerosing adenosis in the subsequent excisional biopsy shown here. (*B*) As with other apocrine lesions, nuclear reactivity for androgen receptor may be seen.

DIFFERENTIAL DIAGNOSIS

The main differential diagnosis of sclerosing adenosis is well-differentiated invasive ductal carcinoma, in particular tubular type. A key to establishing a diagnosis of sclerosing adenosis is recognizing the lobulocentric growth pattern of the lesion. Demonstrating the presence of myoepithelial cells by immunohistochemistry is helpful in difficult cases.

Atypical apocrine adenosis and in situ carcinoma involving sclerosing adenosis have infiltrative appearances that mimic invasive carcinoma. These cases typically lack stromal desmoplasia. Making the distinction between invasive carcinoma and in situ carcinoma in sclerosing adenosis may be challenging in needle core biopsy samples, where the lobulocentric growth pattern of the latter may not be recognizable. In such cases, it is important for pathologists to recognize underlying sclerosing

△△ *Differential Diagnosis*
SMALL GLANDULAR
PROLIFRATIONS

- Sclerosing adenosis
- Radial scar
- Tubular carcinoma
- Microglandular adenosis (MGA)
- Low-grade adenosquamous carcinoma (LGASC)
- Syringomatous adenoma
- Displaced glands from a prior needling procedure

adenosis so the lesion is not misinterpreted as invasive carcinoma. Immunohistochemical stains for myoepithelium help in establishing a diagnosis of in situ carcinoma.

CLINICAL SIGNIFICANCE

Large studies have demonstrated a relative risk of approximately 1.5 to 2 for the development of breast carcinoma in patients with sclerosing adenosis.[1-4] This increase in risk is comparable to the risk seen in patients with other proliferative fibrocystic changes.

The risk of developing carcinoma in patients with atypical apocrine adenosis is less clear. In one study that included 37 patients with a mean follow-up of 8.7 years, the relative risk of developing carcinoma was 5.5.[20] Among patients 60 years or older in the study, the relative risk of developing carcinoma was 14. In another report that studied 51 patients with atypical apocrine sclerosing lesions, no patients developed carcinoma after a mean follow-up of 35 months.[21]

A diagnosis of sclerosing adenosis on needle core biopsy or excision requires no further treatment, provided there is radiologic-pathologic concordance and no associated atypia. Atypical apocrine adenosis diagnosed in needle core biopsy samples should undergo excisional biopsy for further evaluation of the lesion.

RADIAL SCAR

OVERVIEW

Radial scar is a proliferative fibrosclerotic lesion that radiographically, grossly, and microscopically simulates invasive mammary carcinoma. Radial scar has been referred to by a variety of names, including radial sclerosing lesion, sclerosing papillary proliferation, infiltrating epitheliosis, and indurating mastopathy.[24-28] The term *complex sclerosing lesion* refers to a similar lesion that is greater than 1 cm in size, with more irregular architecture and greater proliferative changes, including adenosis and papillary elements.[24-26,29,30]

With the introduction and increased use of mammographic screening, the clinical importance of radial scars has attracted greater interest. Radial scars have been studied in a variety of clinical and radiologic settings to determine their significance. The observed association with malignancy has led some to suggest that radial scar represents a precursor lesion[31]; however, this has not been supported in the literature and most investigators, instead, regard it as an independent risk factor for carcinoma.[26,32] Furthermore, the management of radial scars diagnosed in needle core biopsy samples and the decision to routinely excise these lesions has been debated.

CLINICAL FEATURES

Radial scars occur in a wide age group, with most occurring in women 40 to 60 years of age.[5,25,26,31,33,34] They may be multifocal, multicentric, and bilateral.[26,27,31,35] Most radial scars are discovered incidentally in breast biopsies performed for other abnormalities or are discovered on screening imaging.[30,33] In a mammographically screened population, Cawson and colleagues[34] reported 75 mammographically detected radial scars among 83,066 women (0.09%). Higher frequencies of radial scars have been reported in autopsy series,[26,35] including one study in which 23 of 83 (28%) women were found to have radial scars at autopsy.[35] Infrequently, radial scar presents as a palpable mass.[25,36,37]

IMAGING

With the widespread use of mammographic screening, radial scars have become a well-studied radiographic lesion. On mammography, radial scars present as architectural distortion or a stellate mass with central lucency or are discovered due to the presence of microcalcifications, which may be the only radiographic finding.[25,29,30,34,38] Radial scars characteristically show multiple thin, long spiculations radiating out from the center of the lesion.[34] Because radial scar and invasive mammary carcinoma have similar radiographic features, making the distinction between them on imaging is difficult, and biopsy is required for lesions with their appearance.[33,34,38,39]

GROSS FEATURES

Radial scars typically range in size from 3 mm to 10 mm.[26–28,31,37] The gross appearance of radial scar is similar to that of invasive mammary carcinoma. They are stellate, firm, and show infiltrative edges. The center of a radial scar may show puckering. The cut section is white with a gritty texture and occasional yellow flecks representing elastotic stroma.[29,37] Some radial scars lack a stellate gross configuration and show only an ill-defined area of firmness within the breast parenchyma.[5]

MORPHOLOGIC FEATURES

Radial scar is characterized by a fibroelastotic core containing entrapped and distorted glands, with ducts radiating from the core in a stellate configuration (**Fig. 9**). The glands are invested

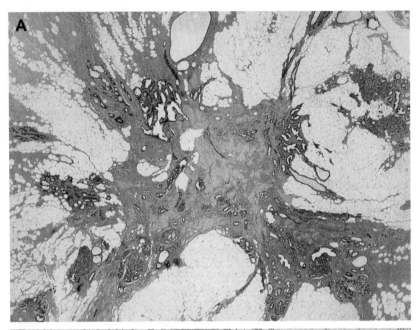

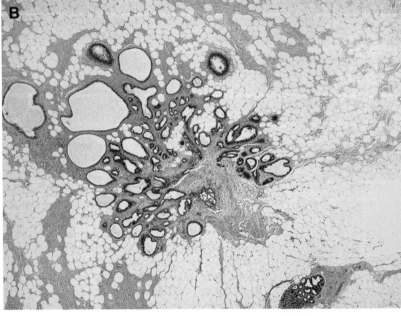

Fig. 9. (*A*) Low-power appearance of a radial scar with a central elastotic nidus. Glands and ductules radiate away from the center in a stellate configuration. (*B*) Another radial scar from the same patient shows a stroma composed predominantly of spindled myofibroblasts without elastosis. Cystically dilated glands are present at the periphery of the lesion.

by a myoepithelial cell layer, which may appear attenuated. The radiating ducts and lobules can show a variety of changes, including adenosis, apocrine metaplasia, duct hyperplasia, and papillomas.[26,27,29] Calcifications may be identified within the radial scar and its associated proliferative elements.[37] The periphery, or corona, of the lesion frequently contains dilated ducts and cysts.[5] As with adenosis, some radial scars show perineural invasion and this feature should not prompt a diagnosis of malignancy.[13]

The stroma of a radial scar is characterized by fibrosis and elastosis, which is most prominent in the central portion of the lesion. Early in the development of a radial scar, the stroma appears more cellular with spindle-shaped myofibroblasts and scattered lymphocytes and plasma cells.[5] The more developed radial scar shows a hypocellular stroma with more abundant fibrosis and elastosis,[5] causing distortion of ducts and lobules and lacking significant inflammation (**Fig. 10**).

Fig. 10. (*A, B*) This radial scar seen in a needle core biopsy sample is characterized by extensive stromal fibrosis, giving the glands an infiltrative appearance.

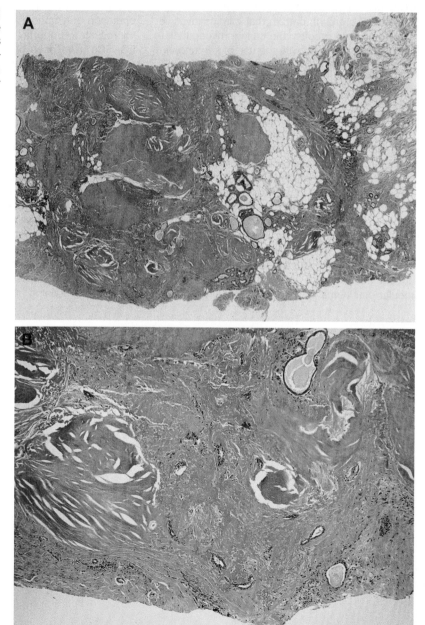

A variety of atypical and malignant lesions can be present in a radial scar and have been observed more frequently at the periphery of the lesion.[24,29] LCIS is the most frequent form of carcinoma present within radial scars.[37,40] Invasive carcinoma, including invasive ductal carcinoma (not otherwise specified), tubular carcinoma, and invasive lobular carcinoma, can be identified within a radial scar and has led some investigators to believe that radial scar is a precursor lesion to invasive carcinoma.[31,37,38] DCIS arising in a radial scar shows cribriform, solid, and micropapillary patterns of various grades. Ducts involved by DCIS are often distorted by the stroma, which gives DCIS a growth pattern that mimics invasive carcinoma.[37] In problematic cases, myoepithelial cells can be identified with the use of immunohistochemical stains.

DIFFERENTIAL DIAGNOSIS

Tubular carcinoma morphologically mimics the distorted glands present within the nidus of a radial scar. Glands in a radial scar emanate away from the central fibroelastotic core in an orderly circumferential fashion, whereas those of tubular carcinoma are distributed in the stroma in a haphazard manner. Glands in the center of a radial scar, however, often show a disorganized growth pattern, mimicking tubular carcinoma (**Fig. 11**). Demonstrating the presence of a myoepithelial cell layer aids in the diagnosis of radial scar without concomitant invasive carcinoma. The glands of tubular carcinoma lack a myoepithelial cell layer,

and this may be demonstrated with the myoepithelial markers, such as p63, smooth muscle myosin heavy chain, and calponin. In densely sclerotic radial scars, however, myoepithelial reactivity may be focal or absent, particularly in the central nidus, and this staining pattern may be misinterpreted as tubular carcinoma arising in a radial scar (**Fig. 12**).

Squamous metaplasia may occur within the glands of a radial scar, sometimes as a result of a prior needling procedure. Squamous metaplasia within a radial scar should be distinguished from low-grade adenosquamous carcinoma (LGASC)[5] and making this distinction may be difficult. The presence of lymphoid aggregates and squamous microcysts supports a diagnosis of LGASC. LGASCs have been observed to arise not infrequently within complex sclerosing lesions and radial scars.[41,42]

CLINICAL SIGNIFICANCE

The clinical significance of radial scars and their relationship with invasive carcinoma have been debated. In the past it was suggested that because the morphologic features of radial scar and tubular carcinoma are similar and that radial scars may harbor carcinoma, they represent precursors to invasive carcinoma.[31] There is little evidence, however, supporting this theory and most investigators consider radial scars a marker for increased risk of cancer.[26]

In a large retrospective analysis, benign breast biopsies containing radial scars from women

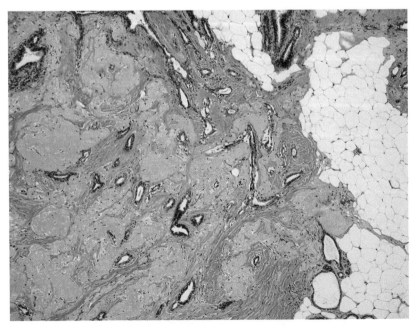

Fig. 11. Central nidus of a radial scar characterized by stromal elastosis and angulated and distorted glands. The growth pattern of the glands can mimic tubular carcinoma, particularly in needle core biopsy material in which only part of the lesion may be sampled.

enrolled in the Nurses' Health Study were reviewed to determine the risk of the subsequent development of breast cancer.[32] Radial scars were present in 7.1% of benign breast biopsies. The investigators found that the risk of developing breast cancer in woman with radial scars was almost double that of woman without radial scars (relative risk, 1.8). In another study, the frequency of radial scars in breasts from women with breast cancer or a history of breast cancer was found significantly higher than in breasts of women of low risk who were studied at autopsy (26% vs 14%).[26]

In an effort to determine which clinical and pathologic factors are associated with the development of malignancy in radial scars, Sloane and Mayers[24] examined 126 radial scars and complex sclerosing lesions from 91 patients. They found a correlation between the presence of atypia or carcinoma and lesion size, patient age, and detection method. Atypia or carcinoma was more likely present in radial scars that were greater than

Fig. 12. (*A*) Glands of a radial scar with angulated contours amid a largely fibrotic stroma. (*B*) A calponin immunostain shows attenuated and focally absent staining for myoepithelial cells around benign glands.

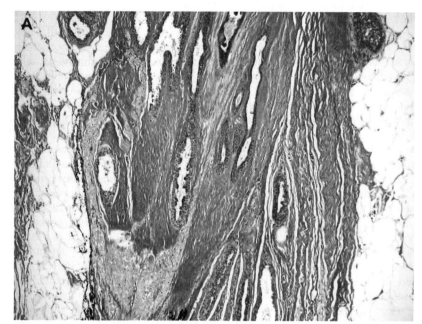

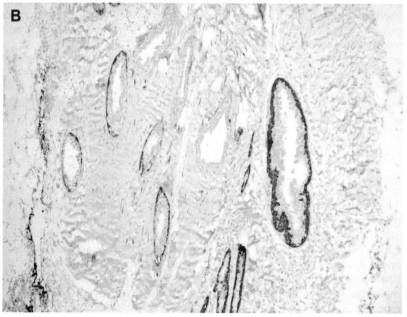

6 mm to 7 mm, in patients older than age 50 years, and in lesions detected by mammography, rather than as incidental findings in breast specimens.

Patients with incidental radial scars found on excision without associated atypia can be managed with routine follow-up. The management of patients diagnosed with radial scars in needle core biopsy samples, however, is unclear. Some investigators recommend routine surgical excision,[25,30] whereas others believe observation is adequate.[28,34] In one study, when an isolated radial scar without atypia was diagnosed on needle core biopsy, 0 of 27 patients had upgraded lesions in the subsequently performed excisions.[33] In a prospective study examining radial scars in a population-based screening program, Cawson and colleagues[34] reported on 63 patients diagnosed with radial scar on needle core biopsy. Of the 62 patients who underwent excision, 4 were diagnosed with malignancy (DCIS) in the excision specimen. All 4 of these patients had either atypical ductal hyperplasia (ADH) or DCIS in the prior needle core biopsy. In a smaller analysis, ADH was found in 4 of 8 radial scars on excision, with 1 of the radial scars showing ADH in the needle core biopsy sample.[38]

The rate of pathologic upgrade to malignancy was found to be higher in patients with atypia associated with radial scars on needle core biopsy in one multi-institutional study.[28] This study examined 157 radial scars diagnosed on needle core biopsy from 152 patients and found carcinoma present on excision in 28% of lesions associated with atypia versus 4% of lesions without atypia.

From these data, it seems reasonable that patients with small isolated radial scars found in needle core biopsies without associated atypia can be followed with clinical and radiologic follow-up, provided there is radiologic-pathologic concordance. Further prospective studies with long-term follow-up in patients with radial scars who undergo surveillance are needed to support this approach. Radial scars with associated atypia should undergo excision.

TUBULAR CARCINOMA

OVERVIEW

Tubular carcinoma is a special type of well-differentiated invasive ductal carcinoma composed of tubular neoplastic glands in virtually the entire tumor. The frequency of tubular carcinoma among invasive breast cancers is 1% to 4%.[43–49] Tubular carcinoma has an excellent prognosis with low rates of axillary lymph node involvement, low recurrence rates, and long overall survival. Molecular,

morphologic, and immunophenotypic studies have shown that tubular carcinomas are clonally related to low-grade precursor lesions, such as columnar cell alterations, lobular neoplasia, and low-grade DCIS, and to exhibit genetic alterations common to low-grade luminal-type breast cancers.[50–52]

Morphologically, tubular carcinoma exhibits low-grade cytoarchitectural features, and difficulty may arise, especially in needle core biopsy samples, in recognizing tubular carcinoma or distinguishing it from benign small glandular proliferations.

CLINICAL PRESENTATION

The clinical and radiologic presentation of tubular carcinoma is not different from conventional invasive ductal carcinoma, with the exception that tubular carcinoma tends to be smaller in size and more likely detected on screening imaging than as a palpable mass.[44–46,53] Tubular carcinoma shows a wide age range at diagnosis, with most cases occurring in women in their 50s and 60s.[44–46,48,54–57] Rare cases have been reported in men.[58,59]

Before the era of screening mammography, tubular carcinoma most often presented as a palpable mass.[54,56] Most cases now present with abnormal mammographic findings.[44,49,53] Sullivan and colleagues[49] reported that 56 of 71 (79%) cases of tubular carcinoma were mammographically detected. In a study examining the method of detection of breast carcinoma, tubular carcinomas of the breast were more likely detected on mammography than invasive ductal carcinomas (not otherwise specified) (83% vs 40%).[53] A biopsy performed for mammographically detected microcalcifications present in an adjacent lesion may lead to the incidental discovery of tubular carcinoma.

Tubular carcinoma can be multifocal, multicentric, and bilateral.[44,54,57] The exact frequency of these parameters is difficult to determine due to the various diagnostic criteria and methods of detection used by different investigators in reports of tubular carcinoma. In one study, tubular carcinoma was found to be multicentric in as high as 56% of mastectomy specimens and significantly more likely to be multicentric compared with tumors of other histologic types.[60] Deos and Norris[54] reported on 90 patients with pure tubular carcinoma of the breast, 29 of whom underwent biopsy or mastectomy of the opposite breast. Contralateral invasive carcinoma was present in 6 of 29 patients (21%) and 2 (6.8%) patients had bilateral tubular carcinomas. Bilateral tubular carcinoma is an infrequent finding in most reports.[49,54]

IMAGING

On mammography, tubular carcinoma presents as an ill-defined spiculated mass or architectural distortion (Fig. 13A).[61–64] A central area of density or lucency is commonly seen.[64] Calcifications identified on mammography may represent those present within the tubular carcinoma or in an adjacent lesion.[62–64] Occasionally, cases of tubular carcinoma show normal mammographic findings.[63]

On sonography, tubular carcinoma has the appearance of a hypoechoic mass with ill-defined margins and posterior acoustic shadowing.[64] Tubular carcinoma has a similar radiographic appearance as radial scar and these 2 lesions cannot be reliably distinguished on imaging.[39,65]

GROSS FEATURES

The gross appearance of tubular carcinoma is that of a firm stellate-shaped mass, not distinguishable from conventional well-differentiated invasive ductal carcinoma (see Fig. 13B). The cut surface is white with occasional yellow flecks or streaks representing elastotic stroma. Compared with conventional invasive ductal carcinoma, pure tubular carcinomas are typically smaller in size, with most tumors measuring 1 cm or less.[44–46,51,54,56,57,66] Larger lesions may represent coalescent multifocal tumors.[5]

MORPHOLOGIC FEATURES

Tubular carcinoma is composed of small open tubular glands arranged in a haphazard manner with an infiltrative growth pattern (see Fig. 13C; Figs. 14 and 15). The tubules are 1 cell layer in thickness with oval or angulated contours, often having a teardrop shape. Luminal cytoplasmic snouts are frequently present. The cells of tubular carcinoma are monotonous with small, low-grade nuclei, resembling the cells of flat epithelial atypia. Mitotic activity is absent or minimal. Lymphovascular invasion is not usually identified. Calcifications may be present within the tubular carcinoma, the associated DCIS, or within the stroma. The stroma of tubular carcinoma is desmoplastic and frequently elastotic, appearing distinct from the surrounding mammary stroma.

DCIS is associated with tubular carcinoma in approximately 50% to 70% of cases[43,44,49,51,54–56,67] and is typically a minor component of the tumor. DCIS is commonly of the micropapillary or cribriform architectural types with low to intermediate nuclear grade. Many cases of tubular carcinoma have coexisting ADH without DCIS.

Tubular carcinoma is frequently associated with lobular neoplasia (atypical lobular hyperplasia and

LCIS) and columnar cell alterations, and the presence of these components should raise awareness to the possibility of a coexisting tubular carcinoma.[46,51,57,67,68] In a study by Rakha and colleagues,[46] columnar cell lesions were found in association with 93% of the reported tubular carcinomas. Lobular neoplasia is associated with tubular carcinoma in approximately half of cases.[46,67,68]

To establish a diagnosis of tubular carcinoma, the majority of the tumor should be composed of tubular glands. Some investigators have suggested that as little as a 75% tubular component constitutes a tubular carcinoma.[48,57] The World Health Organization recommends 90% as a practical cutoff point, and most investigators agree that this proportion should define pure tubular carcinoma.[43,46,66,69] Tumors with less than 90% tubular neoplastic glands, but having a significant tubular component, may be designated a mixed tubular carcinoma or a well-differentiated carcinoma with tubular features. Virtually all tubular carcinomas express estrogen receptors (ERs) and progesterone receptors (PRs) and lack HER-2/neu overexpression by immunohistochemistry.[43,46,49,50,70]

DIFFERENTIAL DIAGNOSIS

The morphologic distinction between tubular carcinoma and benign small glandular proliferations may be challenging, particularly in needle core biopsy material. The differential diagnosis of tubular carcinoma includes radial scar, sclerosing adenosis, MGA, and well-differentiated invasive ductal carcinoma with tubular features.

Features characteristic of tubular carcinoma that aid in the distinction from other small glandular proliferations are the haphazard arrangement of tubules, the absence of a myoepithelial cell layer, and the presence of angulated glands infiltrating adipose tissue. In some cases, the haphazard pattern of neoplastic glands may not be obvious (Fig. 16). The absence of myoepithelial cells in tubular carcinoma can be demonstrated by immunohistochemistry (Fig. 17A,B). An interpretative pitfall in the use of immunohistochemistry is the cross-reactivity of some myoepithelial stains, in particular CD10 and smooth muscle actin, with stromal myofibroblasts (see Fig. 17C). The circumferential pattern of staining can give the false impression of the presence of a myoepithelial cell layer and lead to a mistaken diagnosis of benignity.

Radial scars have an orderly stellate low-power appearance with glands radiating from a central fibroelastotic nidus. The glands are larger and more dilated at the periphery of a radial scar, forming a corona. The stroma of tubular

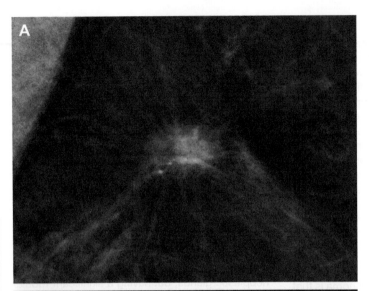

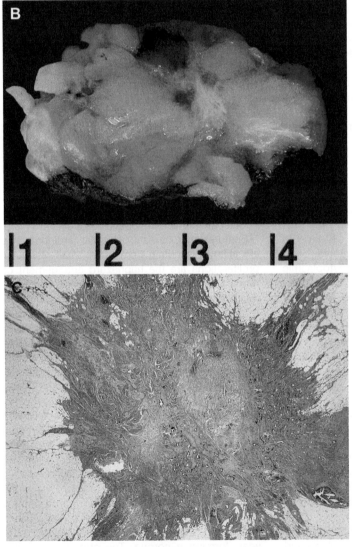

Fig. 13. Mammography and gross and microscopic findings of a case of tubular carcinoma. (A) Mammography showed a spiculated mass. (B) Excisional biopsy of the lesion revealed a stellate-shaped infiltrative mass on gross examination. (C) On low-power microscopic examination, the lesion showed small glands growing in a haphazard pattern with stromal fibrosis and elastosis.

Fig. 14. (*A, B*) Two examples of tubular carcinoma with teardrop-shaped glands growing within a desmoplastic stroma.

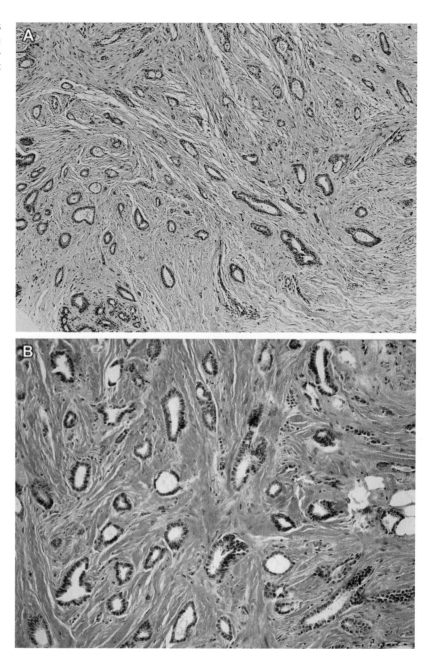

carcinomas and radial scars can be similar in appearance, especially if elastotic in nature. Immunohistochemical stains for myoepithelial cells are useful in making the distinction between 2 entities and highlight myoepithelial cells in the glands of radial scars. Radial scars, however, may harbor tubular carcinoma in some instances (**Fig. 18**).[24,37]

Sclerosing adenosis is characterized by a proliferation of small glands with a lobulocentric appearance that can easily be recognized on low-power examination. The glands of sclerosing adenosis are frequently embedded within a sclerotic stroma. Stromal desmoplasia and elastosis are not typically seen. The lumina of the glands in sclerosing adenosis are frequently compressed or obliterated by intralobular stromal fibrosis, whereas those of tubular carcinoma are open and dilated. Myoepithelial cells can be detected by immunohistochemical stains, such as p63,

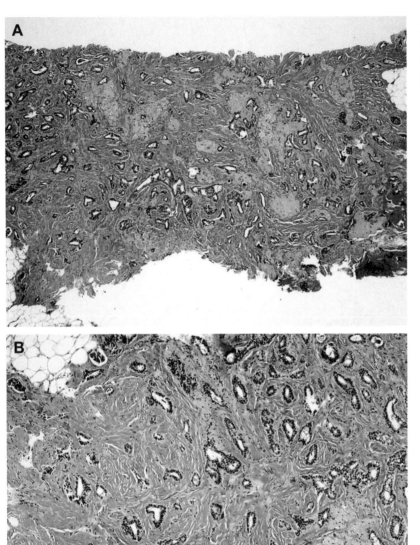

Fig. 15. (A, B) Tubular carcinoma in a needle core biopsy sample showing small glands with low-grade cytoarchitectural features growing within a fibroelastotic stroma.

smooth muscle myosin heavy chain, or calponin in sclerosing adenosis.

MGA, like tubular carcinoma, is a low-grade glandular proliferation with a disorderly growth pattern that infiltrates adipose tissue. Although the glands of tubular carcinoma exhibit angulated contours, those of MGA typically have a uniform rounded shape, although a tubular configuration may be seen. The lumina of glands of MGA contain dense pink secretion, which is not a feature of tubular carcinoma. MGA, like tubular carcinoma, lacks a myoepithelial cell layer but is surrounded by basement membrane, which may be identified on a routine hematoxylin-eosin stain. Immunohistochemical stains, such as laminin and collagen IV, and special stains, such as reticulin, may be

Fig. 16. Tubular carcinoma in a needle core biopsy sample, confirmed by negative staining for myoepithelial markers (not shown), demonstrates glands reminiscent of adenosis. At the top of the image, more typical angulated glands of tubular carcinoma are seen infiltrating adipose tissue.

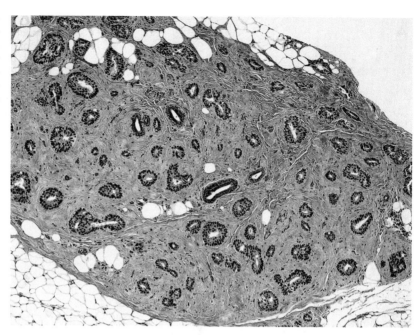

used to highlight the presence of the basement membrane. Strong immunoreactivity for S-100 protein is seen in MGA.[40,43,71,72] Lastly, the coexistence of DCIS supports a diagnosis of tubular carcinoma over MGA.

Tubular carcinoma is distinguished from invasive ductal carcinoma with tubular features or mixed tubular carcinoma based on the larger proportion of tubules present. Invasive ductal carcinoma with tubular features may have slightly higher-grade and contain glands more than 1 cell layer in thickness.

PROGNOSIS

The prognosis of tubular carcinoma is excellent. The reported frequency of axillary lymph node metastasis in patients with tubular carcinoma ranges from 0% to 29%.[45,54–56,62,67,70] This wide range is likely due to the variable diagnostic criteria used in reports of tubular carcinoma. Among pure tubular carcinoma cases (>90% tubular component), Papadatos and colleagues[56] reported a frequency of nodal involvement of 6.6% in a meta-analysis of 244 cases. In another study, the probability of nodal metastasis was significantly lower in pure tubular carcinomas compared with a group of well-differentiated invasive ductal carcinomas (12.9% vs 23.9%).[69] Among a subset of low-risk cases in this analysis, defined as T1 tumors without lymphovascular or perineural invasion, the incidence of axillary metastasis was

lower (7%). In patients with axillary lymph node involvement by tubular carcinoma, the prognosis remains favorable, showing survival rates similar to those of node-negative patients.[45,47,49,55]

The recurrence rate of tubular carcinoma is less than 10% in most studies.[49,55,57,69,70,73] Kader and colleagues[69] reported the rate of local recurrence for tubular carcinomas as significantly lower than in a control group of well-differentiated invasive ductal carcinomas (0.8% vs 4.5%), despite the control group having received more aggressive initial therapy. Survival rates have been shown to be excellent in patients with tubular carcinoma, with rare distant metastases or deaths as a result of the disease.[46,54,57,70] In a study by Rakha and colleagues,[46] 102 patients with tubular carcinoma showed longer disease-free survival and breast cancer–specific survival compared with a group of 212 patients with well-differentiated invasive ductal carcinomas. No patients developed distant metastases or died from breast cancer. Other studies have reported similar findings.[45,48,55] Sullivan and colleagues[49] reported 94.1% 5-year and 81.7% 10-year overall survival rates in a group of 72 patients with tubular carcinoma, which was not significantly different from an aged-matched set of women in the general population (91.3% and 77.6%, respectively). Other reports have also suggested that survival among patients with tubular carcinoma is not different from that of the general population without breast disease,[45,46] which has raised the question of whether adjuvant

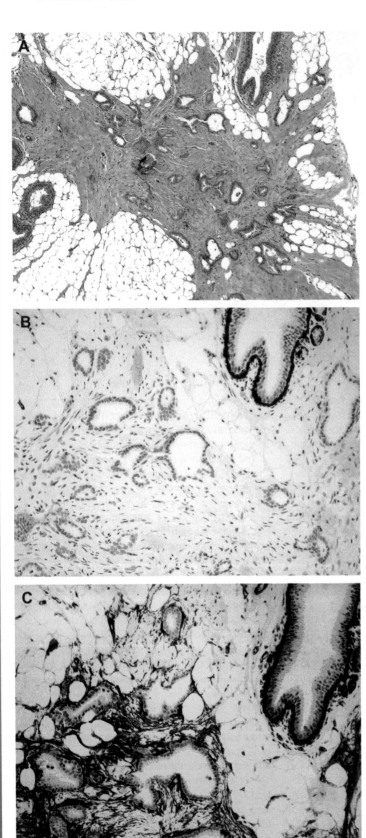

Fig. 17. (*A*) Tubular carcinoma. (*B*) A calponin immunostain demonstrates lack of myoepithelial reactivity in lesional glands. (*C*) An interpretive pitfall in the use of myoepithelial stains is the cross-reactivity with stromal myofibroblasts with some stains, such as smooth muscle actin in this case.

Fig.   18. (*A*) Low-power and (*B*) medium-power views of tubular carcinoma arising within a radial scar. (*C*) The malignant glands show lack of myoepithelial reactivity with a p63 immunostain whereas adjacent benign ducts are positive.

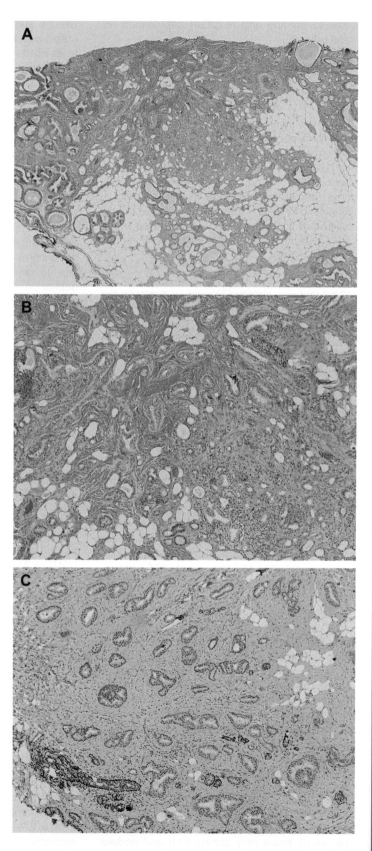

systemic therapy and radiation are needed for these patients.

MICROGLANDULAR ADENOSIS

OVERVIEW

MGA is an uncommon benign proliferative lesion characterized by small uniform glands that infiltrate mammary stroma and adipose tissue. MGA radiographically and histologically mimics invasive mammary carcinoma, in particular, tubular carcinoma. Despite its benign nature, carcinoma may arise within MGA, and there is morphologic, immunohistochemical, and molecular evidence implicating MGA as a precursor lesion to carcinoma.

CLINICAL PRESENTATION

MGA has been reported in women between the ages of 26 and 86 years, with most lesions reported among women in their 40s and 50s.[40,71,74–78] MGA typically presents as a palpable mass or thickening of the breast but may be discovered as an incidental microscopic or radiographic finding.[40,71,74,75,77–80] In some patients, the mass has been reported as painful.[78,79]

IMAGING

There are no specific mammographic findings for MGA; however, the mammogram is frequently abnormal and may be reported as suspicious.[76,78–80] MGA may manifest as an increased density or increased vascularity,[76] and calcifications may be present.[77] In some cases, no mammographic abnormality is detected.[81]

Sonographic and MRI findings of MGA were reported in one case of a woman who was a BRCA1 mutation carrier who underwent more cautious screening.[81] Mammography showed dense breast tissue without any abnormality. High-resolution sonography revealed a hypoechoic, well-defined mass that was more wide than tall and showed irregular borders. MRI of the breast showed a noncircumscribed mass with early and delayed enhancement without washout or rim enhancement. The mass appeared hyperintense on T2-weighted images. These MRI findings were suggestive of a fibroadenoma.

GROSS FEATURES

MGA typically ranges in size from 1 cm to 4 cm[74–77] and has the appearance of an ill-defined and vaguely nodular or circumscribed lesion.[76,82] The breast tissue may appear firm and nodular

with no identifiable abnormality.[71] It is difficult to obtain an exact gross measurement of MGA due to its scattered and discontinuous nature and the presence of coexisting fibrocystic disease.[76] Often the gross measurement underestimates the microscopic extent of disease.[71]

MORPHOLOGIC FEATURES

MGA is characterized by a poorly circumscribed and disorganized proliferation of small glands that infiltrate mammary stroma and adipose tissue (Fig. 19). On low-power examination, multiple clusters of loosely dispersed glands can be identified in a random distribution among pre-existing lobules, and arranged around small ducts.[75] The glands are uniform and round with open lumina, of similar size to or slightly larger than a normal lobular acinus.[74,75] Occasional glands are compressed by surrounding stroma and have closed lumina. The glands are 1 cell layer in thickness and are composed of cuboidal cells with clear to eosinophilic and occasionally granular cytoplasm. The cytoplasm is PAS positive and diastase resistant, due to the presence of cytoplasmic glycogen.[71,74] The cells of MGA have small round uniform nuclei and inconspicuous nucleoli. Mitotic figures are rarely seen.[76] The lumina of the glands contain a dense eosinophilic PAS-positive, diastase-resistant secretion that compresses and flattens the cuboidal cells (Fig. 20A).[71,74,76,79] Calcification of the secretion can be observed.[71,78,79] MGA characteristically lacks a myoepithelial cell layer (Fig. 20B),[75,77,78] a distinctive feature among benign breast lesions. A basement membrane invests the glands of MGA and can be demonstrated with the use of special stains, such as reticulin (Fig. 21A) and PAS,[82] or immunohistochemical stains, such as laminin (Fig. 21B) and collagen IV.[75,83] The stroma surrounding the glands in MGA is made up of adipose tissue or hypocellular and hyalinized fibrous breast tissue.[75,79] A stromal reaction to the infiltrating glands is not present (Fig. 22).[78]

Some cases of MGA, especially those giving rise to carcinoma, have atypical cytologic and architectural features (i.e., atypical MGA) (Fig. 23). In these cases, there is greater architectural complexity of the glands with interconnected glandular units, microcribriform nests, and crowding and obliteration of lumina as well as diminished luminal secretion.[71,77,78] The cells have atypical vesicular nuclei, coarse chromatin, and prominent nucleoli. Mitotic figures can be readily identified.[71,77]

Carcinoma has been shown to arise within MGA in up to 27% of cases[72,77]; however, because most reported cases are seen in consultation, there is

Fig. 19. MGA is characterized by a disorganized proliferation of small glands infiltrating adipose tissue.

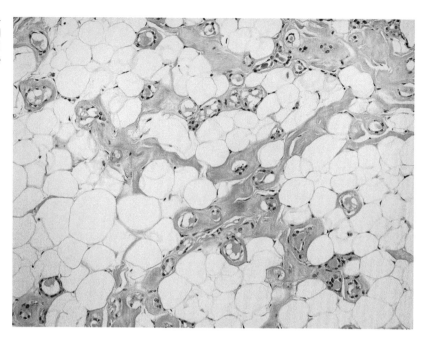

likely some referral bias and the exact frequency is unknown. Although carcinoma may occasionally coexist with and be unrelated to MGA, there is typically a progressive morphologic transition from MGA to carcinoma with atypical MGA present in transitional areas.[77,82,84] Carcinomas arising within MGA frequently resemble MGA and retain its underlying structure[72,82] but may exhibit a variety of morphologic appearances. In situ carcinoma arising in MGA is characterized by solid and cribriform nests of cytologically malignant cells growing in an alveolar or budding pattern, similar to the underlying growth patterns of MGA and atypical MGA.[78,84] Mitotic figures and apoptotic debris are frequent, and comedo-type necrosis may be evident.[71] LCIS has been reported within MGA.[79] Invasive carcinoma arising in MGA is typically high grade and characterized by large coalescent solid nodules, which appear to form from fusing of the alveolar nests of the in situ carcinomatous component.[40,71] A desmoplastic stromal reaction accompanies the invasive carcinoma.[78] In cases of invasive carcinoma arising within MGA, a basement membrane is not present.[82] Other types of carcinoma, including metaplastic (matrix-producing),[77] basaloid,[77,84] and adenoid cystic carcinoma,[77,85] have been described. Clear cell change[78] and chondromyxoid metaplasia have been encountered in some cases of carcinoma arising in MGA.[71,78,84] Rare cases have shown

acinic cell carcinoma–like features with coarse eosinophilic granules reminiscent of intestinal Paneth cells.[78,84,86]

MGA shows strong immunohistochemical staining for S-100 protein[40,71,72,82,83,87] and lacks expression of ER, PR, and HER-2/*neu* protein (**Fig. 24**).[71,77,82,87] A myoepithelial layer is not evident with immunohistochemical staining. In one study, MGA was found to be nonreactive for epithelial membrane antigen and gross cystic disease fluid protein-15.[75] Carcinomas arising within MGA have similar immunohistochemical profiles of typical MGA; however, some may show staining for ER, PR, HER-2/*neu*,[40,71] and epithelial membrane antigen.[80] Increasing Ki-67 and p53 labeling has been observed in the progression from MGA to carcinoma.[40,77,88] Epidermal growth factor receptor (EGFR) expression has been observed in cases of MGA, atypical MGA, and carcinoma arising in MGA.[77,88]

Ultrastructurally, the cells of MGA show an electrolucent cytoplasm with scant organelles, homogenous electron-dense luminal material, and a multilayered electron-dense basement membrane. A myoepithelial cell layer is not present.[75,76] In one report, MGA showed a high degree of villus interdigitation between epithelial cells and abundant apical lysosomal granules.[89]

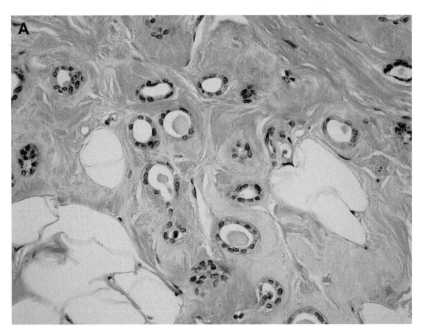

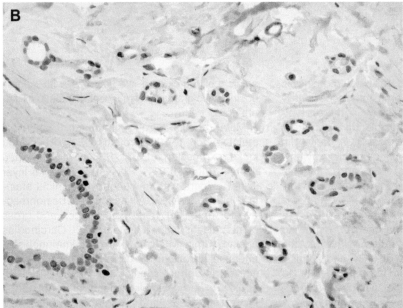

Fig. 20. (*A*) A dense eosinophilic secretion is present in the lumina of the glands of MGA. (*B*) The absence of a myoepithelial cell layer is demonstrated with a p63 immunostain. A benign gland (*left*) shows myoepithelial reactivity for p63.

DIFFERENTIAL DIAGNOSIS

The most important differential diagnosis of MGA is tubular carcinoma. On low-power examination, MGA is multifocal and present as disorganized clusters of glands. Tubular carcinoma is typically unifocal in a given histologic section, although it may be multifocal within the breast. The glands of tubular carcinoma are angulated, are of variable sizes and shapes, and show apical cytoplasmic snouts, whereas those of MGA are small, more uniform in appearance, and lack cytoplasmic snouts. Some lumina of MGA may be closed, whereas virtually all glands in tubular carcinoma

Fig. 21. A basement membrane in MGA can be identified with the use of a reticulin histochemical stain (*A*) or an immunohistochemical stain, such as laminin (*B*).

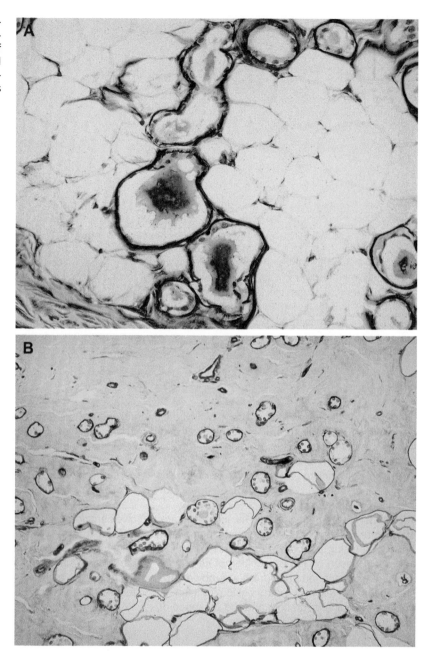

have open dilated lumina.[74] Tubular carcinoma, like MGA, may contain luminal secretion; however, the secretion present in tubular carcinoma is basophilic[74] and not as dense as that of MGA. The stroma of tubular carcinoma is fibroelastotic and desmoplastic, whereas that of MGA is fibrotic and hypocellular with no stromal reaction or consists mainly of adipose tissue. Tubular carcinoma can be associated with ADH or in situ carcinoma, which is not present in uncomplicated MGA. If in situ carcinoma is associated with MGA, it is usually high grade and solid in appearance, whereas that of tubular carcinoma is low grade with micropapillary and cribriform architectural features.[78] A myoepithelial layer is absent in both tubular carcinoma and MGA; however, MGA is

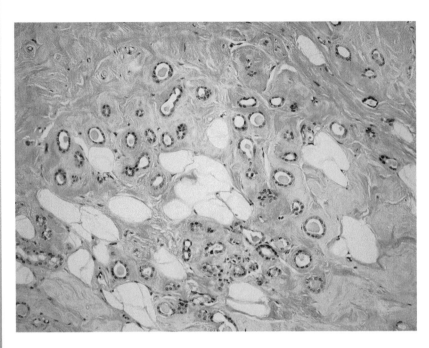

Fig. 22. MGA is present within a hypocellular fibrous stroma with adipose tissue and lacks a desmoplastic stromal reaction.

surrounded by a basement membrane, which can be identified with the use of histochemical and immunohistochemical stains. Almost all tubular carcinomas show reactivity for ER and PR by immunohistochemistry,[44,46] which is typically strong and diffuse, whereas MGA does not express these receptors.

Other forms of adenosis, such as sclerosing adenosis, are included in the differential diagnosis of MGA. Sclerosing adenosis can be distinguished from MGA based on the recognition of its orderly lobulocentric, and often nodular low-power appearance, the frequent compression of glands, the lack of luminal secretion, and the presence of a myoepithelial cell layer.

TREATMENT/PROGNOSIS

MGA is a benign lesion; however, morphologic and molecular observations have supported the concept that MGA is a precursor to in situ and invasive carcinoma. Using high-resolution comparative genomic hybridization (CGH), Shin and colleagues[40] demonstrated a molecular progression from MGA and atypical MGA to carcinoma. The investigators reported some lesions showing little genomic instability, wheras others harbored recurrent genomic copy number changes, including loss of 5q and gain of 8q, the latter corresponding to amplification and gains in the *MYC* oncogene. Geyer and

colleagues[87] reported identical genetic aberrations across the spectrum of MGA lesions, with low-level copy number changes and increasing genetic complexity in the progression from MGA to carcinoma. Their study's investigators proposed the term, *microglandular adenoma*, to reflect the significance of MGA as a nonobligate precursor to invasive carcinoma, akin to colorectal adenomas.

There are few long-term follow-up studies of patients with carcinoma arising within MGA. These carcinomas have been reported, however, to have a favorable course, despite having basal-like features (i.e., lack of ER or PR reactivity, EGFR expression, and high histologic grade).[40,71]

In one series, James and colleagues[71] described 14 cases of MGA with coexisting carcinoma, 13 of which had carcinoma arising within MGA. Six patients (43%) had a family history of breast cancer. Only 1 recurrence was reported in the series, which occurred in a woman who was treated by excision alone. Of the 10 patients treated by mastectomy, none had a recurrence after a median follow-up of 57 months. In 11 cases, axillary lymph node dissection was performed, and 3 patients showed nodal metastasis.

For patients with uncomplicated MGA, treatment with complete local excision and appropriate clinical follow-up is adequate.[76–79] Excisional biopsy is recommended when MGA is found in

Fig. 23. (*A*) Atypical MGA is characterized by glands with crowded lumina infiltrating mammary stroma. High-power view (*inset*) shows glands with enlarged hyperchromatic nuclei with prominent nucleoli. Luminal secretion is diminished. Mitotic figures can be readily identified. (*B*) A basement membrane is retained and is highlighted with a reticulin histochemical stain.

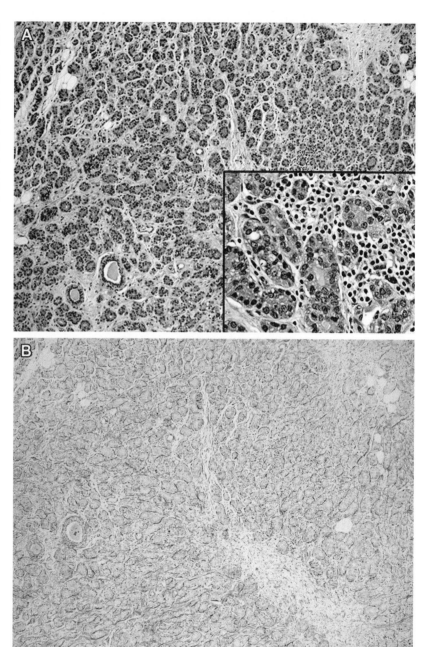

a needle core biopsy.[5] Recurrences of MGA are rare but may occur if excision is incomplete.[75] Re-excision is recommended when excision specimens show atypical MGA present at a surgical margin.[5] Resetkova and colleagues[80] described a patient who underwent excision for carcinoma arising in MGA, in which the carcinoma, but not the MGA, was completely excised. Ten years later, the patient had a recurrence of carcinoma arising within MGA. As illustrated in this case, complete excision may be difficult due to the ill-defined and multifocal nature of MGA and lesions that have not been completely excised may recur in the form of carcinoma.[77,80]

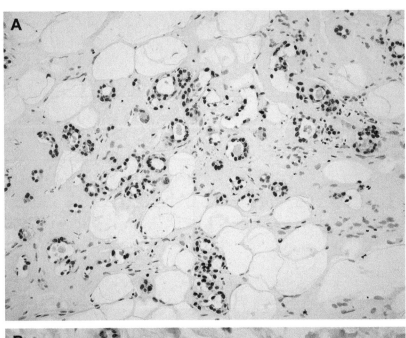

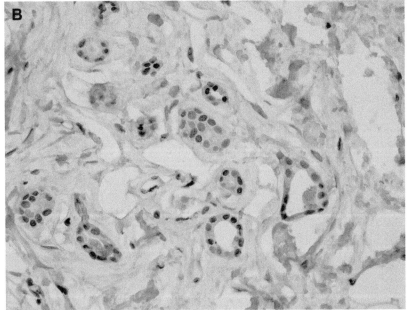

Fig. 24. (A) MGA shows strong nuclear and cytoplasmic expression of S-100 protein and (B) lacks expression of ER.

LOW-GRADE ADENOSQUAMOUS CARCINOMA

OVERVIEW

The Low-grade adenosquamous carcinoma (LGASC) tumor is an uncommon variant of metaplastic carcinoma. Unlike other types of metaplastic carcinomas, LGASC is associated with a favorable prognosis.[90,91]

CLINICAL FEATURES

In 1987, Rosen and Ernsberger[91] published a seminal article describing LGASC as a clinicopathologic entity in 11 patients. Similarly aged to those who develop breast carcinoma of the usual type, these patients commonly present with a palpable unilateral breast mass. On gross examination, the tumor is hard, ill defined, and pale-white to yellow on cut section.[91] A subsequent larger study reported that these tumors were typically found in the upper outer quadrant of the breast.[92] Tumors in the original study ranged in size from 1.5 cm to 3.4 cm[91]; however, a subsequent case of 1 patient with an 8.0 cm tumor was reported.[92] More recently, several examples have come to clinical attention via screening mammography, 1 of which was only 8 mm in size.[93]

MORPHOLOGIC FEATURES

LGASC consists of small cytologically bland glandular structures with variable degrees of squamous differentiation (**Fig. 25**).[90] A moderately intense lymphocytic infiltrate is present either as peripheral aggregates/pseudofollicles or in a dispersed distribution in lesional tissue. The growth pattern of lesional glands is characteristically infiltrative and the glands themselves are elongated, ovoid, or compressed. The neoplastic glands blend subtly with the normal breast parenchyma and insinuate themselves in and around ducts and lobules. Due to their extremely well-differentiated appearance, some lesional glands are indistinguishable from neighboring normal glands. Individual examples of LGASC can differ widely in degree of squamous differentiation, ranging from 10% to 80% of the lesion. Extreme cases of squamous differentiation can show cystic degeneration or calcified keratinous debris,[90,92] whereas less prominent cases may only show luminal keratin debris. Osteocartilagenous metaplasia has been identified in some cases.[91] Transitional areas composed of high-grade metaplastic carcinoma can be concurrently present but is an uncommon finding.[41] The associated stroma is either fibrotic or cellular (**Fig. 26**). Cellular stroma surrounding lesional glands is composed of cytologically bland spindled cells in a fibromyxoid stroma (**Fig. 27**).[91] These stromal cells typically layer around glands of LGASC and can demonstrate histologic merging with adjacent neoplastic glands, lending support that they are neoplastic rather than part of altered benign stroma.[93] Some myoepithelial immunostains, such as smooth muscle myosin heavy chain, have been found to highlight cellular stroma in some cases and demonstrate what has been described as a lamellar pattern of staining.[94] The association of LGASC with pre-existing papillary lesions, such as papillomas,

adenomyoepitheliomas, radial/complex sclerosing lesions, and even collagenous spherulosis, has been well documented.[41,42,92,95]

IMMUNOHISTOCHEMISTRY

Although the clinicopathologic features have been well described since the late 1980s, the immunohistochemical profile of LGASC has largely eluded pathologists, despite the ever-growing array of stains available. This is likely due to the observation that although some immunostains react consistently in LGASC, several that are commonly used for diagnostic purposes show variable staining not only within individual cases but also between cases.

Variable staining, particularly with myoepithelial markers (or evidence of myoepithelium by means other than immunohistochemistry) has been documented by some investigators[92,93]; however, little has been reported about the biologic underpinnings of this phenomenon. Recently, tumors from a cohort of 30 patients were studied for distinctive immunohistochemical staining patterns.[94] The investigators found that myoepithelial stains were variably positive around lesional glands (basal location) as well as in surrounding cellular stroma (**Fig. 28**). The p63 Immunostain additionally stained luminal cells, likely highlighting the degree of squamous differentiation in a given case. In addition, they found that in some cases, there was stronger staining in the luminal epithelial cells (compared with basally located cells) in lesional glands, a pattern the investigators described as core staining and deemed distinctive in LGASC from other small glandular proliferations arising in the breast (**Fig. 29**).[94]

Some immunostains have shown to stain consistently in LGASC. Drudis and colleagues[90] were the first to report in their study of 23 patients that LGASC is characteristically negative for estrogen and progesterone receptors. None had more than 5% of lesional cells staining for either or both receptors. Immunoreactivity for HER-2/neu was also demonstrated in approximately half of studied patients; however, it is unclear whether any met the current American Society of Clinical Oncology/College of American Pathologists standards deemed overexpressed for this protein.[90,96] A more recent study found that none of 5 cases studied showed HER-2/neu overexpression by immunohistochemistry, which was further confirmed in 2 cases by microarray CGH.[97] The study's investigators also found basal markers, cytokeratin (CK)17, CK14, and CK5/6, positive in the epithelial component in all 5 of 5 cases studied

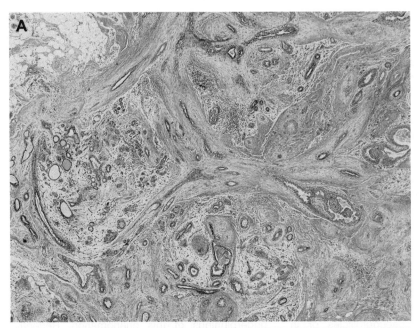

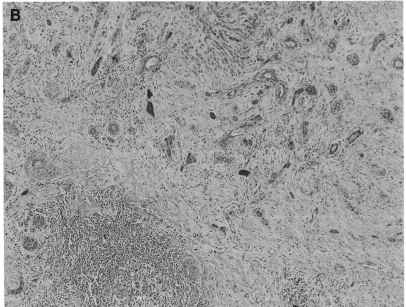

Fig. 25. LGASC. Infiltrating glandular structures with variable degrees of squamous differentiation and associated stroma. Lymphoid aggregates are commonly nearby. Example with little squamous differentiation (A). Example with prominent squamous differentiation (B).

whereas only scattered stromal cells were positive. Furthermore, EGFR was also positive in the epithelial component in 3 of 5 cases. In a separate study, P53 positivity (>10% of tumor cells) was found in a minority (13%) of cases and mostly in the glandular elements.[90]

MOLECULAR STUDIES

Recently, the first genome-wide molecular genetic analysis of LGASC was performed by Geyer and colleagues.[97] They studied 2 cases using high-resolution microarray CGH after microdissection. In the first case, a molecular karyotype comprising

Fig. 26. LGASC. Lesional glands are typically surrounded by fibrotic stroma.

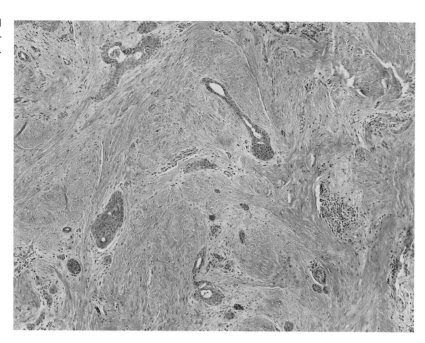

gains of 6p, 7pq, and 8q and losses of 1p, 6p, 6q, 8p, and 9p was seen but no amplifications were identified. In the second case, the genomic profile showed a more complex pattern, consisting of gains in 1q, 5q, 7p, 8q, 12p, 14q, 16p, 16q, and 18pq and losses in 1p, 3q, 8p, 9p, 12q, 17p, 22q, and Xpq. A high level of amplification was detected at 7p11.2, which encompasses the EGFR gene, as well as at 7q11.21. Chromogenic in situ hybridization (CISH) was also performed on these 2 cases for selected regions harboring gains or amplifications. In the first case, CISH for the EGFR gene confirmed that the gains in chromosome 7 detected by CGH showed averages of EGFR and CEP7 copy numbers consistent with gain of copy of chromosome 7 in the epithelial cell clusters and also in the surrounding stromal tumor cells. CISH of the second case revealed that the gains of 7p-q11.21 and high-level amplification of EGFR observed by CGH showed that not only the epithelial cells but also a minority of spindle stromal cells near the epithelial clusters harbored EGFR amplification.

The frequency of BRCA1 mutation in metaplastic carcinomas of the breast has been well documented.[98] Among patients with LGASC specifically, there is only 1 report of a patient harboring a BRCA1 germline mutation.[99] How prevalent this mutation is in patients with LGASC has yet to be determined.

DIFFERENTIAL DIAGNOSIS

Among the other small glandular proliferations found in the breast, LGASC is most commonly confused with radial scar, tubular carcinoma, and syringomatous adenoma. As discussed previously, radial scars infrequently show squamous metaplasia. In addition, LGASC can grow in a stellate, infiltrative pattern much like that of a radial scar and, in rare occasions, can arise within a pre-existing one. LGASC is more commonly misdiagnosed as a radial scar than the converse because radial scars are more frequently encountered in daily practice than is LGASC. Tubular carcinoma and radial scars are typically associated with altered stroma (fibroelastosis or desmoplasia), which can be mistaken for cellular stroma surrounding glands of LGASC. A helpful distinction can be made by immunohistochemistry because tubular carcinomas often show diffuse, strong immunoreactivity for ER and PR whereas LGASC is typically negative for these biomarkers (Fig. 30). A second-chance diagnosis can happen when an initial (mis)diagnosis of tubular carcinoma prompts additional studies to be performed (ER and PR) on a case. The unexpected negativity for these biomarkers should raise suspicion and provoke pathologists to reconsider the diagnosis rendered. In addition to LGASC, other ER/PR negative tumors, such as MGA and syringomatous

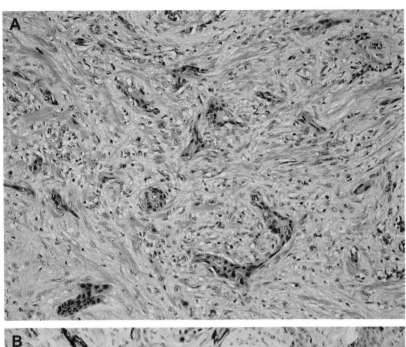

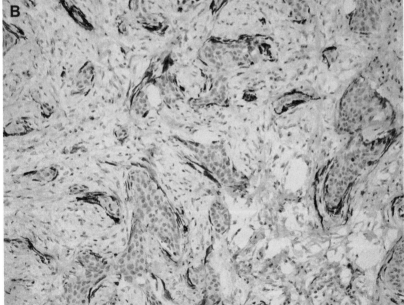

Fig. 27. Cellular stroma surrounding glands of LGASC (A). Lamellar staining pattern is highlighted with smooth muscle myosin heavy chain immunohistochemical stain (B).

adenoma, should be also considered if such a diagnostic scenario should arise.

Most investigators agree that the most difficult morphologic distinction among small glandular proliferations is that of LGASC from syringomatous adenoma. These 2 lesions show significant histologic overlap to the degree that it has been suggested by several investigators that they may represent a single entity.[100,101] It is the authors'

opinion, however, that they are distinct lesions and are discernible from each other in most if not all cases. Although LGASC is an uncommon lesion, syringomatous adenoma in comparison is rare. Clinical correlation is critical in any diagnostically challenging case and it is helpful to know that syringomatous adenomas more commonly arise superficially near the nipple, whereas LGASCs tend to arise in the peripheral and deeper aspects

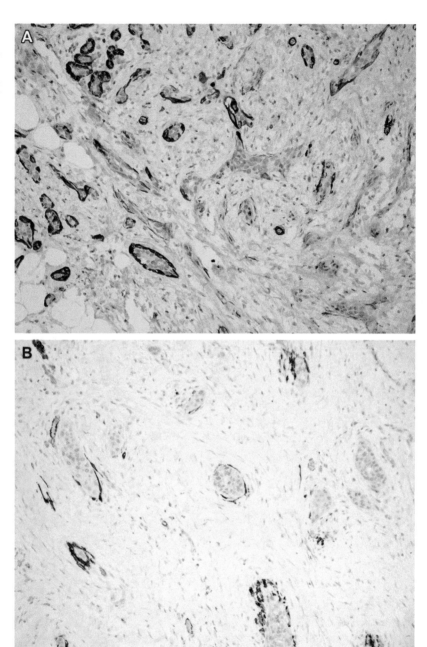

Fig. 28. LGASC. Lesional glands show variable staining with myoepithelial markers. Complete, weak, and discontinuous or absent staining for smooth muscle myosin heavy chain (*A, B*).

of the breast. Also, LGASC is typically associated with chronic inflammation, usually in the form of lymphoid aggregates, whereas syringomatous adenoma arises in uncomplicated mammary stroma. The exception to this distinction is in the case of a ruptured keratin cyst in the latter, which elicits a chronic inflammatory response and foreign body giant cell reaction.

Based up on the findings of both the retention and absence of myoepithelium as demonstrated by various immunohistochemical stains, including p63, smooth muscle myosin heavy chain, smooth muscle actin, and CD10,[94,100,102–108] it seems that syringomatous adenoma exhibits a similarly variable staining pattern in lesional glands with myoepithelial markers to LGASC. The lamellar staining

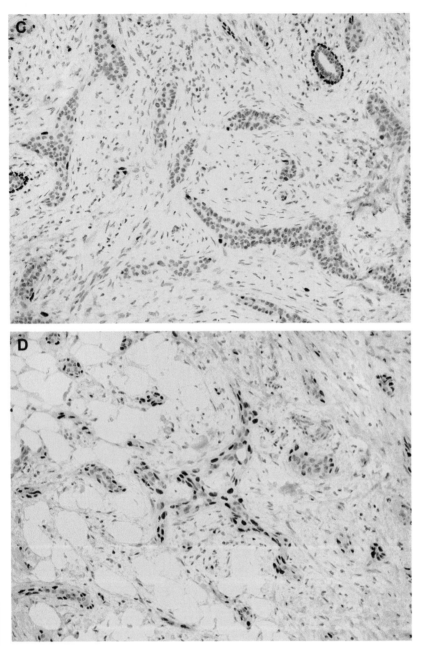

Fig. 28. Negative or discontinuous circumferential staining (C) or luminal staining (D) for p63.

of cellular stroma and core staining of lesional glands recently described in LGASC, however, are likely not seen in syringomatous adenoma. More investigation of the immunohistochemical staining patterns of syringomatous adenoma is needed to confirm this.

TREATMENT/PROGNOSIS

Treatment with local excision and postoperative radiation is sufficient in most cases. Unlike other basal-like or triple-negative breast cancers, LGASC is associated with a favorable prognosis.[109] Nonetheless, the stellate appearance

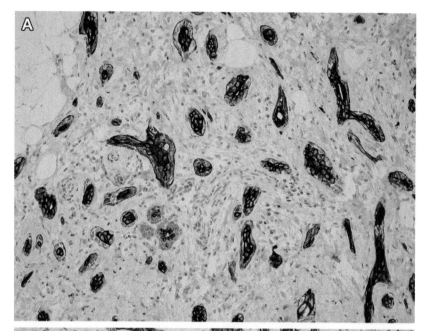

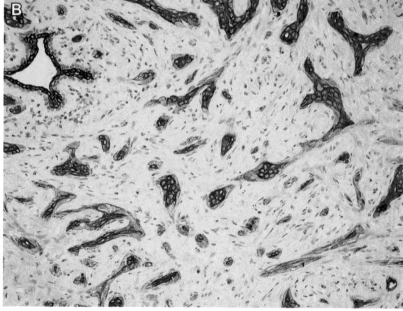

Fig. 29. Cytokeratin staining in LGASC. In some cases, core staining, where stronger staining of luminal cells compared with basally located cells in lesional glands can be seen, by cytokeratin 5/6 in this example (*A*), and by 34βE12 (*B*) in another case.

and many radiating slender extensions of LGASC are features associated with inadequate local excision and high incidence of recurrence.[90] Recurrent tumors tend to recapitulate the adenosquamous pattern of the primary tumor, generally with more prominent squamous features.[91] None of the original 11 patients with LGASC experienced axillary lymph node metastasis or regional or distant metastasis.[91] In the subsequent published series,[92] however, a 40-year-old woman with a 3.5-cm tumor had 1 of 12 axillary lymph nodes involved by metastatic carcinoma. Another 33-year-old female patient with a large tumor (8 cm) developed pulmonary (histologically similar) metastases despite negative axillary lymph nodes.[91,92] LGASC can be considered a locally aggressive tumor with a low incidence of axillary or distant metastases.

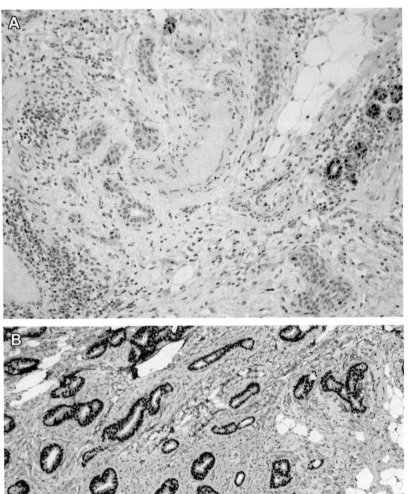

Fig. 30. LGASC. This tumor is characteristically ER/PR negative, which is helpful to distinguish it from invasive well-differentiated duct carcinoma. ER negativity in LGASC (A) in comparison to that of strong, diffuse positivity in tubular carcinoma (B).

SYRINGOMATOUS ADENOMA

OVERVIEW

Syringomatous adenoma is a rare benign but locally infiltrative mammary tumor typically found in the nipple with histologic features similar to that of syringoma of skin adnexal origin.[110] The histologic derivation of this tumor has been debated but likely arises from eccrine structures of the nipple and areola.[103] Before the initial clinicopathologic description of 5 patients by Rosen in 1983,[110] only rare cases resembling syringomatous adenoma were described.[111,112] With the exception of one study consisting of 11 patients,[100] the majority of subsequent reports of patients with this lesion have been described in the form of case reports and small series.[101–108,110,113–125]

Some observers have advocated the term, *syringomatous tumor* over *syringomatous adenoma* to communicate more worrisome features, such as infiltrative growth pattern and, in some cases, the presence of perineural invasion.[101,123] Alternatively, other investigators have suggested the term, *infiltrating syringomatous adenoma*, to connote these more aggressive findings.[100]

CLINICAL FEATURES

With the exception of 1 man,[110] all reported patients have been women.[106] Patients' ages range from 11 to 76 years (average 46 years).[100,110,113] The most common presenting sign is that of a solitary and unilateral mass in the nipple or in the subareolar region.[102,106] Nipple inversion can be concomitantly seen but is not

Fig. 31. Syringomatous adenoma. Biopsy of the nipple/areolar region showing superficial location of infiltrating glands admixed with squamous cysts. Lesional glands surround but do not invade lactiferous ducts (*A*). Infiltrating glands consisting of 1 or 2 layers of cytologically bland squamous or cuboidal epithelium in and around smooth muscle bundles of the nipple (*B*).

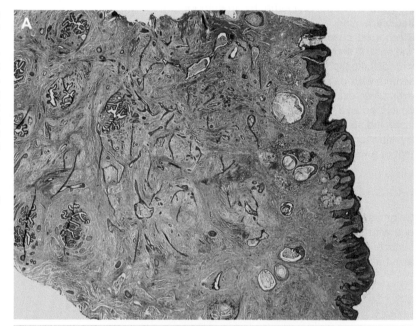

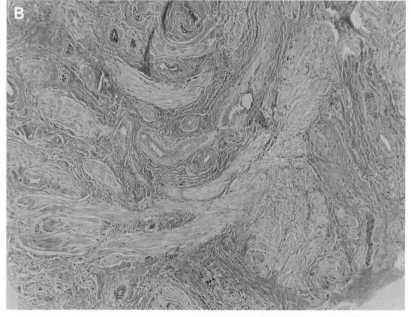

typical. Syringomatous adenomas have been described in supernumerary nipples.[113,119] Affected patients complain of itching, bleeding, pain, or tenderness; however, most report only a painless mass. Nipple discharge can occur and is commonly serous in quality. Erosion and ulceration of the nipple has been reported[111] but is generally considered uncharacteristic of this entity.

IMAGING

Several studies describe the radiologic features of syringomatous adenoma by mammography and ultrasound.[104,105,108,114,116–118,122,124] Of the 6 reported cases with specific mammographic findings, 4 showed a mass, 1 showed a mass with calcifications, and the remaining case presented with calcifications only. The majority of examples evaluated by mammography were described as a "spiculated mass," thus, radiologically indistinguishable from tubular carcinoma. By ultrasound, the most common finding was that of a mass.

GROSS FEATURES

On gross examination, a firm mass, nodule, or plaque with indistinct borders is typical.[100] The cut surface is gray or white. The tumor's size is variable but generally between 1 cm and 3 cm.[100,110]

MORPHOLOGIC FEATURES

Nests, cords, and ducts composed of cytologically bland cells infiltrate around lactiferous ducts (and lobules if they extend into the superficial mammary parenchyma) without direct involvement (Fig. 31). The ducts are well spaced and are classically tadpole-shaped with comma-like tails similar to that of a syringoma (Fig. 32). Some ducts, however, can be compressed or narrowed.[100] The ducts, themselves, are composed of either a flattened single or double cell layer of squamoid or cuboidal-appearing epithelium.[103] Ducts can invade directly into smooth muscle bundles of the nipple as well as peripheral nerves.[100,101,115] Keratin cysts with luminal keratinous debris are common. Focal calcification can be seen in areas of keratinization.[110] The ratio of tubular to squamous components varies from case to case. Connection of lesional structures to the overlying skin has been reported,[101,113] but only pseudoepitheliomatous hyperplasia was described in the original report of 5 cases. The stroma has been described as distinctive and appears either fibrotic or loose and cellular (Fig. 33).[100,101] On low power, cellular stroma form cuffs around epithelial nests, cords, and ducts, which have been found helpful in identifying foci of tumor at low power.[101] A chronic inflammatory background is not characteristic of this entity unless there is focal rupture of a keratinous cyst where foreign body giant cells are also present.

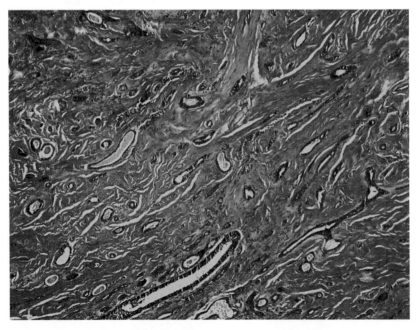

Fig. 32. Syringomatous adenoma. The glands are tadpole-shaped with comma-like tails. Some glands are more compressed. The degree of squamous differentiation seen in these glands is variable.

Fig. 33. Syringomatous adenoma. The stroma surrounding lesional glands is either fibrotic (*A*) or loose and cellular, typically concentrated around neoplastic epithelial structures (*B*).

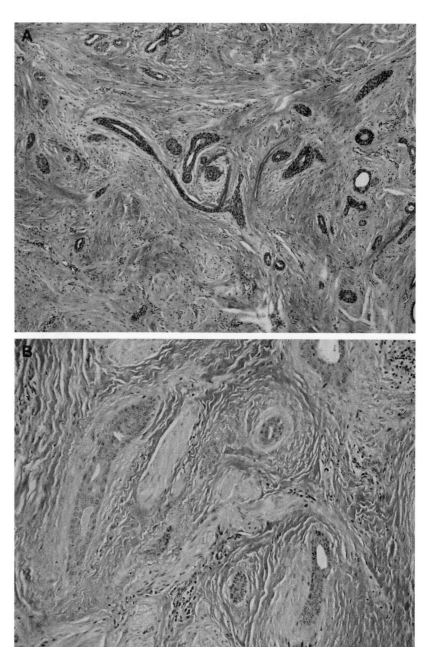

IMMUNOHISTOCHEMISTRY

Due to its rarity, syringomatous adenoma has not been studied extensively by immunohistochemistry. Immunohistochemical stains that react with myoepithelial cells including smooth muscle actin, p63, and calponin have been reported to be variably positive and negative in epithelial structures, confirming (or not) the presence of myoepithelium to these investigators.[100,102–108] The authors have found similarly variable circumferential staining using myoepithelial markers in several cases (unpublished) (**Fig. 34**). Because a recent study has demonstrated similar staining patterns in LGASC,[94] likely myoepithelial markers do not likely distinguish between these 2 entities. Furthermore, although not extensively studied, syringomatous adenomas lack ER/PR expression, much like LGASC.

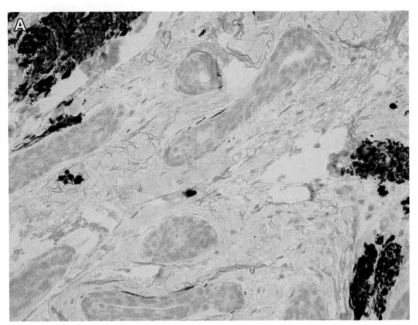

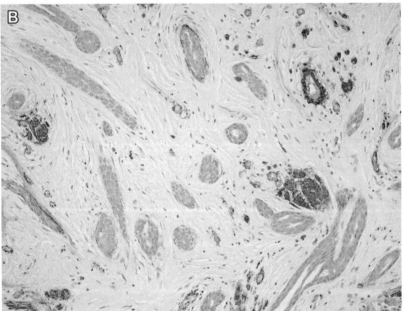

Fig. 34. Syringomatous adenoma. Lesional glands show circumferential, weak and discontinuous or absent staining using myoepithelial immunohistochemical stains. Calponin (*A*). Smooth muscle actin (*B*).

DIFFERENTIAL DIAGNOSIS

Syringomatous adenoma is most commonly mistaken for malignant entities, such as tubular carcinoma or LGASC, both of which lead to over-treatment.[100,103,124] Syringomatous adenoma can be distinguished from tubular carcinoma by several parameters. The ductal structures comprising syringomatous adenoma are typically rounded with smooth contours (tadpole-shaped with comma-like tails) whereas glands of tubular carcinoma are angulated with pointed ends. Moreover, squamous metaplasia/differentiation within lesional glands or keratin cysts is not seen in tubular carcinoma. Although cytologically uniform in both entities, the glands comprising tubular carcinoma are always formed by a single layer whereas those of syringomatous adenoma can be single-layered or double-layered. Tubular carcinoma typically arises deeper in the breast and commonly in the upper outer quadrant compared with syringomatous adenoma, which arises superficially in the nipple or subareolar region. If tubular carcinoma does involve the nipple, nipple retraction and/or Paget disease is expected, both of which are not seen in syringomatous adenoma.[100]

LGASC is morphologically more difficult to discern from syringomatous adenoma than tubular carcinoma. Some investigators believe that these entities are one and the same, the only difference being their relative location within the breast.[100,101] They have many common morphologic features, such as infiltrating ductal structures with varying degrees of squamous differentiation, fibrotic or cellular stroma, and cytologically uniform lesional cells. Clinically, they are both known to be locally infiltrative with a tendency to recur but only rare examples of LGASC have been known to metastasize, which is the reason distinguishing these 2 entities is important.[92] The findings that distinguish LGASC from syringomatous adenoma include the presence of a lymphocytic infiltrate either as scattered aggregates/pseudofollicles or dispersed throughout lesional glands, the deeper location within the breast (away from the nipple), and its tendency to grow in a similar fashion as a radial scar in some cases. Syringomatous adenoma tends to show less squamous differentiation than LGASC and stratification of lesional cysts to small ductules to small cords and nests of cells in syringomatous adenoma is not seen in LGASC.[119]

TREATMENT/PROGNOSIS

Local excision, which may require removal of the nipple, is sufficient treatment. Patients with syringomatous adenoma experience an excellent clinical outcome because this tumor is considered locally infiltrative and recurrent but incapable of metastasis. Incomplete excision can lead to local recurrence and progressive invasive growth of the tumor.[110] In a study by Jones and colleagues,[100] 5 of the 11 (45%) patients developed local recurrence at the site of the index lesion. All of these patients had lesional tissue at the margin in the initial surgical specimen (incomplete excision).

EPITHELIAL DISPLACEMENT BY NEEDLING PROCEDURES

OVERVIEW

Before surgical excision, breast lesions are routinely subjected to a variety of needling procedures, including core biopsy, fine-needle aspiration, local anesthetic injection, suture placement, and needle localization.[126–128] Displacement of benign and malignant epithelium into stroma and lymphovascular channels as a result of these procedures is a recognized phenomenon that can cause significant diagnostic problems.[126,129–131] Displacement of in situ carcinoma into the stroma may be misinterpreted as invasive carcinoma or may lead to an inaccurate assessment of tumor size or margin status.[126,129,132] Displaced epithelium in lymphatic spaces can mimic true lymphovascular channel involvement.[130–133] The incorrect assessment of such parameters has important management implications for patients and may influence decisions regarding additional surgery, radiation, and systemic therapy.[132]

There are potential biologic consequences of the displacement of malignant epithelium during needle procedures. The seeding of a core biopsy tract by carcinomatous epithelium during a biopsy may result in the incomplete removal of carcinoma in a breast-conserving procedure if the entire needle tract is not removed.[127] Recurrences of carcinoma have been reported in the skin as a result of needle core biopsy.[134–136] There is also the theoretic risk of distant tumor dissemination of carcinoma cells via displacement into lymphovascular spaces.[127,129,133] There are limited data addressing the biologic significance of epithelial displacement, and the clinical implications of this phenomenon are currently unknown.[137] No study has demonstrated increased morbidity from tumor seeding, and the risk of tumor recurrence as a result of breast needling procedures seems low.[137–142] The diagnostic problems posed by this phenomenon, however, are significant. This section focuses on the diagnostic issues relevant to epithelial displacement into the stroma manifesting as a small glandular proliferation and the importance of recognizing this artifact commonly found in breast excision specimens.

CLINICAL FEATURES

Epithelial displacement is most often encountered in excisional biopsy specimens but can be observed in needle core biopsy samples from patients without a history of prior needle procedure.[127,129,130] The incidence of epithelial displacement is difficult to ascertain because most needling procedures result in benign diagnoses, which are not followed by excision.[126] Youngson and colleagues[127] found epithelial displacement in 12 of 43 (28%) of excisions or mastectomies from patients with breast carcinoma who had undergone stereotactic core

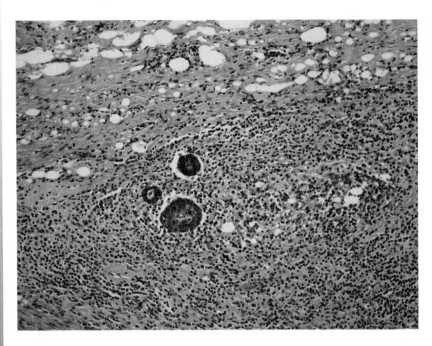

Fig. 35. Displaced glands surrounded by an area of artificial clearing and associated with inflammation and hemorrhage.

biopsy. A similar rate of displacement (32%) was reported among 352 cancer excisions in patients who had undergone large-gauge (11–18–gauge) needle core biopsy.[133]

A variety of benign and malignant breast lesions can be associated with epithelial displacement; however, papillary lesions are most prone to this change.[126,143] In a series reported by Nagi and colleagues,[126] 50/53 (94.3%) cases showing epithelial displacement were associated with some form of underlying benign or malignant papillary lesion. The susceptibility of papillary lesions to epithelial displacement is due to the friability of the papillae, which can be broken off with trauma. It has also been suggested that papillary lesions with a cystic component are prone to

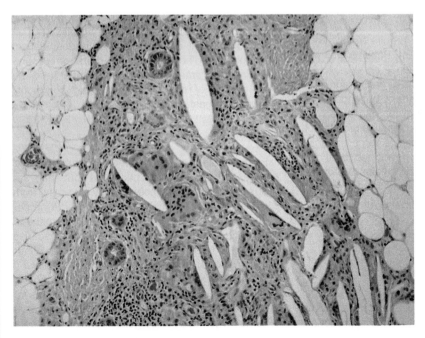

Fig. 36. Biopsy-related changes, including foreign body giant cells, cholesterol clefts, and inflammatory cells, are associated with displaced small glands.

displacement as a result of the intracystic pressure within the lesion, which is released on biopsy, causing spillage of cells into the surrounding tissue.[126,143]

Epithelial displacement can result from virtually any needling procedure but seems to occur less frequently with the use of directional vacuum-assisted biopsy compared with fine-needle aspiration or automated core biopsy.[144] This is likely due to the method in which tissue is obtained with these instruments. Automated core biopsy

needles are fired through the targeted lesion, which may displace lesional cells into the surrounding tissue, whereas vacuum-assisted biopsy needles obtain tissue by firing the needle adjacent to the lesion and use suction to acquire the lesional tissue.[129,144]

Awareness of the time interval between the needling procedure and the excision may be helpful to pathologists. Diaz and colleagues[133] reported a greater likelihood of tumor cell displacement with shorter intervals between core biopsy

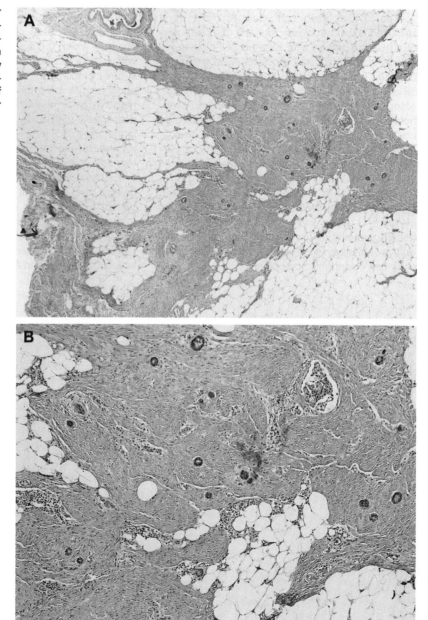

Fig. 37. (*A*) Low-power view and (*B*) medium-power view showing displaced glands within a needle core biopsy tract, which can be identified as a linear area of granulation tissue or scar with inflammation.

and surgical excision. Tumor cell displacement was seen in 42% of patients with an interval of fewer than 15 days, 31% of patients with a 15-day to 28-day interval, and 15% of patients with an interval of greater than 28 days. This suggests that over time, displaced tumor cells lose viability within the inflammatory environment of the biopsy site.[133]

MORPHOLOGIC FEATURES

In excisional biopsies or mastectomies, epithelial displacement may be identified within the biopsy site, in the adjacent stroma, or within lymphatic spaces.[126] Displaced epithelium is most often identified within the biopsy site and can be recognized by the presence of isolated cell clusters or glands in the stroma, associated with traumatic changes from the needle core procedure (Figs. 35 and 36). These changes include hemorrhage, granulation tissue, fat necrosis, inflammation, hemosiderin-laden macrophages, and foreign body giant cell reaction.[126,127,131,144] A needle tract can be identified as a linear area of granulation tissue or scar with inflammatory cells (Fig. 37).[126] Displaced cell clusters are morphologically similar to the primary breast lesion and are often surrounded by an area of artificial clearing.[131] Cells within the biopsy site may undergo squamous metaplasia and show degenerative features, such as pyknotic nuclei and shrunken eosinophilic cytoplasm.[133]

Displaced glands or cell clusters often appear out of place from the surrounding stroma. Postbiopsy stroma has a reactive granulation tissue-like appearance (Fig. 38). This should be distinguished from the stroma of invasive carcinoma, which is desmoplastic and intimately associated with the tumor cells.[127] When displaced epithelium is present in stroma or adipose tissue outside of the biopsy tract, a stromal reaction does not accompany the cell clusters, making the distinction between invasion and displacement more difficult.

The histologic appearance of epithelial displacement varies depending on the time interval between the needling procedure and excision. Biopsy-related changes may be absent in cases in which there was a short time interval, as with needle localization, anesthetic injection, and suture placement.[126,130] In these cases, the changes are minimal and may consist only of hemorrhage or epithelial disruption,[130] sometimes associated with a neutrophilic infiltrate.[126] With longer intervals (>15 days) between the needle procedure and excision, more typical inflammatory and stromal changes are identified.[130]

Epithelial clusters that have been displaced from benign and malignant papillary lesions typically have a micropapillary appearance with cytologic features similar to the primary lesion.[126] Micropapillary features have also been observed in cells displaced from underlying mucinous or cystic lesions, without a primary papillary component.[126]

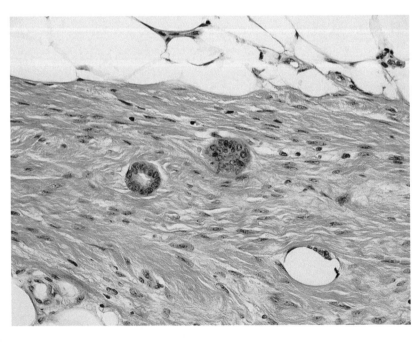

Fig. 38. Displaced glands are present in a reactive stroma without desmoplasia.

Fig. 39. Solid papillary carcinoma with invasion. This growth pattern of invasive carcinoma can mimic epithelial displacement.

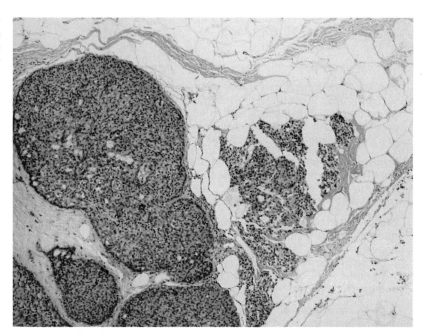

In some cases of solid papillary carcinoma, a pattern of true invasion can mimic epithelial displacement.[5] This pattern is characterized by cohesive sheets of cells that appear as though they were displaced into surrounding adipose tissue without an accompanying stromal reaction (**Fig. 39**).

The use of immunohistochemical stains, such as p63, smooth muscle myosin heavy chain, and calponin may be used to highlight myoepithelial cells when epithelial displacement is suspected. These stains are helpful in establishing displacement only in cases in which a myoepithelial cell layer is present. Staining for myoepithelial cells often shows a pattern of attenuated staining (**Fig. 40**). The myoepithelial cell layer, however, often does not accompany the epithelial fragments that have undergone displacement. This occurs

Fig. 40. Immunostain p63 showing attenuated or absent myoepithelial reactivity in displaced glands.

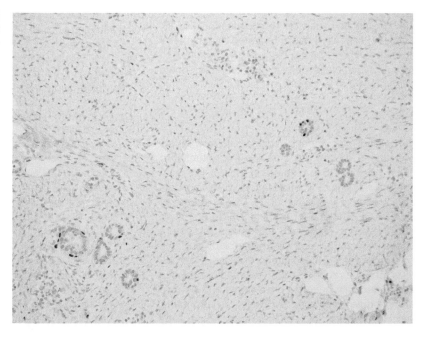

Pitfalls—Morphology
SMALL GLANDULAR PROLIFRATIONS

! Invasion of peripheral nerves may be seen in benign small glandular proliferations, including sclerosing adenosis and radial scar, and this finding should not be interpreted as a sign of malignancy.

! Involvement of sclerosing adenosis with atypical hyperplasia (including apocrine forms) or in situ carcinoma can mimic invasive carcinoma.

! Glands within a radial scar that have undergone squamous metaplasia can simulate the appearance of LGASC. There is, however, a well-documented association of LGASC with radial scars, complex sclerosing lesions, and papillary lesions.

! Tubular carcinoma can arise within a pre-existing radial scar.

! Atypical MGA can mimic invasive ductal carcinoma.

! Epithelial displacement, in and of itself, is a potential diagnostic pitfall, especially with underlying papillary lesions, and can mimic stromal and lymphatic space invasion.

! Invasive carcinoma arising from solid papillary carcinoma often has a "pushed" appearance without a stromal reaction. This may be misinterpreted as epithelial displacement from a prior needling procedure.

Pitfalls—Immunohistochemistry
SMALL GLANDULAR PROLIFRATIONS

! Immunostains for myoepithelial cells can show absent or attenuated reactivity in radial scars (particularly in the sclerotic nidus of the lesion) and in displaced epithelium from a needling procedure.

! Attenuated myoepithelial reactivity may be seen in cases of atypical hyperplasia and in situ carcinoma involving adenosis. This finding can be worrisome for the presence of invasive carcinoma, particularly when apocrine features are present.

! Certain immunostains for myoepithelial cells (smooth muscle actin and CD10) show variable cross-reactivity with stromal myofibroblasts, which can give a false impression of the presence of myoepithelium.

! MGA shows absence of myoepithelial reactivity. A basement membrane can be identified with the use of immunostains, such as laminin and collagen IV.

! The immunohistochemical profile of LGASC is highly variable within each case and between cases.

! LGASC and syringomatous adenoma show similar immunohistochemical staining patterns with myoepithelial markers.

more frequently when the primary lesion is DCIS, which in itself may show attenuated myoepithelial staining without being disrupted.[131] Failure to detect myoepithelial cells in this scenario should not prompt a diagnosis of invasion.

SUMMARY

Epithelial displacement can be caused by a variety of needling procedures and has the potential to cause diagnostic problems in breast excision specimens, including overstaging, overdiagnosis of invasion, and inaccurate assessment of margins. It is helpful for pathologists to be aware of the needling procedure performed, the nature of the lesion that has been sampled, and the time interval from needling to excision. Pathologists should recognize the histologic changes associated with needling procedures and be able to distinguish displacement from true stromal or vascular invasion. Due to their friability, papillary

lesions are particularly prone to displacement by needling procedures and caution should be taken in evaluating papillary lesions that have undergone such procedures. The biologic consequences of epithelial displacement are unknown but seem minimal. Long-term follow-up studies of patients with malignancy who have undergone needling procedures are needed to determine the clinical significance of this phenomenon.[144]

REFERENCES

1. Dupont WD, Page DL. Risk factors for breast cancer in women with proliferative breast disease. N Engl J Med 1985;312:146–51.
2. Jensen RA, Page DL, Dupont WD, et al. Invasive breast cancer risk in women with sclerosing adenosis. Cancer 1989;64:1977–83.
3. Bodian CA, Perzin KH, Lattes R, et al. Prognostic significance of benign proliferative breast disease. Cancer 1993;71:3896–907.
4. Dupont WD, Parl FF, Hartmann WH, et al. Breast cancer risk associated with proliferative breast

disease and atypical hyperplasia. Cancer 1993;71: 1258–65.

5. Rosen PP. Rosen's breast pathology. 3rd edition. Philadelphia: Lippincott Williams & Wilkins; 2009.

6. Taskin F, Koseoglu K, Unsal A, et al. Sclerosing adenosis of the breast: radiologic appearance and efficiency of core needle biopsy. Diagn Interv Radiol 2011;17(4):311–6.

7. Nielsen NS, Nielsen BB. Mammographic features of sclerosing adenosis presenting as a tumour. Clin Radiol 1986;37:371–3.

8. Markopoulos C, Kouskos E, Phillipidis T, et al. Adenosis tumor of the breast. Breast J 2003;9: 255–6.

9. Lanzafame S. Nodular sclerosing adenosis (adenosis tumor) of the breast. An immunohistologic study particularly in reference to the relationship with radial cicatrix and to the differential diagnosis with tubular carcinoma. Pathologica 1989;81:251–66 [in Italian].

10. Gill HK, Ioffe OB, Berg WA. When is a diagnosis of sclerosing adenosis acceptable at core biopsy? Radiology 2003;228:50–7.

11. Jain M, Niveditha SR, Bajaj P, et al. Collagenous spherulosis of breast: diagnosis by FNAB with review of literature. Indian J Pathol Microbiol 2000;43:131–4.

12. Clement PB, Young RH, Azzopardi JG. Collagenous spherulosis of the breast. Am J Surg Pathol 1987;11:411–7.

13. Gobbi H, Jensen RA, Simpson JF, et al. Atypical ductal hyperplasia and ductal carcinoma in situ of the breast associated with perineural invasion. Hum Pathol 2001;32:785–90.

14. Davies JD. Neural invasion in benign mammary dysplasia. J Pathol 1973;109:225–31.

15. Jung WH, Noh TW, Kim HJ, et al. Lobular carcinoma in situ in sclerosing adenosis. Yonsei Med J 2000;41:293–7.

16. Chan JK, Ng WF. Sclerosing adenosis cancerized by intraductal carcinoma. Pathology 1987;19:425–8.

17. Fechner RE. Lobular carcinoma in situ in sclerosing adenosis. A potential source of confusion with invasive carcinoma. Am J Surg Pathol 1981;5:233–9.

18. Rasbridge SA, Millis RR. Carcinoma in situ involving sclerosing adenosis: a mimic of invasive breast carcinoma. Histopathology 1995;27:269–73.

19. Oberman HA, Markey BA. Noninvasive carcinoma of the breast presenting in adenosis. Mod Pathol 1991;4:31–5.

20. Seidman JD, Ashton M, Lefkowitz M. Atypical apocrine adenosis of the breast: a clinicopathologic study of 37 patients with 8.7-year follow-up. Cancer 1996;77:2529–37.

21. Carter DJ, Rosen PP. Atypical apocrine metaplasia in sclerosing lesions of the breast: a study of 51 patients. Mod Pathol 1991;4:1–5.

22. O'Malley FP, Bane AL. The spectrum of apocrine lesions of the breast. Adv Anat Pathol 2004;11:1–9.

23. Tavassoli FA, Norris HJ. Intraductal apocrine carcinoma: a clinicopathologic study of 37 cases. Mod Pathol 1994;7:813–8.

24. Sloane JP, Mayers MM. Carcinoma and atypical hyperplasia in radial scars and complex sclerosing lesions: importance of lesion size and patient age. Histopathology 1993;23:225–31.

25. Patel A, Steel Y, McKenzie J, et al. Radial scars: a review of 30 cases. Eur J Surg Oncol 1997;23:202–5.

26. Wellings SR, Alpers CE. Subgross pathologic features and incidence of radial scars in the breast. Hum Pathol 1984;15:475–9.

27. Andersen JA, Gram JB. Radial scar in the female breast. A long-term follow-up study of 32 cases. Cancer 1984;53:2557–60.

28. Brenner RJ, Jackman RJ, Parker SH, et al. Percutaneous core needle biopsy of radial scars of the breast: when is excision necessary? AJR Am J Roentgenol 2002;179:1179–84.

29. Kennedy M, Masterson AV, Kerin M, et al. Pathology and clinical relevance of radial scars: a review. J Clin Pathol 2003;56:721–4.

30. Shaheen R, Schimmelpenninck CA, Stoddart L, et al. Spectrum of diseases presenting as architectural distortion on mammography: multimodality radiologic imaging with pathologic correlation. Semin Ultrasound CT MR 2011;32:351–62.

31. Linell F, Ljungberg O, Andersson I. Breast carcinoma. Aspects of early stages, progression and related problems. Acta Pathol Microbiol Scand Suppl 1980;(272):1–233.

32. Jacobs TW, Byrne C, Colditz G, et al. Radial scars in benign breast-biopsy specimens and the risk of breast cancer. N Engl J Med 1999;340:430–6.

33. Sohn VY, Causey MW, Steele SR, et al. The treatment of radial scars in the modern era—surgical excision is not required. Am Surg 2010;76:522–5.

34. Cawson JN, Malara F, Kavanagh A, et al. Fourteen-gauge needle core biopsy of mammographically evident radial scars: is excision necessary? Cancer 2003;97:345–51.

35. Nielsen M, Jensen J, Andersen JA. An autopsy study of radial scar in the female breast. Histopathology 1985;9:287–95.

36. Wallis MG, Devakumar R, Hosie KB, et al. Complex sclerosing lesions (radial scars) of the breast can be palpable. Clin Radiol 1993;48:319–20.

37. Alvarado-Cabrero I, Tavassoli FA. Neoplastic and malignant lesions involving or arising in a radial scar: a clinicopathologic analysis of 17 cases. Breast J 2000;6:96–102.

38. Philpotts LE, Shaheen NA, Jain KS, et al. Uncommon high-risk lesions of the breast diagnosed at stereotactic core-needle biopsy: clinical importance. Radiology 2000;216:831–7.

39. Frouge C, Tristant H, Guinebretiere JM, et al. Mammographic lesions suggestive of radial scars: microscopic findings in 40 cases. Radiology 1995; 195:623–5.

40. Shin SJ, Simpson PT, Da Silva L, et al. Molecular evidence for progression of microglandular adenosis (MGA) to invasive carcinoma. Am J Surg Pathol 2009;33:496–504.

41. Denley H, Pinder SE, Tan PH, et al. Metaplastic carcinoma of the breast arising within complex sclerosing lesion: a report of five cases. Histopathology 2000;36:203–9.

42. Gobbi H, Simpson JF, Jensen RA, et al. Metaplastic spindle cell breast tumors arising within papillomas, complex sclerosing lesions, and nipple adenomas. Mod Pathol 2003;16:893–901.

43. Tavassoli F, Devilee P, editors. Tumours of the breast and female genital organs. Lyon (France): IARC Press; 2003.

44. Holland DW, Boucher LD, Mortimer JE. Tubular breast cancer experience at Washington University: a review of the literature. Clin Breast Cancer 2001;2:210–4.

45. Diab SG, Clark GM, Osborne CK, et al. Tumor characteristics and clinical outcome of tubular and mucinous breast carcinomas. J Clin Oncol 1999; 17:1442–8.

46. Rakha EA, Lee AH, Evans AJ, et al. Tubular carcinoma of the breast: further evidence to support its excellent prognosis. J Clin Oncol 2010;28:99–104.

47. McBoyle MF, Razek HA, Carter JL, et al. Tubular carcinoma of the breast: an institutional review. Am Surg 1997;63:639–44 [discussion: 44–5].

48. Carstens PH, Greenberg RA, Francis D, et al. Tubular carcinoma of the breast. A long term follow-up. Histopathology 1985;9:271–80.

49. Sullivan T, Raad RA, Goldberg S, et al. Tubular carcinoma of the breast: a retrospective analysis and review of the literature. Breast Cancer Res Treat 2005;93:199–205.

50. Abdel-Fatah TM, Powe DG, Hodi Z, et al. Morphologic and molecular evolutionary pathways of low nuclear grade invasive breast cancers and their putative precursor lesions: further evidence to support the concept of low nuclear grade breast neoplasia family. Am J Surg Pathol 2008;32:513–23.

51. Aulmann S, Elsawaf Z, Penzel R, et al. Invasive tubular carcinoma of the breast frequently is clonally related to flat epithelial atypia and low-grade ductal carcinoma in situ. Am J Surg Pathol 2009; 33:1646–53.

52. Waldman FM, Hwang ES, Etzell J, et al. Genomic alterations in tubular breast carcinomas. Hum Pathol 2001;32:222–6.

53. Newcomer LM, Newcomb PA, Trentham-Dietz A, et al. Detection method and breast carcinoma histology. Cancer 2002;95:470–7.

54. Deos PH, Norris HJ. Well-differentiated (tubular) carcinoma of the breast. A clinicopathologic study of 145 pure and mixed cases. Am J Clin Pathol 1982;78:1–7.

55. Cabral AH, Recine M, Paramo JC, et al. Tubular carcinoma of the breast: an institutional experience and review of the literature. Breast J 2003;9:298–301.

56. Papadatos G, Rangan AM, Psarianos T, et al. Probability of axillary node involvement in patients with tubular carcinoma of the breast. Br J Surg 2001; 88:860–4.

57. Peters GN, Wolff M, Haagensen CD. Tubular carcinoma of the breast. Clinical pathologic correlations based on 100 cases. Ann Surg 1981;193:138–49.

58. Taxy JB. Tubular carcinoma of the male breast: report of a case. Cancer 1975;36:462–5.

59. Heller KS, Rosen PP, Schottenfeld D, et al. Male breast cancer: a clinicopathologic study of 97 cases. Ann Surg 1978;188:60–5.

60. Lagios MD, Rose MR, Margolin FR. Tubular carcinoma of the breast: association with multicentricity, bilaterality, and family history of mammary carcinoma. Am J Clin Pathol 1980;73:25–30.

61. Zandrino F, Calabrese M, Faedda C, et al. Tubular carcinoma of the breast: pathological, clinical, and ultrasonographic findings. A review of the literature. Radiol Med 2006;111:773–82.

62. Elson BC, Helvie MA, Frank TS, et al. Tubular carcinoma of the breast: mode of presentation, mammographic appearance, and frequency of nodal metastases. AJR Am J Roentgenol 1993;161:1173–6.

63. Leibman AJ, Lewis M, Kruse B. Tubular carcinoma of the breast: mammographic appearance. AJR Am J Roentgenol 1993;160:263–5.

64. Sheppard DG, Whitman GJ, Huynh PT, et al. Tubular carcinoma of the breast: mammographic and sonographic features. AJR Am J Roentgenol 2000;174:253–7.

65. Vega A, Garijo F. Radial scar and tubular carcinoma. Mammographic and sonographic findings. Acta Radiol 1993;34:43–7.

66. Leikola J, Heikkila P, von Smitten K, et al. The prevalence of axillary lymph-node metastases in patients with pure tubular carcinoma of the breast and sentinel node biopsy. Eur J Surg Oncol 2006; 32:488–91.

67. Brandt SM, Young GQ, Hoda SA. The "Rosen Triad": tubular carcinoma, lobular carcinoma in situ, and columnar cell lesions. Adv Anat Pathol 2008;15:140–6.

68. Abdel-Fatah TM, Powe DG, Hodi Z, et al. High frequency of coexistence of columnar cell lesions, lobular neoplasia, and low grade ductal carcinoma in situ with invasive tubular carcinoma and invasive lobular carcinoma. Am J Surg Pathol 2007;31: 417–26.

69. Kader HA, Jackson J, Mates D, et al. Tubular carcinoma of the breast: a population-based study of

nodal metastases at presentation and of patterns of relapse. Breast J 2001;7:8–13.

70. Javid SH, Smith BL, Mayer E, et al. Tubular carcinoma of the breast: results of a large contemporary series. Am J Surg 2009;197:674–7.

71. James BA, Cranor ML, Rosen PP. Carcinoma of the breast arising in microglandular adenosis. Am J Clin Pathol 1993;100:507–13.

72. Salarieh A, Sneige N. Breast carcinoma arising in microglandular adenosis: a review of the literature. Arch Pathol Lab Med 2007;131:1397–9.

73. Goldstein NS, Kestin LL, Vicini FA. Refined morphologic criteria for tubular carcinoma to retain its favorable outcome status in contemporary breast carcinoma patients. Am J Clin Pathol 2004; 122:728–39.

74. Clement PB, Azzopardi JG. Microglandular adenosis of the breast—a lesion simulating tubular carcinoma. Histopathology 1983;7:169–80.

75. Eusebi V, Foschini MP, Betts CM, et al. Microglandular adenosis, apocrine adenosis, and tubular carcinoma of the breast. An immunohistochemical comparison. Am J Surg Pathol 1993;17:99–109.

76. Tavassoli FA, Norris HJ. Microglandular adenosis of the breast. A clinicopathologic study of 11 cases with ultrastructural observations. Am J Surg Pathol 1983;7:731–7.

77. Khalifeh IM, Albarracin C, Diaz LK, et al. Clinical, histopathologic, and immunohistochemical features of microglandular adenosis and transition into in situ and invasive carcinoma. Am J Surg Pathol 2008;32:544–52.

78. Rosenblum MK, Purrazzella R, Rosen PP. Is microglandular adenosis a precancerous disease? A study of carcinoma arising therein. Am J Surg Pathol 1986;10:237–45.

79. Rosen PP. Microglandular adenosis. A benign lesion simulating invasive mammary carcinoma. Am J Surg Pathol 1983;7:137–44.

80. Resetkova E, Flanders DJ, Rosen PP. Ten-year follow-up of mammary carcinoma arising in microglandular adenosis treated with breast conservation. Arch Pathol Lab Med 2003;127:77–80.

81. Sabate JM, Gomez A, Torrubia S, et al. Microglandular adenosis of the breast in a BRCA1 mutation carrier: radiological features. Eur Radiol 2002;12: 1479–82.

82. Shui R, Yang W. Invasive breast carcinoma arising in microglandular adenosis: a case report and review of the literature. Breast J 2009;15:653–6.

83. Diaz NM, McDivitt RW, Wick MR. Microglandular adenosis of the breast. An immunohistochemical comparison with tubular carcinoma. Arch Pathol Lab Med 1991;115:578–82.

84. Koenig C, Dadmanesh F, Bratthauer GL, et al. Carcinoma Arising in Microglandular Adenosis: an immunohistochemical analysis of 20 intraepithelial

and invasive neoplasms. Int J Surg Pathol 2000;8: 303–15.

85. Acs G, Simpson JF, Bleiweiss IJ, et al. Microglandular adenosis with transition into adenoid cystic carcinoma of the breast. Am J Surg Pathol 2003; 27:1052–60.

86. Huo L, Bell D, Qiu H, et al. Paneth cell-like eosinophilic cytoplasmic granules in breast carcinoma. Ann Diagn Pathol 2011;15:84–92.

87. Geyer FC, Kushner YB, Lambros MB, et al. Microglandular adenosis or microglandular adenoma? A molecular genetic analysis of a case associated with atypia and invasive carcinoma. Histopathology 2009;55:732–43.

88. Geyer FC, Weigelt B, Natrajan R, et al. Molecular analysis reveals a genetic basis for the phenotypic diversity of metaplastic breast carcinomas. J Pathol 2010;220:562–73.

89. Kay S. Microglandular adenosis of the female mammary gland: study of a case with ultrastructural observations. Hum Pathol 1985;16:637–41.

90. Drudis T, Arroyo C, Van Hoeven K, et al. The pathology of low-grade adenosquamous carcinoma of the breast. An immunohistochemical study. Pathol Annu 1994;29(Pt 2):181–97.

91. Rosen PP, Ernsberger D. Low-grade adenosquamous carcinoma. A variant of metaplastic mammary carcinoma. Am J Surg Pathol 1987;11:351–8.

92. Van Hoeven KH, Drudis T, Cranor ML, et al. Low-grade adenosquamous carcinoma of the breast. A clinocopathologic study of 32 cases with ultrastructural analysis. Am J Surg Pathol 1993;17: 248–58.

93. Ho BC, Tan HW, Lee VK, et al. Preoperative and intraoperative diagnosis of low-grade adenosquamous carcinoma of the breast: potential diagnostic pitfalls. Histopathology 2006;49:603–11.

94. Kawaguchi K, Shin SJ. Immunohistochemical staining characteristics of low-grade adenosquamous carcinoma of the breast. Am J Surg Pathol 2012; 36(7):1009–20.

95. Pastolero GC, Bowler L, Meads GE. Intraductal papilloma associated with metaplastic carcinoma of the breast. Histopathology 1997;31:488–90.

96. Wolff AC, Hammond ME, Schwartz JN, et al. American Society of Clinical Oncology/College of American Pathologists guideline recommendations for human epidermal growth factor receptor 2 testing in breast cancer. J Clin Oncol 2007;25: 118–45.

97. Geyer FC, Lambros MB, Natrajan R, et al. Genomic and immunohistochemical analysis of adenosquamous carcinoma of the breast. Mod Pathol 2010; 23:951–60.

98. Turner NC, Reis-Filho JS. Basal-like breast cancer and the BRCA1 phenotype. Oncogene 2006;25: 5846–53.

99. Noel JC, Buxant F, Engohan-Aloghe C. Low-grade adenosquamous carcinoma of the breast–A case report with a BRCA1 germline mutation. Pathol Res Pract 2010;206:511–3.

100. Jones MW, Norris HJ, Snyder RC. Infiltrating syringomatous adenoma of the nipple. A clinical and pathological study of 11 cases. Am J Surg Pathol 1989;13:197–201.

101. Ward BE, Cooper PH, Subramony C. Syringomatous tumor of the nipple. Am J Clin Pathol 1989;92:692–6.

102. Biernat W, Jablkowski W. Syringomatous adenoma of the nipple. Pol J Pathol 2000;51:201–2.

103. Carter E, Dyess DL. Infiltrating syringomatous adenoma of the nipple: a case report and 20-year retrospective review. Breast J 2004;10:443–7.

104. Odashiro M, Lima MG, Miiji LN, et al. Infiltrating syringomatous adenoma of the nipple. Breast J 2009;15:414–6.

105. Oliva VL, Little JV, Carlson GW. Syringomatous adenoma of the nipple—treatment by central mound resection and oncoplastic reconstruction. Breast J 2008;14:102–5.

106. Oo KZ, Xiao PQ. Infiltrating syringomatous adenoma of the nipple: clinical presentation and literature review. Arch Pathol Lab Med 2009;133:1487–9.

107. Riaz N, Khan SM, Idrees R, et al. Infiltrating syringomatous adenoma of nipple. J Coll Physicians Surg Pak 2008;18:438–9.

108. Yosepovich A, Perelman M, Ayalon S, et al. Syringomatous adenoma of the nipple: a case report. Pathol Res Pract 2005;201:405–7.

109. Rakha EA, Elsheikh SE, Aleskandarany MA, et al. Triple-negative breast cancer: distinguishing between basal and nonbasal subtypes. Clin Cancer Res 2009;15:2302–10.

110. Rosen PP. Syringomatous adenoma of the nipple. Am J Surg Pathol 1983;7:739–45.

111. Doctor VM, Sirsat MV. Florid papillomatosis (adenoma) and other benign tumours of the nipple and areola. Br J Cancer 1971;25:1–9.

112. Handley RS, Thackray AC. Adenoma of nipple. Br J Cancer 1962;16:187–94.

113. Azita N, Hana S. Syringomatous adenoma occurring within a supernumerary nipple. Indian J Dermatol Venereol Leprol 2011;77:730.

114. Coulthard A, Liston J, Young JR. Case report: infiltrating syringomatous adenoma of the breast—appearances on mammography and ultrasonography. Clin Radiol 1993;47:62–4.

115. Hwang TS, Ham EK, Kim JP. Syringomatous adenoma of nipple–a case report. J Korean Med Sci 1987;2:263–5.

116. Kim HM, Park BW, Han SH, et al. Infiltrating syringomatous adenoma presenting as microcalcification in the nipple on screening mammogram: case report and review of the literature of radiologic features. Clin Imaging 2010;34:462–5.

117. Kubo M, Tsuji H, Kunitomo T, et al. Syringomatous adenoma of the nipple: a case report. Breast Cancer 2004;11:214–6.

118. Ku J, Bennett RD, Chong KD, et al. Syringomatous adenoma of the nipple. Breast 2004;13:412–5.

119. Page RN, Dittrich L, King R, et al. Syringomatous adenoma of the nipple occurring within a supernumerary breast: a case report. J Cutan Pathol 2009;36:1206–9.

120. Sarma DP, Stevens T. Infiltrating syringomatous eccrine adenoma of the nipple: a case report. Cases J 2009;2:9118.

121. Singh SS, Velusami SD. Syringomatous adenoma of the nipple: report of a case. Indian J Pathol Microbiol 2007;50:808–11.

122. Slaughter MS, Pomerantz RA, Murad T, et al. Infiltrating syringomatous adenoma of the nipple. Surgery 1992;111:711–3.

123. Suster S, Moran CA, Hurt MA. Syringomatous squamous tumors of the breast. Cancer 1991;67:2350–5.

124. Toyoshima O, Kanou M, Kintaka N, et al. Syringomatous adenoma of the nipple: report of a case. Surg Today 1998;28:1196–9.

125. Wadhwa N, Mishra K, Agarwal S. Syringomatous adenoma of the nipple: a case report. Pathology 2003;35:271–2.

126. Nagi C, Bleiweiss I, Jaffer S. Epithelial displacement in breast lesions: a papillary phenomenon. Arch Pathol Lab Med 2005;129:1465–9.

127. Youngson BJ, Liberman L, Rosen PP. Displacement of carcinomatous epithelium in surgical breast specimens following stereotaxic core biopsy. Am J Clin Pathol 1995;103:598–602.

128. Youngson BJ, Cranor M, Rosen PP. Epithelial displacement in surgical breast specimens following needling procedures. Am J Surg Pathol 1994;18:896–903.

129. Koo JS, Jung WH, Kim H. Epithelial displacement into the lymphovascular space can be seen in breast core needle biopsy specimens. Am J Clin Pathol 2010;133:781–7.

130. Tardivon AA, Guinebretiere JM, Dromain C, et al. Histological findings in surgical specimens after core biopsy of the breast. Eur J Radiol 2002;42:40–51.

131. Rosen PP, Hoda SA. Breast pathology, diagnosis by needle core biopsy. 3rd edition. Philadelphia: Wolters Kluwer Health/Lippincott Williams & Wilkins; 2010.

132. Phelan S, O'Doherty A, Hill A, et al. Epithelial displacement during breast needle core biopsy causes diagnostic difficulties in subsequent surgical excision specimens. J Clin Pathol 2007;60:373–6.

133. Diaz LK, Wiley EL, Venta LA. Are malignant cells displaced by large-gauge needle core biopsy of the breast? AJR Am J Roentgenol 1999;173: 1303–13.

134. Stolier A, Skinner J, Levine EA. A prospective study of seeding of the skin after core biopsy of the breast. Am J Surg 2000;180:104–7.

135. Uriburu JL, Vuoto HD, Cogorno L, et al. Local recurrence of breast cancer after skin-sparing mastectomy following core needle biopsy: case reports and review of the literature. Breast J 2006; 12:194–8.

136. Chao C, Torosian MH, Boraas MC, et al. Local recurrence of breast cancer in the stereotactic core needle biopsy site: case reports and review of the literature. Breast J 2001;7:124–7.

137. Liebens F, Carly B, Cusumano P, et al. Breast cancer seeding associated with core needle biopsies: a systematic review. Maturitas 2009;62: 113–23.

138. Loughran CF, Keeling CR. Seeding of tumour cells following breast biopsy: a literature review. Br J Radiol 2011;84:869–74.

139. Knight R, Horiuchi K, Parker SH, et al. Risk of needle-track seeding after diagnostic image-guided core needle biopsy in breast cancer. JSLS 2002;6:207–9.

140. Kopans DB, Gallagher WJ, Swann CA, et al. Does preoperative needle localization lead to an increase in local breast cancer recurrence? Radiology 1988;167:667–8.

141. Fitzal F, Sporn EP, Draxler W, et al. Preoperative core needle biopsy does not increase local recurrence rate in breast cancer patients. Breast Cancer Res Treat 2006;97:9–15.

142. Chen AM, Haffty BG, Lee CH. Local recurrence of breast cancer after breast conservation therapy in patients examined by means of stereotactic core-needle biopsy. Radiology 2002;225:707–12.

143. Douglas-Jones AG, Verghese A. Diagnostic difficulty arising from displaced epithelium after core biopsy in intracystic papillary lesions of the breast. J Clin Pathol 2002;55:780–3.

144. Liberman L. Clinical management issues in percutaneous core breast biopsy. Radiol Clin North Am 2000;38:791–807.

VASCULAR LESIONS OF THE BREAST

Brooke Howitt, MD[a], Alessandra F. Nascimento, MD[b],*

KEYWORDS

- Angiolipoma • Hemangioma • Atypical vascular lesion • Angiosarcoma • Radiation-associated

ABSTRACT

Vascular lesions represent a minority of tumors originating in the breast. The most common entities are benign and include hemangiomas and angiolipomas. Malignant vascular lesions (angiosarcomas) are rare and may be primary or secondary to radiation. Also appreciated in association to radiotherapy is the development of cutaneous atypical vascular lesion affecting the skin of the breast. The relationship of the latter to radiation-associated angiosarcoma is controversial and remains to be elucidated. This article reviews the most likely encountered vascular lesions in the breast, with emphasis on key pathologic diagnostic features and potential diagnostic pitfalls.

ANGIOLIPOMA

OVERVIEW

Angiolipoma is a common, benign tumor that affects primarily young and middle-aged adults and arises primarily within the subcutaneous tissue of the limbs. Lesions may be solitary or multiple. When in the breast, angiolipoma may affect subcutis and mammary parenchyma. Similar to angiolipomas elsewhere on the body, patients with subcutaneous lesions arising on the skin of the breast present with a painful well-circumscribed nodule. When arising within the parenchyma of the breast, this neoplasm shows a wide age distribution and presents as a small and painless nodule.[1] Although angiolipoma has been considered to represent a variant of lipomas,

cytogenetic studies to date have shown essentially all angiolipomas to have normal karyotype.[2,3]

GROSS FEATURES

Angiolipoma is usually small (<2 cm) and well circumscribed and often encapsulated. The cut surface typically is yellow and somewhat lobulated, indistinguishable from a conventional lipoma. As the vascular component increases in angiolipomas, tumors may appear more firm and/or red in color.

MICROSCOPIC FEATURES

Angiolipoma is well demarcated from the surrounding breast parenchyma and is characterized by a proliferation of mature adipocytic tissue admixed with varying amounts of small-caliber capillary vessels showing prominent intravascular fibrin microthrombi (**Fig. 1**A, B). The adipocytic component is benign appearing with no atypia, hyperchromasia, or pleomorphism. The small vessels tend to

> ***Pathologic Key Features***
> OF **ANGIOLIPOMA**
>
> Mixed mature adipose tissue and small-caliber, thick-walled vessels
>
> Fibrin microthrombi, predominant at the periphery of the lesion
>
> Absence of cellular atypia
>
> Low mitotic activity

[a] Department of Pathology, Brigham and Women's Hospital, Harvard Medical School, 75 Francis Street, Boston, MA 02115, USA
[b] Department of Pathology, Baptist Hospital of Miami, 8900 N Kendall Drive, Miami, FL 33176, USA
* Corresponding author.
E-mail address: AlessandraFN@bapisthealth.net

Surgical Pathology 5 (2012) 645–659
http://dx.doi.org/10.1016/j.path.2012.06.002
1875-9181/12/$ – see front matter © 2012 Published by Elsevier Inc

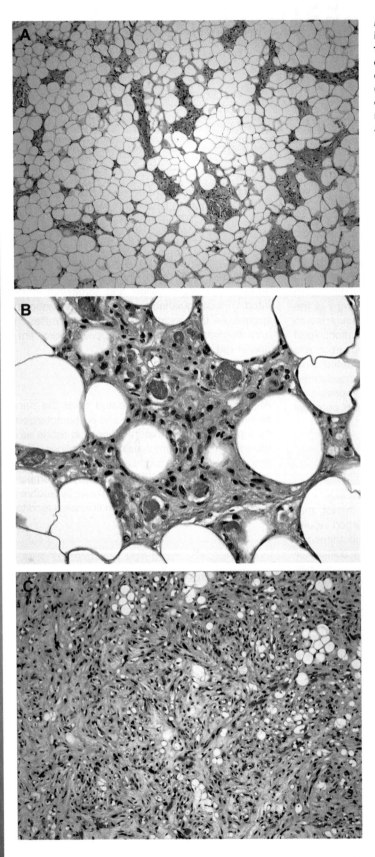

Fig. 1. (*A*) Angiolipoma is characterized by a variable mixture of adipose tissue and small vessels. (*B*) Small-caliber vessels in angiolipoma typically contain fibrin microthrombi. (*C*) Cellular angiolipoma show a dominance of the vascular component with minimal or no admixed adipose tissue.

Differential Diagnosis
OF ANGIOLIPOMA

Adipocytic-predominant angiolipoma	Lipoma Atypical lipomatous tumor
Vascular-predominant angiolipoma	Hemangioma Angiosarcoma

Pitfall
OF ANGIOLIPOMA

! Fibrin microthrombi must be present in the absence of changes suggestive of trauma to the lesion.

be thick walled and more densely located at the periphery of the lesion. In cellular examples of angiolipoma, the vascular component predominates with little to no admixed adipose tissue (see **Fig. 1C**). Mitotic activity is typically low, although in cellular angiolipomas there may be focal high mitotic activity. Cytologic atypia is absent.

DIFFERENTIAL DIAGNOSIS

Although angiolipoma is usually a straightforward diagnosis, in some instances, such as small core biopsies, the correct diagnosis may be difficult.

Adipocytic-predominant angiolipoma should be distinguished from lipoma and atypical lipomatous tumor (ALT). Although lipomas are also well circumscribed, often with a delicate fibrous capsule, they have limited vascularity. Fibrin microthrombus is not a feature of lipomas. ALT shows variation in adipocyte size and shape, cellular fibrous septae containing hyperchromatic atypical cells, and, occasionally, lipoblasts. Immunostains for MDM2 and CDK4 show nuclear staining in more than 95% of ALTs.[4]

Cellular angiolipomas have only a minimal adipocytic component and, therefore, may be mistaken for a hemangioma or angiosarcoma. In contrast to angiolipoma, hemangioma shows vessels of various calibers and absence of fibrin microthrombi. Angiosarcoma shows angulated vascular channels with dissecting architecture, nuclear atypia, and pleomorphism (discussed later). Immunohistochemistry in angiolipoma and angiosarcoma shows vessels to be positive for markers, such as CD31 and CD34; however, in contrast to angiolipoma, angiosarcoma lacks smooth muscle actin–positive pericytes surrounding vascular channels.

PROGNOSIS

Angiolipoma is benign and simple excision is curative. There is no potential for local recurrence or metastasis.

PERILOBULAR HEMANGIOMA

OVERVIEW

Perilobular hemangioma is a benign lesion that affects patients in a wide age range and is often an incidental finding, present in 1.3% to 10% of patients undergoing breast biopsies, excisions, or mastectomies for unrelated reasons and in autopsy studies.[5,6] It may be solitary or multiple, unilateral or bilateral.

GROSS AND MICROSCOPIC FEATURES

Perilobular hemangioma is macroscopically and radiologically inconspicuous, smaller than 5 mm. It is often associated with lobules and/or ducts; however, this relationship is not necessarily seen (**Fig. 2**). It is characterized by a well-defined proliferation of benign-appearing vascular channels containing red blood cells. The blood vessels are thin walled, with absent muscular coating, and anastomosing with minimal dissection of the surrounding stroma. The endothelial cells lining these spaces are flat and show no hyperchromasia or atypia.

Pathologic Key Features
OF PERILOBULAR HEMANGIOMA

Benign-appearing vessels containing red blood cells

Often, but not always, associated with lobules and/or ducts

No nuclear atypia, hyperchromasia, or multi-layering

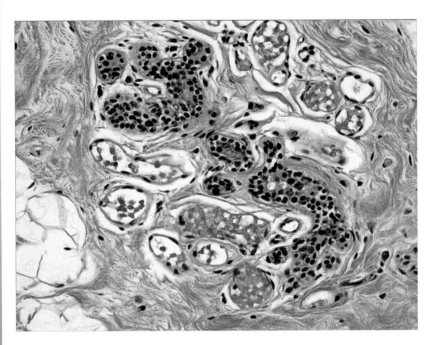

Fig. 2. Perilobular hemangioma is often associated with lobules and/or ducts and shows no cytologic atypia.

DIFFERENTIAL DIAGNOSIS

The diagnosis of perilobular hemangioma is often straightforward and requires no additional immunostains. Pseudoangiomatous stromal hyperplasia (PASH) may morphologically overlap with perilobular hemangioma; however, in contrast to hemangiomas, the cells lining the spaces in PASH are fibroblasts and myofibroblasts and do not express vascular markers, such as CD31, nor are the spaces filled with blood. Other types of hemangiomas of the breast are often larger (>2 cm) and not closely associated with the lobular unit. In a few specimens, the possibility of angiosarcoma may be raised; however, in contrast to perilobular hemangioma, vessels composing angiosarcoma show a prominent dissecting growth pattern around breast parenchyma and in adipose tissue, and endothelial cells display nuclear atypia, multilayering and hyperchromasia (discussed later).

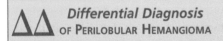

Differential Diagnosis
OF PERILOBULAR HEMANGIOMA

PASH

Other hemangiomas

Angiosarcoma

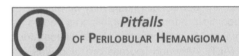

Pitfalls
OF PERILOBULAR HEMANGIOMA

! The lesion is unencapsulated and shows anastomosing small vessels.

! Vascular channels may show a dissecting growth pattern but it is limited.

PROGNOSIS

Perilobular hemangioma is a benign condition that requires no treatment.

HEMANGIOMA

OVERVIEW

Hemangiomas of the breast are a benign group of lesions with a broad morphologic spectrum and are potentially diagnostically challenging in small core biopsies. Overall, they affect patients in a wide age range and may arise within breast parenchyma or subcutaneous tissue of the breast. For the purpose of this article, only hemangiomas arising within the breast parenchyma are discussed.

Hemangioma is often palpable and/or detected by imaging studies. Rarely, this lesion may diffusely involve the breast and is descriptively referred to as *angiomatosis*.

GROSS FEATURES

Macroscopically, hemangioma is a lobulated, well-circumscribed lesion, albeit unencapsulated, located within the breast parenchyma and measuring up 5 cm.[7] The cut surface is soft, dark red, or brown and hemorrhagic.

MICROSCOPIC FEATURES

Histologically, hemangioma of the breast can often be subclassified into 3 main categories, namely, cavernous, capillary, or complex (or mixed). Cavernous hemangioma (**Fig. 3**A) is characterized by proliferation of large dilated vessels separated by fibrous septae. Occasionally, areas of thrombosis, infarction, and revascularization may be present. Within these areas, increased numbers of mitoses may be present as well as calcifications and micropapillary structures, consistent with recanalization. When thrombosis and recanalization are extensive, it is often difficult to appreciate the presence of a pre-existing hemangioma, and these lesions are often referred to as intravascular papillary endothelial hyperplasia or Masson tumor.[8]

Capillary hemangioma is composed of small vessels with muscular walls (see **Fig. 3**B). A larger feeding vessel is often identified at the periphery of the lesion. In complex hemangioma, there is a mixture of large, thin-walled, dilated vessels and small capillary-sized vessels.

 Differential Diagnosis OF HEMANGIOMA

Low-grade and intermediate-grade primary mammary angiosarcoma

Cytologically, the neoplastic cells lining hemangioma vessels are flat and show some degree of hyperchromasia; however, there is no appreciable nuclear atypia or multilayering (see **Fig. 3**C).

DIFFERENTIAL DIAGNOSIS

The differential diagnosis of hemangiomas is primary mammary angiosarcoma of low and intermediate histologic grade, particularly in small core biopsies. In contrast to hemangioma, angiosarcoma usually demonstrates a dissecting growth pattern as well as cytologic atypia. In small samples, however, it may be difficult to appreciate the edge of the neoplasm and excision of the lesion may be necessary for further evaluation of the lesion. In areas of Masson tumor, there may be increased cellularity and mitotic activity, similar to what is seen in intermediate-grade angiosarcoma; however, frank nuclear atypia is not present.

Although immunoperoxidase studies are not helpful in this differential, it has been suggested that Ki-67 index in these 2 lesions may be useful.[9] In one study, hemangiomas showed positivity for MIB-1 in 1.7% of neoplastic nuclei, whereas in angiosarcomas, 40.3% of the nuclei are positive.[9] The applicability of this stain in core biopsy specimens, however, remains to be validated.

PROGNOSIS

Hemangioma is a benign and marginal surgical excision is curative.

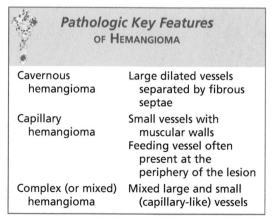 **Pathologic Key Features** OF HEMANGIOMA

Cavernous hemangioma	Large dilated vessels separated by fibrous septae
Capillary hemangioma	Small vessels with muscular walls. Feeding vessel often present at the periphery of the lesion
Complex (or mixed) hemangioma	Mixed large and small (capillary-like) vessels

 Pitfall OF HEMANGIOMA

! Areas of thrombosis and revascularization may contain increased mitotic activity and formation of intralesional papillary structures (Masson tumor).

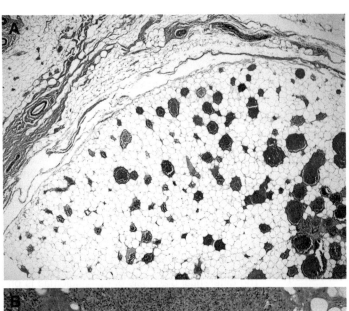

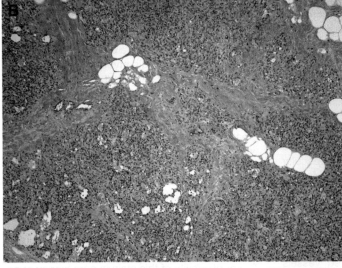

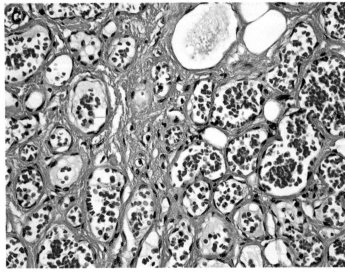

Fig. 3. (*A*) Hemangioma is well circumscribed and distinct from surrounding breast parenchyma. (*B*) Capillary hemangioma is characterized by a proliferation of small vessels. (*C*) Endothelial cells in hemangiomas are flat with hyperchromasia but no nuclear atypia or multilayering.

CUTANEOUS ATYPICAL VASCULAR LESIONS

OVERVIEW

Cutaneous atypical vascular lesions (AVLs) are radiation-associated lesions, first described by Fineberg and Rosen in 1994,[10] arising in patients after conservative treatment of breast carcinoma. Although it has been suggested that AVL is a precursor lesion for the development of angiosarcoma, the majority of AVLs show benign clinical behavior.[10–14] Patient median age at presentation is 55 to 59 years and lesions invariably develop in the field of radiation, typically 3 to 5 years after exposure.[10–14]

GROSS FEATURES

AVLs present clinically as small, erythematous, painless papules or nodules on the irradiated skin, almost always less than 1 cm in greatest dimension.

MICROSCOPIC FEATURES

Histologically, AVLs are characterized by a proliferation of thin-walled, dilated, anastomosing vascular channels. The lesion tends to be well circumscribed within the dermis and is often wedge-shaped (Fig. 4A). Extension into subcutaneous fat or breast parenchyma is not a feature of this lesion.

Cytologically, the vessels are lined by a single layer of hyperchromatic endothelial cells with or without hobnailing (see Fig. 4B). There is no nuclear pleomorphism or atypia and no endothelial multilayering. Focally, the formation of small papillary tufts of endothelial cells extending into the vessel lumen, however, may be seen.

Differential Diagnosis
OF CUTANEOUS ATYPICAL VASCULAR LESIONS

Cutaneous hemangioma

Low-grade radiation-associated cutaneous angiosarcoma

DIFFERENTIAL DIAGNOSIS

In the appropriate clinical context, the differential diagnosis for AVL is cutaneous hemangioma and radiation-associated low-grade cutaneous angiosarcoma. Cutaneous hemangioma is usually well circumscribed and shows no evidence of dissection of dermal collagen as well as absent nuclear atypia. In contrast to AVL, cutaneous angiosarcoma shows a less-circumscribed tumor area with infiltration into deep dermis and subcutaneous tissue and dissecting growth patterns. In addition, low-grade angiosarcoma is characterized by nuclear atypia, hyperchromasia, and multilayering. The distinction between these 2 entities is based on histologic finding; however, recently, molecular studies have shown that amplification of *MYC* and *FLT4* genes is present in radiation-associated angiosarcoma (RAS) and not seen in AVLs.[15]

PROGNOSIS

The clinical course of AVLs is benign in the majority of cases. Although AVLs may recur and patients may develop new lesions, progression to angiosarcoma is rare, occurring in less than 1% of reported cases.[4] Surgical excision is the main therapy; however, patients require long-term follow-up to monitor future recurrences.

Pathologic Key Features
CUTANEOUS ATYPICAL VASCULAR LESIONS

Wedge-shaped lesion limited to the dermis

Thin-walled anastomosing vessels

Hyperchromatic cells with or without hobnailing but no atypia

Small intraluminal papillary formations

Pitfalls
OF CUTANEOUS ATYPICAL VASCULAR LESIONS

! Extension of the lesion into subcutaneous tissue warrants the diagnosis of low-grade angiosarcoma.

! Although there seems to be minimal relationship between AVLs and angiosarcoma, close follow-up should be recommended.

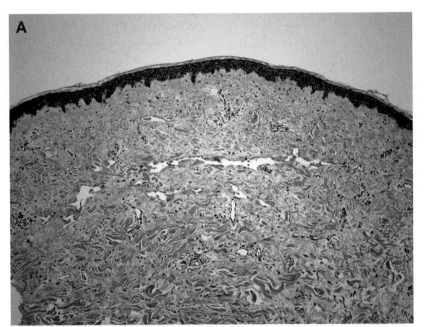

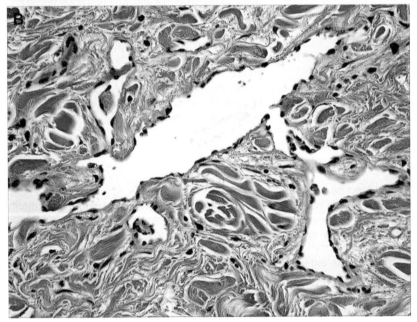

Fig. 4. (*A*) AVL is a wedge-shaped lesion limited to upper dermis in patients with prior exposure to radiation. (*B*) Lesional cells often show hyperchromasia and hobnailing, but there is no evidence of endothelial multilayering or pleomorphism.

RADIATION-ASSOCIATED CUTANEOUS ANGIOSARCOMA

OVERVIEW

Radiation-associated cutaneous angiosarcoma is a rare but well-established complication occurring in patients treated conservatively for breast carcinoma. The estimated incidence RAS is approximately 0.16%.[16] Patients are typically postmenopausal and are distinctly older than the population affected by primary mammary angiosarcoma (average age at diagnosis for RAS is 70 years).[16–19] The interval between exposure to radiation and the development of RAS is approximately 5 to 6 years.[16,18,20]

GROSS FEATURES

Grossly, RAS presents in previously irradiated skin and may have a varied appearance in regard to size and color. Usually angiosarcomas are larger than 1 cm and not uncommonly may present as large or multifocal lesions. Skin often shows a reddish discoloration or ecchymosis-like pattern.

MICROSCOPIC FEATURES

RAS is a mostly dermal-based lesion frequently showing involvement of underlying subcutaneous tissue and, less likely, underlying breast parenchyma. Similarly to soft tissue angiosarcomas, RAS can morphologically be classified into 3 histologic grades:

1. Grade I (low grade)
2. Grade II (intermediate grade)
3. Grade III (high grade)

Fig. 5. (*A*) RAS shows a prominent dissecting pattern within the dermis and subcutaneous tissue. Nuclear atypia is a common finding in RAS (*B*) as well as multi-layering of neoplastic cells (*C*).

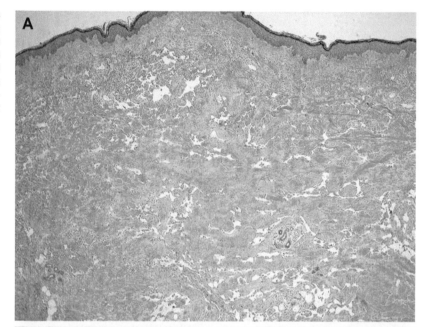

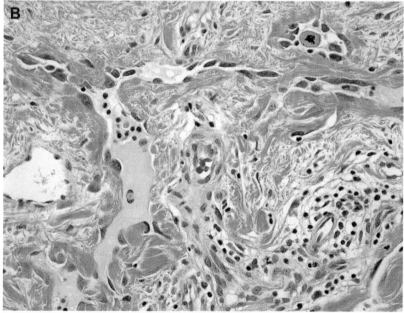

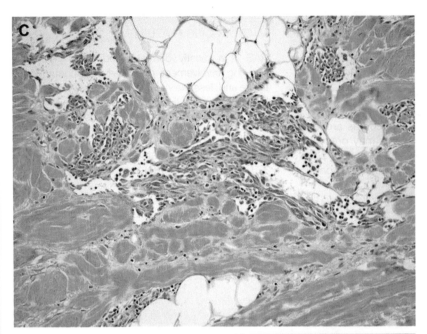

Fig. 5. (*D*) Epithelioid RAS shows a sheet-like growth pattern often overlapping histologically with carcinoma and malignant melanoma.

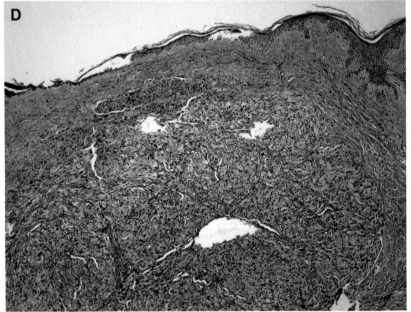

Pathologic Key Features	
OF RADIATION-ASSOCIATED CUTANEOUS ANGIOSARCOMA	
Low-grade RAS	Dermal-based lesion with frequent extension into subcutaneous tissue
	Thin-walled vessels with prominent dissecting growth pattern
	Prominent nuclear atypia and hyperchromasia
Intermediate-grade RAS	Increased cellularity with formation of papillae
High-grade RAS	Sheet-like growth of neoplastic cells
	Frequent necrosis and mitosis
Epithelioid RAS	Sheets of neoplastic cells with round nuclei, prominent nucleoli, and palely eosinophilic cytoplasm

Low-grade RAS is characterized by an ill circumscribed proliferation of thin-walled anastomosing vessels, showing a dissecting growth pattern (Fig. 5A). High-grade RAS shows a sheet-like proliferation of spindled tumor cells with little to no vasoformative areas. Occasionally, blood lakes lined by tumor cells may be noted. Mitoses and necrosis are often conspicuous in high-grade RAS. Intermediate-grade RAS demonstrates evidence of vascular differentiation, but it is more cellular than low-grade RAS and shows papillary proliferations into the lumen of vascular channels. Neoplastic cells in RAS are hyperchromatic with prominent nuclear atypia (see Fig. 5B, C). Finally, high-grade RAS may also show epithelioid morphology, with round nuclei, prominent nucleoli, and moderately abundant palely eosinophilic cytoplasm (see Fig. 5D).

Immunoperoxidase studies show a heterogenous pattern of staining of vascular markers (ie, CD31, CD34, and D2-40) in RAS. In a small subset of cases, in particular those showing epithelioid morphology, there may be expression of cytokeratins.

Overall, angiosarcomas are characterized molecularly by upregulation of vascular-specific receptor tyrosine kinases. Recently, it has been shown that RAS contains 8q24 gains due to amplification of MYC.[15]

DIFFERENTIAL DIAGNOSIS

The differential diagnosis of low-grade and intermediate-grade RAS includes cutaneous hemangioma and AVL, whereas high-grade and epithelioid RAS must be differentiated from poorly differentiated carcinoma and malignant melanoma. Cutaneous hemangioma is a superficial, well-circumscribed vascular proliferation lacking nuclear atypia or dissecting growth pattern. AVL, as described previously, is limited to the upper dermis. Although hyperchromasia may be present, there is no nuclear atypia or endothelial multilayering.

Poorly differentiated carcinoma and malignant melanoma show a solid growth pattern and may involve dermis and subcutaneous tissue of the breast, histologically resembling high-grade and

Differential Diagnosis
OF RADIATION-ASSOCIATED
CUTANEOUS ANGIOSARCOMA

Low-grade and intermediate-grade RAS	Cutaneous hemangioma AVLs
High-grade and epithelioid RAS	Poorly differentiated carcinoma Malignant melanoma

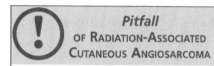

Pitfall
OF RADIATION-ASSOCIATED
CUTANEOUS ANGIOSARCOMA

! Expression of vascular markers by immunoperoxidase stains is variable in angiosarcoma and a comprehensive panel may be applied to these lesions, including CD31, CD34, D2-40, cytokeratins (AE1/AE3, Pan-K, CAM 5.2), S100, and other melanocytic markers.

epithelioid RAS. Poorly differentiated carcinoma of cutaneous origin as well as malignant melanoma may show evidence of an in situ or junctional component, aiding in the differential. Immunoperoxidase stains can be useful in the differential diagnosis. Although RAS is positive for vascular markers, poorly differentiated carcinoma is at least focally positive for cytokeratins, and melanoma is positive for S-100 protein and other melanocytic markers.

PROGNOSIS

The mainstay of treatment of RAS is surgical resection with wide margins. The utility of chemotherapy and radiation remains uncertain in this entity. RAS is a locally aggressive neoplasm regardless of tumor grade, with a tendency for local recurrence and, less often, distant metastasis. The rate of local recurrence is reportedly between 40% and 80%.[16–19] The median survival for patients with RAS is 33.5 to 37.4 months.[17,18]

PRIMARY ANGIOSARCOMA

OVERVIEW

Primary angiosarcoma of the breast accounts for less than 0.05% of all breast malignancies. In contrast to RAS, there is no prior history of exposure to radiation therapy in the majority of patients who develop primary angiosarcoma. In rare cases, however, there may be history of radiation exposure.[20] There is a wide age range, but generally, patients are approximately 10 years younger compared with those developing RAS.[20,21] Patients often present with a painless, palpable mass or breast fullness, with no cutaneous involvement. In rare cases, tumor is bilateral, synchronously or metachronously, raising the possibility of locoregional metastases.[20]

GROSS FEATURES

Grossly, primary angiosarcoma presents as an intramammary, red, hemorrhagic mass with fairly well defined borders. Focally, there might be extension into overlying skin.

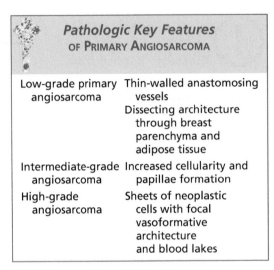

Pathologic Key Features
OF PRIMARY ANGIOSARCOMA

Low-grade primary angiosarcoma	Thin-walled anastomosing vessels Dissecting architecture through breast parenchyma and adipose tissue
Intermediate-grade angiosarcoma	Increased cellularity and papillae formation
High-grade angiosarcoma	Sheets of neoplastic cells with focal vasoformative architecture and blood lakes

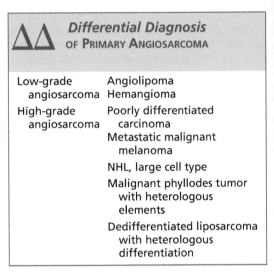

Differential Diagnosis
OF PRIMARY ANGIOSARCOMA

Low-grade angiosarcoma	Angiolipoma Hemangioma
High-grade angiosarcoma	Poorly differentiated carcinoma Metastatic malignant melanoma NHL, large cell type Malignant phyllodes tumor with heterologous elements Dedifferentiated liposarcoma with heterologous differentiation

MICROSCOPIC FEATURES

Similarly to RAS of the breast and soft tissue angiosarcoma, primary mammary angiosarcoma can be histologically graded as in 3 categories, namely, low, intermediate, or high.

Low-grade primary mammary angiosarcoma is characterized by a proliferation of thin-walled vascular channels with a prominent dissecting architecture throughout the breast parenchyma and adipose tissue (**Fig. 6**A). Focally, endothelial multilayering may be seen. Intermediate-grade angiosarcoma shows areas of increased cellularity and papillae formation of neoplastic cells (see **Fig. 6**). Frequent mitoses and focal necrosis may be present. High-grade angiosarcoma is characterized by the proliferation of neoplastic cells in solid sheets with focal formation of blood lakes (see **Fig. 6**). Additionally, angiosarcoma can demonstrate epithelioid morphology with tumor cells showing round nuclei and moderate amount of palely eosinophilic cytoplasm (see **Fig. 6**). Within a single tumor, there may be great variability in grading, with low-grade morphology often apparent at the periphery of the tumor mass.

DIFFERENTIAL DIAGNOSIS

The main differential diagnosis of low-grade mammary angiosarcoma is benign hemangioma and angiolipoma. In the latter 2 entities, there is no infiltration and dissection of surrounding breast parenchyma and adipose tissue. In addition, atypia is not seen in hemangioma and angiolipoma. In small biopsies, the distinction can be difficult and complete excision of the lesion may be recommended for definitive diagnosis.

High-grade and/or epithelioid angiosarcoma may overlap morphologically with poorly differentiated carcinoma, metastatic melanoma to the breast, and non-Hodgkin lymphoma (NHL), large cell type. In poorly differentiated carcinoma, neoplastic cells grow in sheet and there may be focal degenerating areas mimicking a vascular proliferation. Immunoperoxidase studies are of great utility for the differential. Poorly differentiated carcinoma is positive for at least one cytokeratin although negative for vascular markers. Metastatic malignant melanoma also shows sheets of neoplastic cells with round nuclei and prominent eosinophilic nucleoli. Vasoformative architecture is not a feature of melanoma. Immunostain for S-100 protein and other melanocytic markers may aid in the distinction. NHL, large cell type, is often a discohesive proliferation of large atypical cells lacking a vasoformative appearance. As part of the panel of stains, leukocyte common antigen as well as specific markers for T lymphocytes and B lymphocytes, such as CD20, BSAP, and CD3, among others, may be added for the diagnosis and subclassification of NHL.

Finally, rarely, angiosarcoma may also be present as part of other malignant mesenchymal neoplasm involving the breast, such as malignant phyllodes tumor or dedifferentiated liposarcoma with heterologous differentiation. The presence of leaflet-like architecture as well as the existence of other heterologous elements, such as chondrosarcomatous or osteosarcomatous components, is helpful in the diagnosis of phyllodes tumor. Dedifferentiated liposarcoma involving breast parenchyma is a rare phenomenon and may demonstrate the presence of heterologous elements. In addition to identifying a well-differentiated adipocytic component to the tumor, MDM2 and CDK4 may aid in the recognition of dedifferentiated liposarcoma; however, these markers may also be expressed in other neoplasms.[4] Appropriate sampling of the neoplasm is

Fig. 6. (*A*) Low-grade primary angiosarcoma of the breast is characterized by a florid dissecting architecture within mammary parenchyma. (*B*) Intermediate-grade angiosarcoma shows increased cellularity and formation of papillary structures within the lumen of the vascular channels.

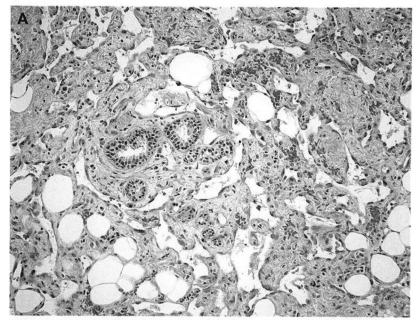

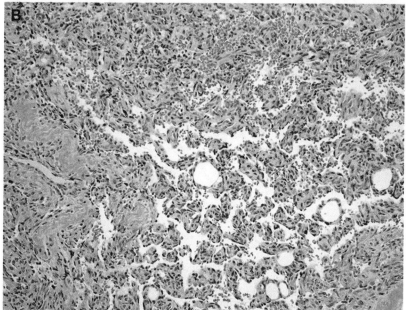

pivotal for the correct diagnosis of either phyllodes tumor or dedifferentiated liposarcoma.

PROGNOSIS

Surgery with wide uninvolved margins (ie, mastectomy) is the mainstay of treatment of primary mammary angiosarcoma. The prognosis is similar to angiosarcoma arising in other soft tissue sites, including RAS, and is independent

Pitfalls
OF PRIMARY ANGIOSARCOMA

! Primary angiosarcoma may rarely be associated with history of prior radiation exposure.

! Definitive diagnosis and histologic grading of angiosarcoma may require complete excision of the lesion.

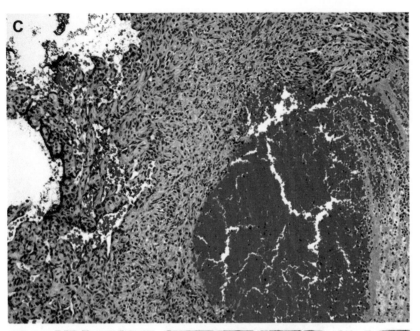

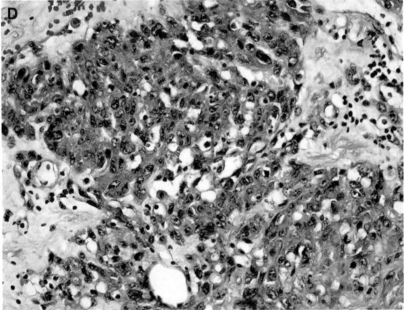

Fig. 6. (C) High-grade angiosarcoma typically demonstrates a solid growth pattern of spindled cells and occasional blood lakes can be present. (D) High-grade angiosarcoma often demonstrated a sheet like proliferation of neoplastic cells with epithelioid morphology.

of histologic tumor grade.[20,21] Approximately 25% of patients develop local recurrence and 60% have evidence of distance metastasis.[20] The most common sites for the development of metastatic disease are lung, liver, skin, and bones.[20]

REFERENCES

1. Kryvenko ON, Chitale DA, VanEgmond EM, et al. Angiolipoma of the female breast: clinicopathological correlation of 52 cases. Int J Surg Pathol 2011;18: 35–43.

2. Fletcher CD, Akerman M, Dal Cin P, et al. Correlation between clinicopathological features and karyotype in lipomatous tumors. A report of 178 cases from the Chromosomes and Morphology (CHAMP) Collaborative Study Group. Am J Pathol 1996;148:623–30.

3. Sciot R, Akerman M, Dal Cin P, et al. Cytogenetic analysis of subcutaneous angiolipoma: further evidence supporting its difference from ordinary pure lipomas: a report of the CHAMP Study Group. Am J Surg Pathol 1997;21:441–4.

4. Binh MB, Sastre-Garau X, Guillou L, et al. MDM2 and CDK4 immunostainings are useful adjuncts in diagnosing well-differentiated and dedifferentiated liposarcoma subtypes: a comparative analysis of 559 soft tissue neoplasms with genetic data. Am J Surg Pathol 2005;29:1340–7.

5. Rosen PP, Ridolfi RL. The perilobular hemangioma. A benign microscopic vascular lesion of the breast. Am J Clin Pathol 1977;68:21–3.

6. Lesueur GC, Brown RW, Bhathal PS. Incidence of perilobular hemangioma in the female breast. Arch Pathol Lab Med 1983;107:308–10.

7. Jozefczyk MA, Rosen PP. Vascular tumors of the breast. II. Perilobular hemangiomas and hemangiomas. Am J Surg Pathol 1985;9:491–503.

8. Branton PA, Lininger R, Tavassoli FA. Papillary endothelial hyperplasia of the breast: the great impostor for angiosarcoma. A clinicopathologic review of 17 cases. Int J Surg Pathol 2003;11:83–7.

9. Shin SJ, Lesser M, Rosen PP. Hemangiomas and angiosarcomas of the breast. Diagnostic utility of cell cycle markers with emphasis on Ki-67. Arch Pathol Lab Med 2007;131:538–44.

10. Fineberg S, Rosen PP. Cutaneous angiosarcoma and atypical vascular lesions of the skin and breast after radiation therapy for breast carcinoma. Am J Clin Pathol 1994;102:757–63.

11. Sener SF, Milos S, Feldman JL, et al. The spectrum of vascular lesions in the mammary skin, including angiosarcoma, after breast conservation treatment for breast cancer. J Am Coll Surg 2001;193:22–8.

12. Brenn T, Fletcher CD. Radiation-associated cutaneous atypical vascular lesions and angiosarcoma: clinicopathologic analysis of 42 cases. Am J Surg Pathol 2005;29:983–96.

13. Gengler C, Coindre JM, Leroux A, et al. Vascular proliferations of the skin after radiation therapy fro breast cancer: clinicopathologic analysis of a series in favor of a benign process: a study from the French Sarcoma Group. Cancer 2007;109:1584–98.

14. Patton KT, Deyrup AT, Weiss SW. Atypical vascular lesions after surgery and radiation of the breast: a clinicopathologic study of 32 cases analyzing histologic heterogeneity and association with angiosarcoma. Am J Surg Pathol 2008;32:943–50.

15. Guo T, Zhang L, Chang NE, et al. Consistent MYC and FLT4 gene amplification in radiation-induced angiosarcoma but not in other radiation-associated atypical vascular lesions. Genes Chromosomes Cancer 2011;50:25–33.

16. Strobbe LJ, Peterse HL, van Tinteren H, et al. Angiosarcoma of the breast after conservation therapy for invasive cancer, the incidence and outcome. An unforeseen sequela. Breast Cancer Res Treat 1998;47:101–9.

17. Billings SD, McKenney JK, Folpe AL, et al. Cutaneous angiosarcoma following breast-conserving surgery and radiation: an analysis of 27 cases. Am J Surg Pathol 2004;28:781–8.

18. Biswas T, Tang P, Muhs A, et al. Angiosarcoma of the breast: a rare clinicopathological entity. Am J Clin Oncol 2009;32:582–6.

19. Scow JS, Reynolds CA, Degnim AC, et al. Primary and secondary angiosarcoma of the breast: the Mayo Clinic experience. J Surg Oncol 2010;101:401–7.

20. Nascimento AF, Raut CP, Fletcher CD. Primary angiosarcoma of the breast: clinicopathologic analysis of 49 cases, suggesting that grade is not prognostic. Am J Clin Pathol 2008;32:1896–904.

21. Hodgson NC, Bowen-Wells C, Moffat F, et al. Angiosarcomas of the breast: a review of 70 cases. Am J Clin Oncol 2007;30:570–3.

COMBINED EPITHELIAL-MYOEPITHELIAL LESIONS OF THE BREAST

Rola H. Ali, MD, FRCPC[a],
Malcolm M. Hayes, MMed Path, FRCPath, FRCPC[a,b,*]

KEYWORDS

- Fibrocystic breast disease adenoma • Pleomorphic adenomyoepithelioma carcinoma
- Adenoid cystic spherulosis • Adenomyoepithelial adenosis

ABSTRACT

Epithelial-myoepithelial proliferations of the breast are a heterogeneous poorly defined group of lesions characterized morphologically by dual differentiation into ductal (luminal) and myoepithelial cells. They include neoplastic and non-neoplastic entities that have overlapping morphologic features that may give rise to diagnostic difficulty. Many of these entities are low grade or of uncertain malignant potential but the biology of some of these rare lesions remains to be elucidated. This article discusses the differential diagnosis of epithelial-myoepithelial lesions of the breast and highlights the morphologic features of some of these entities.

OVERVIEW

Epithelial-myoepithelial lesions of the breast (also known as adenomyoepithelial lesions of breast) comprise a heterogeneous group of entities, some of which are rare. Their clinical behavior shows a spectrum ranging from benign through borderline to malignant. Currently, no unifying classification system exists and precise definitions of some of the various nosologic entities are lacking. Problems with existing classifications include overlapping morphologic features between hyperplastic and neoplastic disorders, diverse morphology within each diagnostic category, description of the same entity under different names in the literature, and

poor clinical follow-up data available due to the rarity of many of these lesions. The current World Health Organization (WHO) classification of breast tumors lists most of these lesions as "epithelial-myoepithelial" lesions,[1] with myoepithelial carcinoma also included in the category of metaplastic carcinoma. This review discusses the differential diagnosis of epithelial-myoepithelial lesions of the breast (Box 1), excluding lesions composed exclusively of cells of myoepithelial lineage. Because even normal breast tissue is composed of both epithelial and myoepithelial cells, and so too are many of the common well-defined benign proliferative entities familiar to most pathologists (papilloma, fibrocystic changes, fibroadenoma, tubular adenoma [TA], and so forth), these processes are excluded from this review.

ADENOSIS AND ADENOMYOEPITHELIAL ADENOSIS

OVERVIEW

Adenosis of common, or usual, type is a localized exaggerated synchronous hyperplasia of both ductal luminal cells and myoepithelial cells out of step with the surrounding breast tissue. It affects a wide age range but is more common after the fourth decade. Adenosis of usual type is seen as an incidental finding in the context of fibrocystic changes, sclerosing adenosis, and adenosis nodules (ANs) and within papillomas and fibroadenomas.

The authors have nothing to disclose.
[a] Department of Pathology, University of British Columbia and Consultant Pathologist, BC Cancer Agency, 600 West 10th Avenue, Vancouver, BC V5Z 4E6, Canada
[b] Pathology and Laboratory Medicine, University of British Columbia, Vancouver, BC V6T 2B5, Canada
* Corresponding author. Department of Pathology, University of British Columbia and Consultant Pathologist, BC Cancer Agency, 600 West 10th Avenue, Vancouver, BC V5Z 4E6, Canada.
E-mail address: mhayes@bccancer.bc.ca

Surgical Pathology 5 (2012) 661–699
http://dx.doi.org/10.1016/j.path.2012.06.003
1875-9181/12/$ – see front matter © 2012 Elsevier Inc. All rights reserved.

GROSS FEATURES

No specific gross features have been described because AMEA is usually an incidental microscopic finding. Occasionally, it presents as a localized focus of thickening, a nodular or multinodular mass lesion. AMEA usually presents along with a gross nodule of AME but a single case of AMEA presented as an irregular spiculated mass on mammography.[7]

MICROSCOPIC FEATURES

Adenosis of usual type is encountered commonly in breasts containing fibrocystic changes and sclerosing adenosis and goes largely unnoticed in routine pathology. The morphology of usual-type adenosis is well known and is not discussed further. The distinct entity of AMEA is characterized by a proliferation of tubular glands along with myoepithelial hyperplasia sometimes forming multiple layers around the tubule (**Fig. 1**). A thick basal lamina is constantly present. The luminal epithelial cells may have apocrine features acquiring abundant eosinophilic granular cytoplasm often associated with apical cytoplasmic blebs.[4] The myoepithelial cells are often enlarged, have abundant clear cytoplasm, and encircle the crowded tubular acini. The high-power features closely resemble those of the well-differentiated epithelial-myoepithelial carcinoma of salivary gland or the tubular variant of AME of the breast. At low magnification, however, the lesion lacks the mass effect of AME. Nevertheless, some cases are associated with an adjacent AME, suggesting that AMEA is either a variant growth pattern of AME or a precursor lesion.

Immunohistochemical staining of AMEA highlights the dual epithelial and myoepithelial composition. The luminal ductal epithelial component stains for low molecular weight keratins, Cam

Thus, it presents clinically as mammographically detected calcifications, increased stromal density, or a mass detected on imaging studies or by palpation. The authors regard this usual type of adenosis as part of the spectrum of fibrocystic changes rather than as a specific entity. Other specific variants of adenosis are listed in **Box 1**. A full discussion of all of these variants is outside the scope of this review. This discussion focuses on a distinct rare subtype of adenosis, termed *AMEA*, that is reported to occur in association with AME,[2–6] but whether or not it is a hyperplastic or neoplastic disorder, a precursor lesion for AME, or a variant of tubular AME is unclear. Unfortunately, there is little attention paid to AMEA in the current WHO classification of breast tumors.[1]

Key Features
ADENOMYOEPITHELIAL ADENOSIS

- AMEA is an incidental microscopic finding usually occurring in association with AME.
- There is a prominent layer of myoepithelial cells with clear cytoplasm.
- Thick basement membranes are a key feature of AMEA.
- Apocrine differentiation of the luminal cells is typical.
- AMEA may be the precursor lesion of AME.

Fig. 1. AMEA (*A, B*). Tubular glands lined by luminal cells showing apocrine differentiation surrounded by a prominent layer of myoepithelial cells. Thick basement membranes encircle the tubules. ("A" *Courtesy of Professor Vincenzo Eusebi MD, University of Bologna.*)

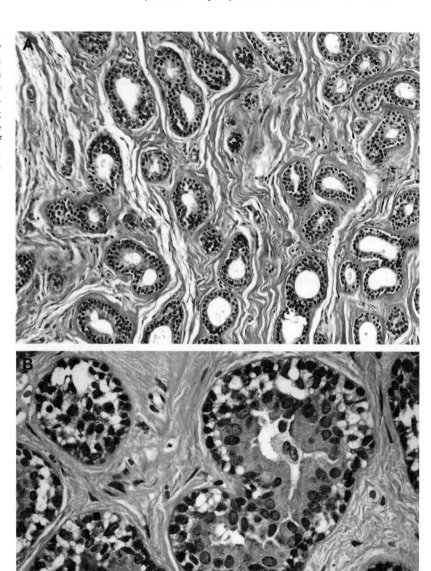

5.2, CK7, CK8/18, EMA, and GCDFP-15. The myoepithelial cells are positive for a variety of immunostains that include p63; CD10; myoid markers, such as smooth muscle actin, muscle specific actin, calponin, and smooth muscle heavy chain (SMHC) myosin; and high molecular weight keratins, CK5/6 and CK14. Immunostains for estrogen receptors (ER) and progesterone receptors (PR) are variably positive in a patchy pattern in usual-type adenosis but are negative in AMEA. AMEA adjacent to AME has been shown to have a high proliferative rate based on a high labeling index for proliferating cell nuclear antigen.[8]

DIAGNOSIS AND DIFFERENTIAL DIAGNOSIS

AMEA can be confused with other types of adenosis, in particular microglandular adenosis. Both have an infiltrative growth pattern and have thick basement membranes. Microglandular adenosis, however, shows small, more uniform glandular structures that lack a myoepithelial layer and lack apocrine differentiation. Tubular carcinoma, another mimic, also lacks myoepithelial cells. It features angulated glands with open lumina and apical snouts, lacks thick basement membranes, and is associated with a desmoplastic reaction. The tubular variant of AME (discussed later) is distinguished from AMEA by distortion of normal breast architecture with formation of a focal mass lesion surrounded by a pseudocapsule of compressed collagen.

PROGNOSIS

Because most cases of AMEA are incidental findings in biopsies performed for more significant lesions, the prognosis relates to that of the index lesion. AMEA may progress to AME.[5,8]

ADENOSIS NODULE

OVERVIEW

AN or tumor is one of the most commonly encountered lesions. Similar to other forms of adenosis, it is frequently seen as part of the spectrum of fibrocystic changes and sclerosing adenosis. It is a form of adenosis that gives rise to a distinct mass detected clinically by palpation or by imaging studies. It may be nonpalpable and associated with clustered calcifications[9] that are often interpreted as indeterminate calcifications on mammogram, so may be subjected to core biopsy. ANs typically arise in the third and fourth decades.[10]

GROSS FEATURES

ANs are usually multiple and[11] small and often are well circumscribed on imaging. Rarely, ANs are solitary. Most measure less than 1 cm in diameter. They may show cystic or granular areas grossly.

MICROSCOPIC FEATURES

On low power, ANs are characterized by a well-circumscribed nodular proliferation of small compressed glands surrounded by a fibrotic stroma. They may have irregular borders, however, with a pseudoinfiltrative pattern. They usually evolve in synchrony with hyperplasia of the adjacent breast parenchyma. Typically, the proliferating glands are small and compressed, although a mixture of other glandular patterns is not uncommon, including round glands with open lumina (tubular pattern), markedly distorted glands with spindle cell pattern, and a blunt duct adenosis-like pattern.[10] A myoepithelial cell layer is invariably present but is often flattened and inconspicuous on hematoxylin-eosin staining but is readily identified by immunohistochemical staining. Associated histologic features may include cysts, apocrine metaplasia, papillary hyperplasia, fibroelastosis, calcifications, and histiocytes.[10] When present, the apocrine metaplastic cells may be cytologically atypical and can contain mitoses giving rise to a worrisome picture (termed, *atypical apocrine adenosis*). Sometimes spindle cells are prominent in the stroma of AN and these cells can show myofibroblastic or smooth muscle differentiation.[12]

DIAGNOSIS AND DIFFERENTIAL DIAGNOSIS

AN may mimic AME; however, the latter is usually greater than 1 cm in size and has more numerous and larger myoepithelial cells (discussed later). TA can be difficult to distinguish from AN on a core biopsy, a distinction that may not be of value because both are benign lesions. In excision biopsies, TA is readily separated from AN because of its compressed pseudocapsule and uniform distribution of patent tubular glands arranged in a distinctly lobular architecture set in a loose stroma. AN, alternatively, has a multinodular patchy arrangement of compressed glands within a sclerotic stroma with distortion of the underlying lobular architecture. The compressed distorted glands, inconspicuous myoepithelial cells, and irregular borders of AN may also mimic invasive carcinoma, in particular invasive lobular carcinoma in core biopsies.

△△ *Differential Diagnosis*
ADENOSIS NODULE

- AME
- TA
- Invasive carcinoma (especially lobular type)

Immunostains may be necessary to highlight the myoepithelial cells in order to rule out malignancy.

PROGNOSIS

Adenosis nodule is benign, requiring simple excision only. In rare instances, low-grade adenosquamous carcinoma (LGAS), mucoepidermoid carcinoma, or metaplastic carcinomas of squamous or spindle cell type arise within ANs.

COLLAGENOUS SPHERULOSIS

OVERVIEW

CS, first described by Clement et al in 1987,[13] is a variant of intraductal hyperplasia associated with the production of nodular deposits of hyaline basement membrane material. Occasionally CS presents as a density or microcalcifications detected by mammography[14,15] but is usually discovered incidentally in excision specimens performed for other reasons.

GROSS FEATURES

CS is usually an incidental unifocal or multifocal microscopic finding[13] that is not evident grossly except in rare instances.[15–17]

MICROSCOPIC FEATURES

On low-power examination, there is usually a background of fibrocystic changes and many cases of CS are associated with a radial sclerosing lesion or sclerosing papilloma. The normal breast ductal and lobular architecture is maintained with no evidence of an infiltrative pattern. Medium-sized ducts, terminal ducts, and lobular units are distended by a proliferation of epithelial and myoepithelial cells arranged in a pseudocribriform pattern. The pseudospaces contain spherical masses of hyaline basement membrane material[18] that show a concentric lamination or a spider-like fibrillary appearance radiating from a central dense focus (Fig. 2).[13] Sometimes the collagen within the pseudospaces has a watery mucoid quality (the so-called mucinous variant of CS or mucinous spherulosis)[19] and may be almost

Key Features
COLLAGENOUS SPHERULOSIS

- Incidental microscopic finding or "innocent bystander" but may be present in breast containing malignancy
- Commonly associated with florid benign proliferative changes (eg, sclerosing adenosis and sclerosing papilloma/radial scar)
- Not evident grossly except in rare instances
- Has a characteristic cribriform pattern with myoepithelial cell–lined spaces containing basement membrane material
- Not precancerous

invisible on hematoxylin-eosin stains. On careful examination under high magnification, a basement membrane of variable thickness, sometimes partly retracted from the adjacent myoepithelial cells, is detected at the periphery of the pseudolumens. Rarely, CS-like areas are seen in association with atypical ductal hyperplasia, ductal carcinoma in situ (DCIS), and even ACC.[20,21] Colonization of CS by in situ lobular neoplasia is known to occur and can prove a diagnostic challenge because it closely simulates atypical ductal hyperplasia or cribriform DCIS (Fig. 3).

Immunostaining with p63, SMHC myosin, calponin, and other myoepithelial markers shows that the pseudospaces containing the hyaline globules are covered by myoepithelial cells.[22] In contrast, the true duct lumens are lined by ductal epithelial cells. This is confirmed by ultrastructural studies.[23] Stains for CK14 and CK5/6 highlight both the myoepithelial cells and many of the hyperplastic ductal cells.

DIAGNOSIS AND DIFFERENTIAL DIAGNOSIS

The key features of CS are small size, lack of an infiltrative growth pattern, lack of cytologic atypia in the epithelial component, presence of a thin collagenous cuticle lining the pseudolumina, and the fibrillary quality of some of the hyaline globules under high-power examination. In contrast to CS, cribriform DCIS shows true secondary lumen formation with ductal cells directly abutting and polarized around the lumen without interposed basement membrane or myoepithelial cells. Furthermore, cribriform DCIS exhibits uniformly intense positive staining for ER in contrast to the mottled staining pattern in CS, and shows negative immunostaining for myoepithelial markers in the intraductal proliferating cells with preservation

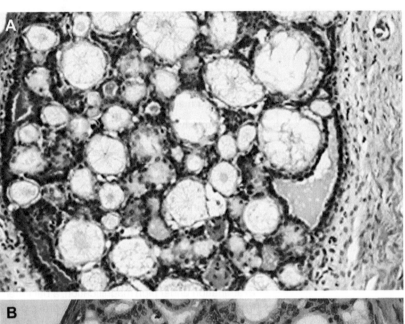

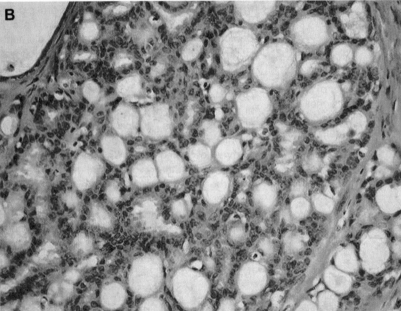

Fig. 2. CS. (*A*) Note the spider-like pattern of the collagen and the partly retracted basement membrane and (*B*) the separation of the myoepithelial cells by a thick basement membrane from the central mucinous component of the spherules.

of a myoepithelial layer at the periphery of the duct. CS can be secondarily over-run by lobular carcinoma in situ (LCIS), or lobular neoplasia, which also results in an impression of cribriform DCIS.[17,24] Attention to the discohesive property of the cells, the contents of lumens, positive myoepithelial markers around the pseudolumens, and lack of E-cadherin immunostaining of the epithelial component is a guide to the correct diagnosis of CS colonized by LCIS.

CS can also be confused with low-grade invasive cribriform carcinoma. The latter is frankly invasive, showing irregular infiltrating masses of cribriform epithelium with infiltrative margins and a desmoplastic stromal reaction. Lack of immunostaining for myoepithelial cell markers both within the cribriform masses and at the periphery of the cell groups is key in making the diagnosis of carcinoma. Cribriform carcinoma may also show a minor component of invasive tubular carcinoma. Similar to cribriform DCIS, invasive cribriform carcinoma is strongly and diffusely ER positive.

Distinction of CS from ACC is more problematic (**Fig. 4**). Both lesions have a cribriform pattern with

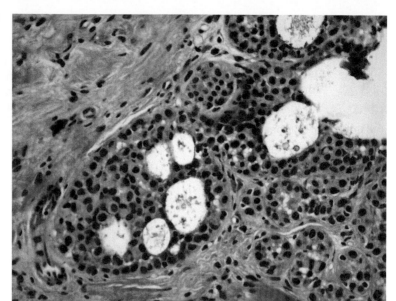

Fig. 3. LCIS (LIN2) involving the mucinous variant of CS.

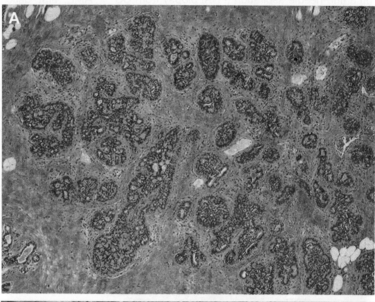

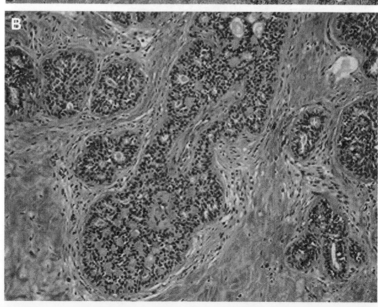

Fig. 4. CS (*A, B*) with a growth pattern simulating ACC.

2 types of lumina, namely lumina lined by epithelial cells producing epithelial mucins and pseudolumina lined by cells with myoepithelial differentiation and producing basement membrane material.[18,22] In particular, the identification of hyaline globules on a fine-needle aspiration (FNA) biopsy from CS can lead to an erroneous diagnosis of ACC (**Fig. 5**).[25–30] In contrast to CS, ACC usually presents as a palpable mass. Unlike CS, which grows within pre-existing ducts, ACC exhibits stromal invasion.[31] Finally, the myoepithelial component predominates in the cribriform variant of ACC whereas the ductal cell component predominates in CS. Although both lesions contain myoepithelial cells, a recent study has reported calponin and SMHC myosin to be expressed only in CS, whereas CD117 marked the ductular epithelium in ACC but not in CS.[32] In the authors' experience, however, calponin and SMHC myosin are not infrequently positive in ACC and CD117 may be weakly positive in CS. On FNA, the cell groups of CS are more cohesive than those of ACC, the dual cell type is more evident, and the collagenous spherules are smaller and more irregular in outline than those of ACC.

PROGNOSIS

CS is a benign incidental finding. Although CS-like areas can rarely be seen adjacent to malignancy,[20,21] it is not considered precancerous.

ADENOMYOEPITHELIOMA

OVERVIEW

AME, first described by Hamperl in 1970,[33] is a biphasic neoplasm composed of ductal and myoepithelial cells that is identical to epithelial-myoepithelial carcinoma of the salivary gland and lacks the features of other specific diagnostic categories of related neoplasms.[34,35] AME is most common after the fifth decade but is seen occasionally in younger women.[36,37] The commonest presentation is a mass lesion detected either clinically or on imaging.[38–40] Occasionally AME arises within a fibroadenoma or phyllodes tumor[41] AME is rarely seen in men.[42] Although the relationship between AME and ductal adenoma is controversial,[43–48] many authorities currently regard these lesions as synonymous.

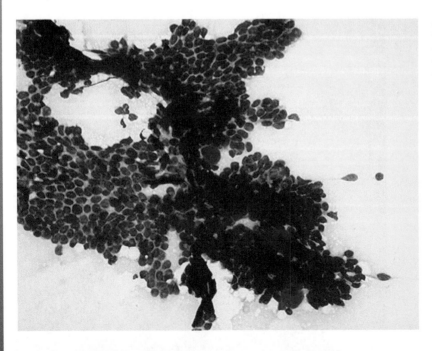

Fig. 5. CS. The presence of hyaline globules on a FNA biopsy from CS can lead to an erroneous diagnosis of ACC.

GROSS FEATURES

AME usually presents as a solitary circumscribed multilobated nodule exceeding 1 cm in size. It occasionally shows a cystic component or may be predominantly cystic.[49–51]

MICROSCOPIC FEATURES

On low-power examination, most AMEs are expansile multilobulated masses lacking a capsule but separated sharply from the normal surrounding breast tissue.[6,37,52] Microscopic satellite nodules may occur at the periphery of the main mass. Central sclerosis of the tumor is common. Classical AME has a uniform admixture of small ducts and surrounding conspicuous myoepithelial cells, often with clear cytoplasm, identical to epithelial-myoepithelial carcinoma of salivary gland. Based on architecture and growth pattern, AME can be lobulated, papillary, tubular, or intraductal or show mixed patterns (Fig. 6). Cytologically, the myoepithelial cells are polygonal or spindle in shape and frequently have abundant clear cytoplasm (Fig. 7A, B).[53] They can also have abundant eosinophilic cytoplasm imparting a myoid

Fig. 6. AME. (*A*) Multilobulated and (*B*) papillary patterns of AME.

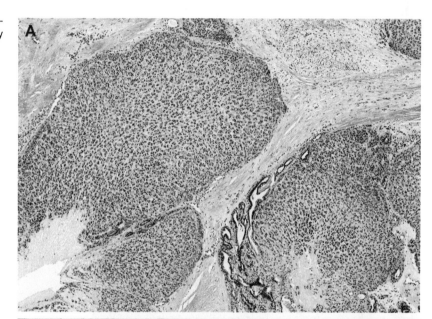

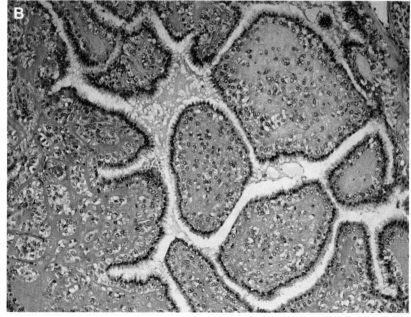

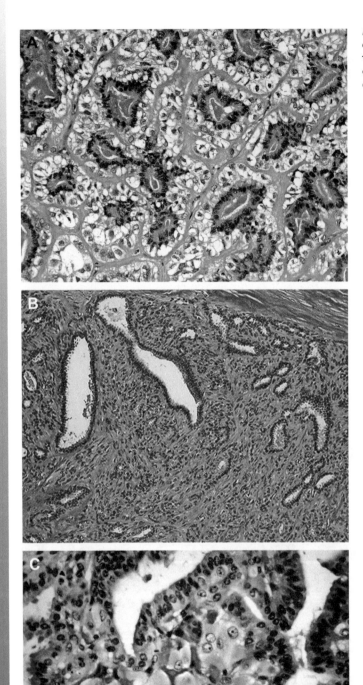

Fig. 7. AME. (*A*) Myoepithelial cells with clear cytoplasm surrounding ductal structures. (*B*) Spindle-shaped myoepithelial cells. (*C*) Myoid-looking myoepithelial cells.

appearance simulating a leiomyoma (see **Fig. 7C**) or can have a plasmacytoid appearance with eccentric nuclei and glassy cytoplasm resembling the hyaline cells seen in PA of salivary gland. The myoepithelial cells in AME are usually more numerous and larger than those seen in normal breast lobules, ANs, or simple papillomas, and they can overgrow the ductal elements. Mitoses are identified in both the ductal and myoepithelial cells of AME. Dense sclerotic collagenous matrix material is common.[54] The matrix may also be myxoid or chondroid reminiscent of that seen in PA (**Fig. 8**).

The lobulated variant of AME is composed of nests of clear cells or eosinophilic myoepithelial cells surrounding compressed epithelial-lined spaces. The tubular pattern of AME has well-formed, rounded, epithelial-lined tubular structures surrounded by prominent myoepithelial cells. The spindle cell variant shows a predominance of spindle-shaped myoepithelial cells with few epithelial-lined lumens.[55] The nuclei may be arranged in palisades simulating a schwannoma. Other features that may be encountered in an AME include a papillary component,[53] apocrine metaplasia of the luminal cells,[53] squamous metaplasia,[56] focal sebaceous differentiation (**Fig. 9**),[53,56] and rarely CS.[57,58] AME is sometimes associated with AMEA, which is believed the precursor lesion (discussed previously).[7,8]

Immunohistochemical staining of AME highlights its dual epithelial and myoepithelial composition.[59,60] A variety of immunostains can be used to highlight the myoepithelial cells (**Fig. 10**)

Key Features
ADENOMYOEPITHELIOMA

- Seen in postmenopausal women; rare before fifth decade
- Solitary circumscribed nodule >1 cm
- Architectural patterns: lobulated, tubular, papillary, intraductal, mixed
- Myoepithelial cytologic patterns: polygonal, spindled, clear cell, myoid, hyaline cell
- IHC: demonstrates dual population of epithelial and myoepithelial cells
- Biomarkers: ER negative to weak; Her2/neu negative
- Slow growing, recurs locally but low metastatic potential
- Potential for malignant progression

although the pattern of staining varies from case to case and in different areas within the same tumor. These include p63 (nuclear stain); the myoid markers, smooth muscle actin, muscle-specific actin, calponin, and SMHC myosin (cytoplasmic)[61–63]; and high molecular weight keratins, CK5/6 and CK14 (cytoplasmic). Other myoepithelial markers are S-100 protein, GFAP, CD10, CD109, maspin,[64] caveolin 1, p75, and 14-3-3 σ.[65] The spindle cell variant of AME is typically

Fig. 8. AME with chondroid matrix resembling PA.

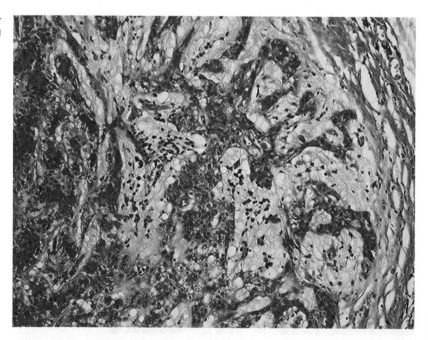

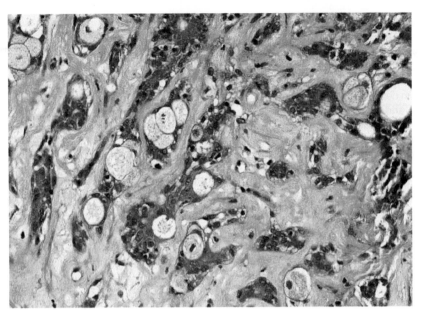

Fig. 9. AME with sebaceous metaplasia.

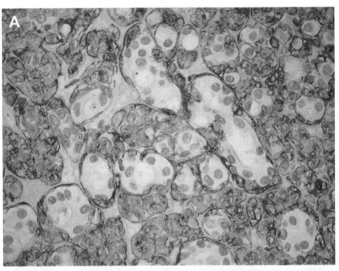

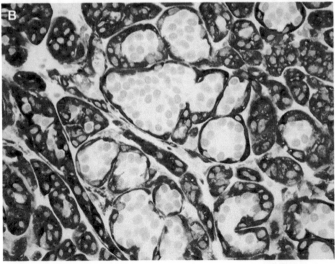

Fig. 10. Myoepithelial markers in AME. Immunostaining for CK5/6 (*A*), CK14 (*B*), p63 (*C*), and SMHC myosin (*D*) highlights the numerous myoepithelial cells.

Fig. 10. (continued)

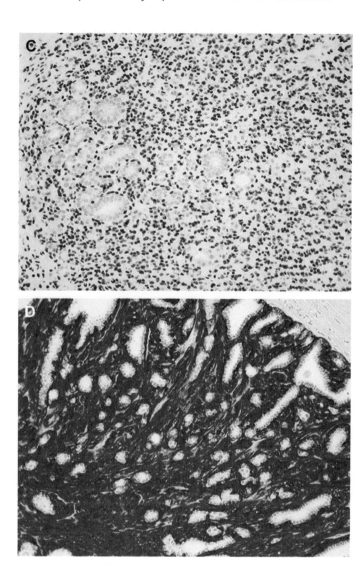

strongly positive for S-100 protein. The luminal epithelial cells stain for low molecular weight keratins Cam 5.2, CK7, and CK8/18 as well as EMA. Often, the luminal cells also stain weakly for high molecular weight keratins in contrast to the more intense staining of the myoepithelial component, and in addition, foci of squamous metaplasia also stain intensely with high molecular weight keratins and p63. Thus, the immunophenotypic distinction between ductal and myoepithelial cells in AME is often much more subtle than in normal breast tissue. The Ki-67 proliferative index may be higher in the myoepithelial cells than in the ductal cells.[61] AMEs are usually negative or weakly positive for ER and PR. Her2/neu is negative for amplification and overexpression.

DIAGNOSIS AND DIFFERENTIAL DIAGNOSIS

Several benign conditions can mimic AME, including ANs, simple papillomas, TA, ductal adenoma, and PA. Usually, the myoepithelial cells in AME are more numerous and larger than those seen in these mimics. ANs are usually smaller than 1 cm, arise in the third to fourth decades, are usually multiple, and evolve in synchrony with the hyperplasia of the adjacent breast. They usually exhibit compressed or distorted glands at least focally with an attenuated or inconspicuous myoepithelial layer. Their distinction from AME, however, may be impossible in core biopsy samples. Similarly, TA can be difficult to distinguish from AME on a core biopsy. The former is

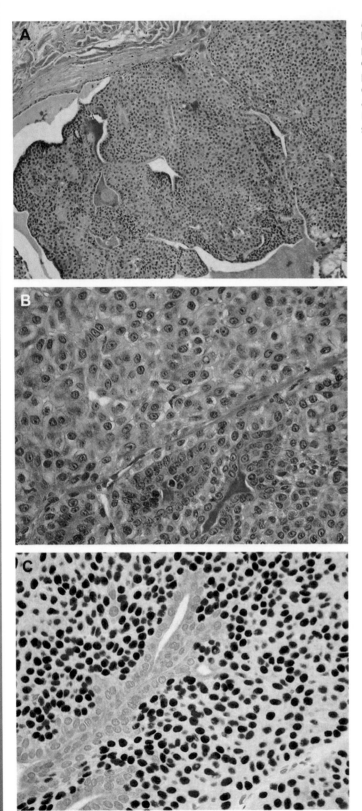

Fig. 11. Clear cell hidradenoma of the breast. The lesion at low power is partly cystic and has a focal papillary configuration (*A*). It is composed predominantly of polygonal squamoid cells with focal ductal differentiation, a picture reminiscent of AME (*B*). p63 Immunostaining is positive in the squamoid cells (*C*).

composed of closely packed glands arranged in a regular lobular architecture that is lacking in AME. TA has a much less prominent myoepithelial layer than AME. When a papillary architecture predominates in an AME, it may be difficult to separate from intraductal papilloma with myoepithelial hyperplasia (myoepitheliosis).[53] If the myoepithelial cell hyperplasia is florid, however, exceeding one layer in thickness, and involves the lesion diffusely rather than focally, the lesion is better regarded as an AME. Ductal adenoma, regarded as a variant of AME by many pathologists, is characterized by the presence of a capsule containing elastic fibers derived from the underlying duct wall and lacks the multilobated architecture of AME.[43,44] PA of the breast can also show overlapping features with AME, especially when the latter contains chondromyxoid matrix. Although PA is characterized by a more prominent chondromyxoid matrix and often bone, the dividing line between these lesions is somewhat arbitrary. Rosen[66] considers AME, PA, and ductal adenoma variants of intraductal papilloma. Fibroadenomas or phyllodes tumors can have AME-like areas but features diagnostic of fibroadenoma or phyllodes always predominate. Myoepithelioma of the breast shares the same myoepithelial morphologic spectrum seen in AME but is a monophasic lesion lacking the ductal component. Rarely, the cutaneous adnexal neoplasm clear cell hidradenoma occurs in the breast[67–69] and can be confused with AME. Typically, hidradenoma occurs in the superficial subcutaneous tissue of the breast but is

occasionally located deeper in the breast parenchyma. Like the cutaneous counterpart, clear cell hidradenoma of breast is a well-circumscribed solid/cystic lesion, with a partly papillary configuration (Fig. 11A). It is composed predominantly of uniform polygonal squamoid cells with clear or eosinophilic cytoplasm and distinct cell borders and lacking cytologic atypia (see Fig. 11B). Focal eccrine ductal differentiation is seen. An eosinophilic collagenous matrix identical to that of AME is commonly seen. The squamoid component is diffusely positive for p63, CK5/6, and CK14 but the foci of ductal differentiation are negative (see Fig. 11C). Thus, the immunophenotype partly overlaps with that of AME, but smooth muscle actin, SMHC myosin, and calponin are negative in hidradenoma.[69] Hidradenoma of the breast shows at (11;19) translocation that has not been demonstrated in AME.[70]

AME can also be confused with some malignant breast tumors. AME, with its bilayered tubular structures composed of ductal and myoepithelial cells, may resemble ACC of the breast (Fig. 12), but the latter neoplasm has infiltrative borders and a characteristic cribriform architecture with hyaline spherules in most cases. Furthermore, the myoepithelial cells of ACC are smaller, more hyperchromatic, and basaloid-looking with much less cytoplasm than those of AME. AME can also be mistaken for other carcinomas, especially on a core biopsy, such as LGAS, low-grade invasive ductal carcinoma not otherwise specified (NOS) (Fig. 13), or glycogen-rich clear cell carcinoma (GRC). The

Fig. 12. AME with foci resembling ACC. The rest of the tumor (not shown) is typical for AME.

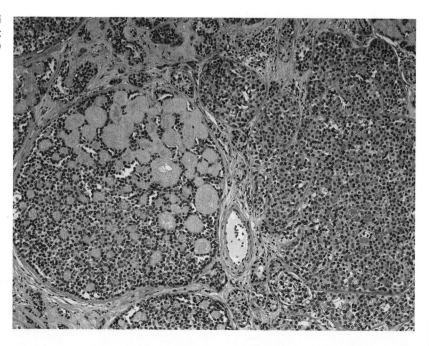

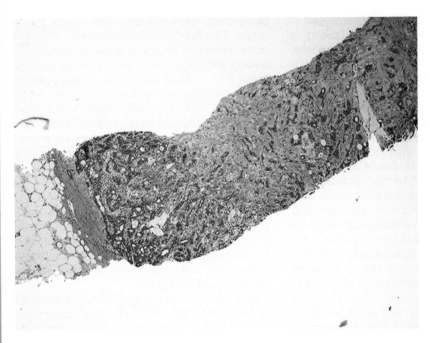

Fig. 13. AME misdiagnosed as invasive carcinoma on core biopsy. Note the circumscribed border of the lesion.

GRC enters the differential diagnosis when the clear-type myoepithelial cells predominate in an AME. Carcinomas, however, show obvious stromal infiltration and abundant desmoplastic stroma and, apart from LGAS, lack a myoepithelial component. Weak ER staining is a helpful clue that is in favor of AME because most low-grade invasive ductal carcinomas are strongly positive for ER. Myoepithelial markers should be negative in conventional carcinoma NOS and clear cell carcinoma, but p63 and CK5/6 are expected to be expressed in the squamous component of LGAS carcinoma, and calponin and SMHC myosin mark the myoepithelial cells present at the periphery of the infiltrating tubules and nests of this neoplasm.

PROGNOSIS

AMEs are usually slow growing neoplasms with a low metastatic potential. Despite the bland histologic features, however, local recurrence can occur. Therefore, complete excision is recommended.[6] Local recurrence is probably related to the multinodular growth and intraductal extension of the lesion, which can form satellite nodules away from the main tumor mass. Metastasis of histologically benign AME is rare[71,72] but the metastatic potential increases significantly with malignant progression (discussed later).

ADENOMYOEPITHELIOMA WITH MALIGNANT PROGRESSION

OVERVIEW

Malignant AMEs usually arise from a pre-existing benign AME although some arise de novo in the absence of a precursor low-grade lesion. Malignant AME typically presents as a long-standing breast mass followed by a phase of rapid growth.

△△ **Differential Diagnosis**
ADENOMYOEPITHELIOMA

- AN and sclerosing adenosis with myoid differentiation
- Papilloma with myoepithelial hyperplasia (myoepitheliosis)
- TA
- Ductal adenoma
- PA
- Fibroadenoma or phyllodes tumor with AME-like areas
- Myoepithelioma
- Clear cell hidradenoma of breast
- ACC
- LGAS
- Invasive ductal carcinoma NOS or clear cell type

GROSS FEATURES

These tumors are often large. They are usually deceptively well circumscribed but are infiltrative on microscopic examination. Cystic degeneration and necrosis may be seen.

MICROSCOPIC FEATURES

The tumor has 2 components: a benign/low-grade AME component and a malignant component. The latter often shows an infiltrative growth pattern, marked cytologic atypia, and a high mitotic rate and may be associated with necrosis. The malignant component can show ductal differentiation, myoepithelial differentiation, or both,[5,73–77] and the histologic grade of this malignant component can range from low grade to high grade.[37,78] The ductal component can give rise to a large spectrum of carcinomas, including conventional invasive ductal carcinoma NOS (**Fig. 14**), undifferentiated carcinoma,[79,80] and metaplastic carcinoma. The myoepithelial component can give rise to malignant myoepithelioma that may be of spindle, epithelioid, or clear cell morphology[77,81,82] or a mixture of these patterns (**Fig. 15A**). When the malignant transformation differentiates along both epithelial and myoepithelial cell lineages, the tumor has a biphasic composition, with both elements having a malignant appearance, resembling poorly differentiated epithelial-myoepithelial carcinoma of salivary gland (see **Fig. 15B, C**).[5,59] This can occur de novo or as the result of malignant progression of a benign AME. Biphasic epithelial and myoepithelial malignant

transformation can also occur in the form of low-grade ACC.[83] A variety of metaplastic carcinomas can develop within AME. These include the spindle cell variant of squamous carcinoma, acantholytic variant of squamous carcinoma, LGAS,[84–86] mucoepidermoid carcinoma, and metaplastic carcinoma with heterologous chondrosarcomatous and osteosarcomatous differentiation.[87–89]

DIAGNOSIS AND DIFFERENTIAL DIAGNOSIS

The differential diagnosis depends on the differentiation lineage of the malignant components. When the malignant component differentiates along an

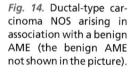

Fig. 14. Ductal-type carcinoma NOS arising in association with a benign AME (the benign AME not shown in the picture).

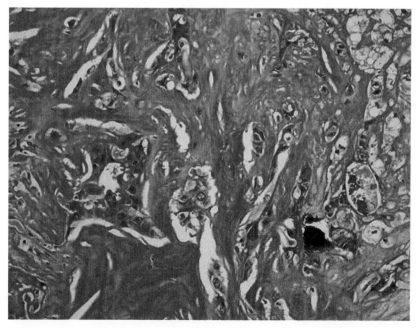

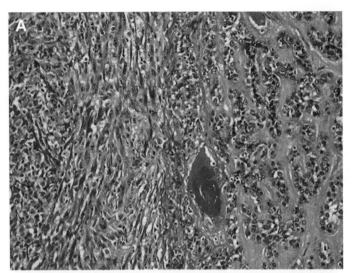

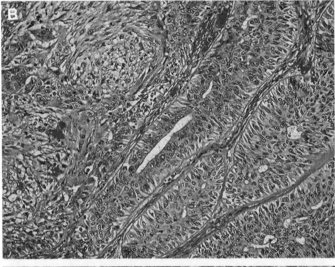

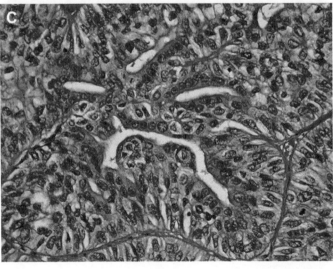

Fig. 15. Malignant AME. (*A*) Malignant myoepithelial component showing a mixture of epithelioid (*right*) and spindle cell sarcomatoid morphology (*left*) imparting a biphasic appearance. (*B*) Malignant AME (*right*) showing bilayered tubules of epithelial and myoepithelial cells, with a sarcomatoid component to the left. (*C*) On higher power, the bilayered tubules are better appreciated resembling epithelial-myoepithelial carcinoma of salivary gland. (*Courtesy of* Malcolm M Hayes. Adenomyoepithelioma of the breast: a review stressing its propensity for malignant transformation. J Clin Pathol 2011;64:477–84; with permission.)

Fig. 16. AME with sarcomatoid malignant progression. (*A*) Typical benign AME (*left*) adjacent to a sarcomatoid spindle cell area (*right*). The sarcomatoid area is positive for SMHC myosin immunostain (*B*) but negative for wide spectrum keratin (*C*) This immunophenotype favors myoepithelial sarcoma (arising from AME) over spindle cell metaplastic carcinoma.

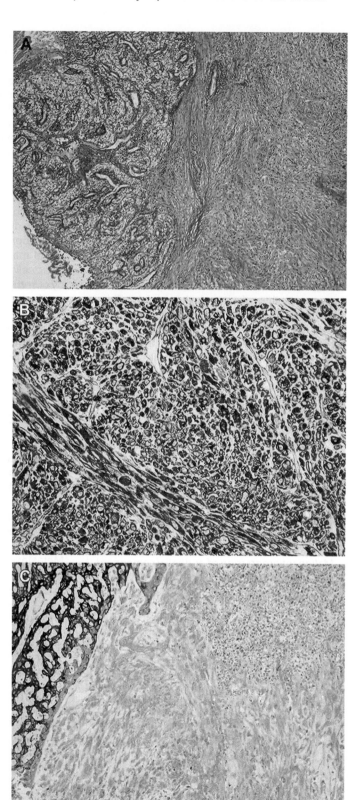

epithelial lineage, the tumor can resemble invasive ductal carcinoma NOS. The transformed component can outgrow the myoepithelial component. In such cases, the identification of residual benign or low-grade AME within or adjacent to the tumor is the clue to the correct diagnosis.

When the malignant component differentiates along a myoepithelial lineage with a spindle cell sarcomatoid morphology, the tumor becomes difficult to separate from metaplastic spindle cell (sarcomatoid) carcinoma. These two tumors probably overlap but positive immunostaining for the myoepithelial markers, calponin and SMHC myosin, and absence of low molecular weight keratin immunostaining in the spindle cell component favor malignant AME over spindle cell carcinoma (Fig. 16). Again, identification of a low-grade component of AME is required in order to separate these lesions with certainty. This is particularly so for spindle cell squamous carcinoma, which shows immunohistochemical features of myoepithelial differentiation in more than a third of cases.[90] Malignant phyllodes tumor with stromal overgrowth can resemble malignant AME, but this usually shows a nodular fibroepithelial component reminiscent of fibroadenoma and/or a leaf-like growth pattern at least focally. Spindle cell sarcoma, especially leiomyosarcoma, is another differential diagnosis, but primary spindle cell sarcomas of the breast are so rare that metaplastic carcinoma, malignant AME, and malignant phyllodes tumor should always be excluded before rendering this diagnosis. Besides, leiomyosarcoma should be diffusely positive for the smooth muscle markers, desmin and h-caldesmon, in addition to calponin and SMHC myosin and negative for high molecular weight keratins.

When the myoepithelial cells show a clear cell morphology[82] the differential diagnosis includes other clear cell tumors, such as GRC and lipid-rich carcinoma of the breast. GRC has abundant clear cytoplasm that is periodic acid-schiff (PAS)-positive diastase labile. Most GRCs have a luminal immunophenotype and are negative for myoepithelial markers. Lipid-rich carcinomas also show clear cells, but these contain lipid demonstrated by oil red O or Sudan black methods and are negative for mucin and myoepithelial markers.

AME transformed to matrix-producing carcinoma can mimic metaplastic carcinoma with matrix production. The presence of an identifiable benign or low-grade component of AME is required for the correct diagnosis.[87] Finally, in situ carcinoma is usually absent in malignant AME.

PROGNOSIS

Malignant AME has a greater potential to recur locally and to metastasize than benign AME. The metastatic potential is probably related to the grade of the malignant component with metastases typically occur in patients who have high-grade malignant transformation of AME. Most metastases involve the lungs[91,92] but can also involve the liver,[93] bone, brain, and other sites. Metastasis to lymph nodes is unusual and, therefore, axillary lymph node dissection is not indicated unless there is clinically detected lymphadenopathy.[53] The role of radiotherapy and chemotherapy is unknown.

PLEOMORPHIC ADENOMA (MIXED TUMOR OF THE BREAST)

OVERVIEW

PA is a neoplasm of ductal and myoepithelial cells associated with chondromyxoid matrix material identical to PA of salivary gland.[94] It is commonly located in the central subareolar zone related to a major duct and may be regarded as a variant of intraductal papilloma.[66] The majority of patients are postmenopausal. Occasionally, it occurs in men.[95] PA presents as a mass, often containing calcifications, that can simulate carcinoma on clinical examination and imaging studies.[96,97] Some

△△ **Differential Diagnosis**
ADENOMYOEPITHELIOMA WITH MALIGNANT PROGRESSION

Malignant progression of epithelial component
- Invasive ductal carcinoma, NOS

Malignant progression of myoepithelial component
- Metaplastic carcinoma with or without matrix production
- Malignant phyllodes tumor with stromal overgrowth
- Spindle cell sarcomas—leiomyosarcoma, fibrosarcoma
- Glycogen-rich carcinoma
- Lipid-rich carcinoma

Malignant progression of both epithelial and myoepithelial components
- Metaplastic carcinoma of carcinosarcoma type
- ACC

investigators question the existence of PA as a distinct entity and regard it as a variant of intraductal papilloma.[98,99]

GROSS FEATURES

PA can occur as a single or multifocal lesion.[100] It is usually a well-circumscribed lobulated rubbery mass.

MICROSCOPIC APPEARANCE

PA of the breast resembles that of salivary gland.[34,100-104] It is a circumscribed encapsulated tumor composed of epithelial and myoepithelial elements forming benign ductal structures, acini, trabeculae, and islands, associated with an abundant hyalinized collagenous matrix showing chondromyxoid change (Fig. 17). The myoepithelial cells usually merge with or melt into the surrounding chondromyxoid elements. The myoepithelial cells can show a range of appearances, including clear cell, spindle cell, plasmacytoid, and myoid. They are arranged singly, or in cords, sheets, or nests. Radially dispersed crystals may be seen surrounded by myoepithelial cells.[100] Mature hyaline-type cartilage with or without enchondral ossification to form lamellar bone may be seen (Fig. 18). Squamous and sebaceous metaplasia may also occur. The cytologic features are identical to those of the salivary gland counterpart,[105,106] but, especially in core biopsies, may be misinterpreted because carcinoma particularly of mucinous or metaplastic types.[101,107,108]

Key Features
PLEOMORPHIC ADENOMA

- Subareolar in location

- Solitary, rarely multifocal

- Microscopic features: epithelial and myoepithelial elements surrounded by chondromyxoid matrix

- IHC: highlights dual population of epithelial and myoepithelial cells

- Biomarkers: ER negative or weak; Her2/neu negative

- Benign but may recur locally if incompletely excised

- Rarely shows malignant progression

Immunohistochemical and ultrastructural studies confirm the dual epithelial-myoepithelial phenotype (Fig. 19).[104,109] Typically, ER stains are negative or weak but rare cases show more impressive ER staining.[110]

DIAGNOSIS AND DIFFERENTIAL DIAGNOSIS

Metaplastic breast carcinoma with chondroid matrix is the most important differential diagnosis that should be considered. Unlike PA, metaplastic carcinoma shows overt invasion with foci of

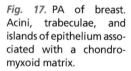

Fig. 17. PA of breast. Acini, trabeculae, and islands of epithelium associated with a chondromyxoid matrix.

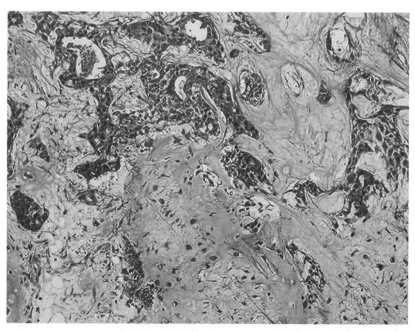

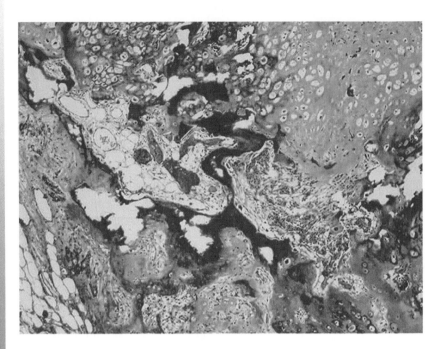

Fig. 18. PA of breast with hyaline cartilage undergoing enchondral ossification to form lamellar bone.

conventional poorly differentiated ductal carcinoma, lacks the dual composition of epithelial and myoepithelial cells, and shows overtly malignant cytologic features. In contrast to PA, an associated component of in situ carcinoma is often present. Mucinous carcinoma is another mimic of PA because it is cytologically bland and contains abundant myxoid matrix[102] but, unlike PA, mucinous carcinoma lacks a myoepithelial cell component. When stained with alcian blue, the staining of the mucin is not obliterated by pretreatment with hyaluronidase (ie, mucinous carcinoma has epithelial-type mucin rather than hyaluronic acid). In contrast to PA, mucinous carcinoma is strongly positive for ER. Malignant phyllodes tumor may contain foci of heterologous cartilaginous differentiation

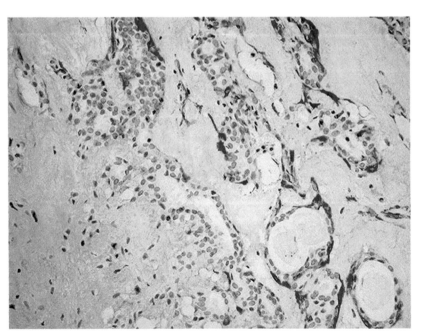

Fig. 19. PA of breast. Immunostain for smooth muscle actin demonstrates a periductal myoepithelial cell layer.

Differential Diagnosis
PLEOMORPHIC ADENOMA

- Metaplastic carcinoma with matrix production
- Mucinous carcinoma
- Phyllodes tumor with heterologous cartilaginous differentiation
- Ductal adenoma with chondromyxoid change
- AME with chondromyxoid change
- Mammary hamartoma with chondroid elements

resembling the chondroid matrix of PA but the diagnostic features of malignant phyllodes tumor (leaf-like architecture, cellular stroma, atypia, and mitoses) are always evident. Occasionally ductal adenomas[46] and AMEs have a chondromyxoid matrix, but in PA the chondromyxoid matrix is more prominent and the myoepithelial elements merge and blend with the surrounding matrix. Ductal adenoma has a capsule containing elastic fibers derived from the underlying duct wall. The distinction of these lesions, however, may be arbitrary and Rosen regards PA and ductal adenoma as variants of intraductal papilloma and AME.[66] Other investigators have also noted the association between PA and intraductal papillomas.[34,98,99] Mammary hamartoma is another breast lesion that can contain cartilage. It is a circumscribed tumor composed of a mixture of mature fat, fibrous stroma, and normal ducts and lobules and sometimes contains smooth muscle and mature hyaline cartilage.

PROGNOSIS

The prognosis of PA is excellent. Most PAs are cured by conservative surgical excision but local recurrence may occur as it does in the salivary gland.[99] Therefore, excision of the lesion with a cuff of normal tissue, as is the practice in the salivary gland, is recommended.[111] Malignant progression is rare. Separation of malignant PA from metaplastic carcinoma with matrix production[112] depends on the identification of a benign component of PA.

PLEOMORPHIC ADENOMA WITH MALIGNANT PROGRESSION

OVERVIEW

Malignant transformation of PA is well known to occur in salivary glands, giving rise to a variety of

histologic types of malignancy. In the breast, malignant PA is rare. Only 3 cases have been described so far.[112] Potentially, PA can dedifferentiate along several lines,[113–115] namely epithelial, myoepithelial, and mesenchymal. Accordingly, it can give rise to carcinoma (equivalent to carcinoma ex PA of salivary gland), myoepithelial carcinoma, true malignant mixed tumor (carcinosarcoma), or sarcoma ex PA.

GROSS FEATURES

No specific gross features are described.

MICROSCOPIC FEATURES

PA with malignant progression is composed of a benign PA component and a histologically malignant infiltrative component with a gradual or abrupt transition between the 2 components. The 3 cases reported by Hayes and colleagues[112] all showed a benign PA with gradual transition to high-grade malignant areas, unlike the abrupt transition seen in salivary glands. The low-grade element must show areas in which both epithelial and myoepithelial cells are distributed in an organized fashion and have a low proliferative rate. Potentially, the malignant elements can be a high-grade carcinoma, myoepithelial carcinoma, biphasic carcinosarcoma, or a pure sarcoma. The cases described hitherto, however, showed either high-grade ductal carcinoma NOS or/and metaplastic carcinoma with chondroid matrix production. Regardless of the histologic type, the malignant component shows an overtly infiltrative growth pattern, high-grade cytologic features, and high mitotic rate, with or without necrosis (**Fig. 20**). Furthermore, the high-grade component loses the organized relationship between the

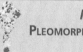 *Key Features*
PLEOMORPHIC ADENOMA WITH MALIGNANT PROGRESSION

- Presents as a breast mass with an accelerated growth phase.
- A low-grade (benign) component is a prerequisite.
- The malignant component can be epithelial, myoepithelial, mesenchymal, or a mixture.
- Shows overlapping features with matrix-producing metaplastic carcinoma.
- Behavior: the paucity of the literature prevents any meaningful conclusions.

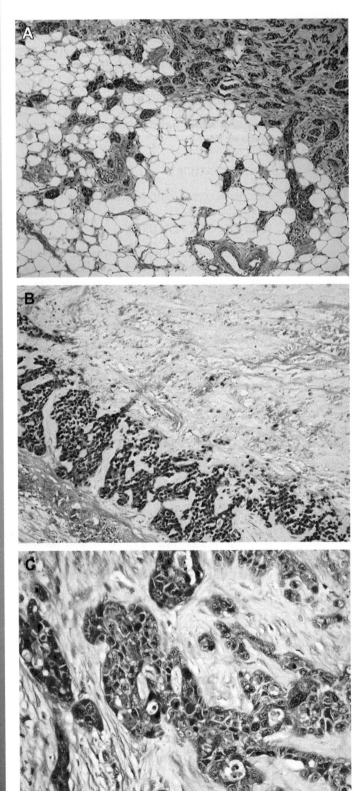

Fig. 20. Malignant PA: high-grade component showing infiltrative margins (*A*), zonal tumor necrosis (*B*), and cytologic atypia with a high mitotic count (*C*).

epithelial and myoepithelial components that is seen in the low-grade PA component.

Myoepithelial markers are positive in the benign PA areas but are negative in the malignant areas (**Fig. 21**). MIB-1 immunostaining shows scanty positive nuclei in the benign areas but numerous positive nuclei in the malignant areas (**Fig. 22**). p53 Immunostain highlights some nuclei in the malignant areas. Unlike the salivary gland counterparts, Her2/neu is not overexpressed.[112]

DIAGNOSIS AND DIFFERENTIAL DIAGNOSIS

The differential diagnosis includes matrix-producing metaplastic carcinoma, but this variant of metaplastic carcinoma is typically uniformly high grade and does not contain benign areas with a periductal myoepithelial cell layer resembling PA (see **Fig. 21**).[112] Although malignant AME occasionally shows matrix production, the benign component of this tumor does not look like a PA. The high-grade basaloid variant of ACC

Fig. 21. Myoepithelial markers in malignant PA. p63 Immunostain is positive in the benign PA areas in an organized periductal pattern (*A*) but is almost negative in the malignant areas (*B*).

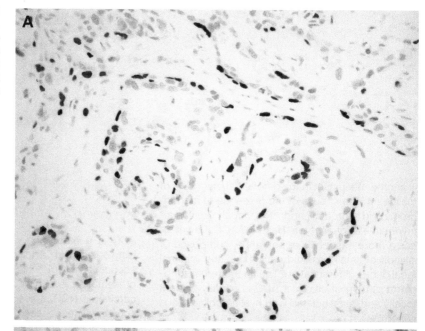

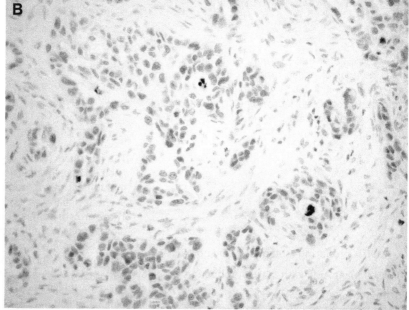

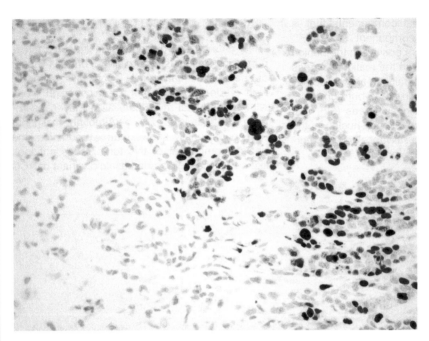

Fig. 22. MIB-1 immunostain shows increased proliferative index in the malignant PA component (*right*) compared to the benign PA component (*left*).

is another neoplasm in the differential diagnosis of malignant PA because of the presence of a chondromyxoid stroma and the dual epithelial-myoepithelial phenotype. Basaloid ACC, however, has a more basophilic appearance, composed of islands of small basaloid cells exhibiting minimal focal ductal differentiation. The characteristic cribriform pattern of classical ACC is usually evident focally and is associated with hyaline collagenous spherules.

PROGNOSIS

Outcome data of these tumors are limited by the small number of cases reported in the literature and short clinical follow-up. In salivary glands, important prognostic factors include tumor size, grade, stage, proliferation index, and extent of invasion.[116]

 Differential Diagnosis
PLEOMORPHIC ADENOMA WITH
MALIGNANT PROGRESSION

- Matrix-producing metaplastic carcinoma
- Malignant AME with matrix production
- High-grade ACC

ADENOID CYSTIC CARCINOMA

OVERVIEW

ACC is a carcinoma of low malignant potential, histologically similar to its salivary gland counterpart, accounting for 0.1% of all breast carcinomas. Age at presentation is similar to that for invasive ductal carcinoma NOS. It presents as a discrete nodule, sometimes tender, located in the periareolar/subareolar region in approximately 50% of cases. Occasionally ACC is seen in children and in men.

GROSS FEATURES

ACC presents as circumscribed mass with or without microcysts. Occasionally, the margin is partly irregular.

MICROSCOPIC FEATURES

The infiltrative nature of ACC is better appreciated microscopically than is evident grossly. Usually, the tumor has a dominant central nodule with a subtle infiltrative component at the periphery. Three growth patterns have been recognized: cribriform (most characteristic), trabecular-tubular, and solid (**Fig. 23**), but most ACCs contain all of these patterns in variable proportions.[117–121] The solid pattern predominates in higher-grade ACCs, especially the basaloid variant. An in situ component is difficult to find or absent.

Fig. 23. ACC. (*A*) Typical cribriform pattern. (*B*) Tubular (*upper left*) and solid (*lower right*) growth patterns.

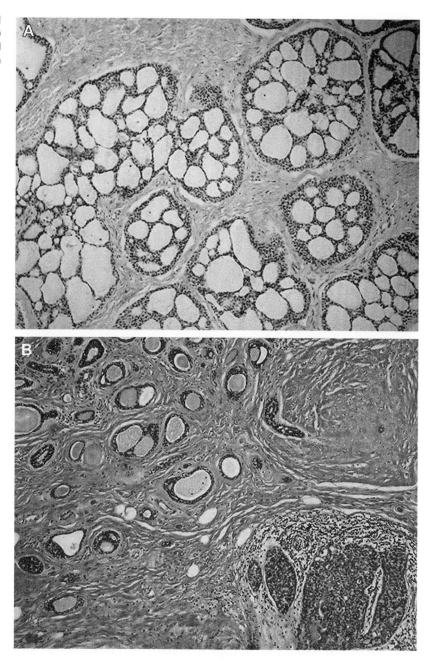

The tumor is composed of two cell types, epithelial and myoepithelial.[34,122] The myoepithelial cells usually predominate. These have small dark nuclei and scanty cytoplasm, and form cribriform structures (Swiss cheese pattern), bilayered tubular structures, and nests. The myoepithelial cells produce a dense eosinophilic matrix material forming ball-like structures within the cribriform pseudoglandular spaces. Some of the spaces contain acid mucin (alcian blue positive at pH2.5). Thick glassy membranes are also seen around cell groups and these may coalesce to form irregular stromal masses. This membranous material is metachromatic on Giemsa-stained preparations in FNA samples.[123–125] Rarely, metaplastic cartilage and bone may be seen in the stroma, simulating PA.

Often, the epithelial cells have a striking eosinophilic cytoplasm and paler nuclei than the myoepithelial cells (**Fig. 24**). These epithelial cells form

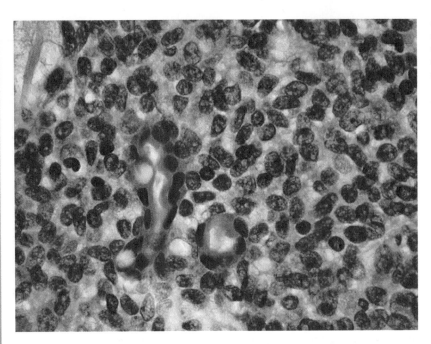

Fig. 24. The epithelial cells in ACC often have a striking eosinophilic cytoplasm, whereas the surrounding myoepithelial cells have scanty cytoplasm and a basaloid appearance.

true ductal spaces, which may contain neutral mucin (mucicarmine and PAS-diastase both positive). The ducts may be tiny glandular spaces lying within the sheets of basaloid myoepithelial cells (see **Fig. 24**), round cystic ducts, or elongated irregular syringomatous ducts. Occasionally, sebaceous as well as squamous cells are encountered as in AME. Mitotic figures vary in number and are seen most often in the myoepithelial cell component. Necrosis may occur in the solid areas. Rarely, metaplastic cartilage and bone may be seen in the stroma simulating PA.

Perineural invasion is uncommon in the breast, in contrast to ACC of salivary gland. Lymphatic invasion is unusual and must be differentiated from shrinkage artifact.

Ro et al[126] proposed a 3-tier grading system for ACC based on the percentage of the solid component: grade 1, no solid component; grade 2, less than 30% solid; and grade 3, greater than 30% solid. The prognostic value of grading of ACC, however, is controversial.[127] High-grade solid basaloid variant of ACC (**Fig. 25**) with necrosis, atypia, and numerous mitoses probably has a higher metastatic potential than the lower grades of ACC but this is not universally believed.[128–130]

Some cases of ACC have a subtle pattern of infiltrating tubules at their periphery, which can cause problems in determining the adequacy of excision (**Fig. 26**).[131] This is because the tubules of ACC may be well differentiated and resemble normal terminal ducts. Keys to their recognition

include the abnormal architecture (abnormal distribution of ducts) on low-power examination and the hyperchromasia of the lining cells. In addition, the immunostain for p63 sometimes shows a double layer of myoepithelial cells in the neoplastic ducts (**Fig. 27**) and larger myoepithelial cell nuclei compared with those present in the adjacent normal benign ducts.

The immunoprofile of ACC is variable both within individual tumors and between different cases. In particular, the high-grade solid basaloid variant of ACC often lacks most of the expected markers of ductal and myoepithelial cells. In most cases of ACC, the myoepithelial cells show positive immunostaining for p63, CK5/6, CK14, and CK34βE12 and patchy inconsistent staining for S-100 protein, SMA, calponin, and SMHC myosin.[132,133] The epithelial cells show a range of differentiation from pure basal (CK5/6+, CK14+, and CK34βE12+) through luminal cells (CK7+, CK8/18+, and Cam 5.2+), with many cells showing combined staining patterns. CD117 immunostain is positive in most cases[134,135] but the specificity of this stain is unknown because it is positive in many grade 3 ductal carcinomas, especially basal-type carcinomas. ER staining is usually weakly and focally positive but some cases are negative for ER.[136,137] The newly described ER-α36, however, an isoform of ER-α, is frequently expressed in ACC, which may potentially be useful for targeted therapy.[138] Her2/neu is negative. Collagen IV and laminin are positive in the

Fig. 25. ACC, high-grade solid variant showing irregular nests of basaloid cells in a dense and vaguely chondroid stroma reminiscent of metaplastic carcinoma.

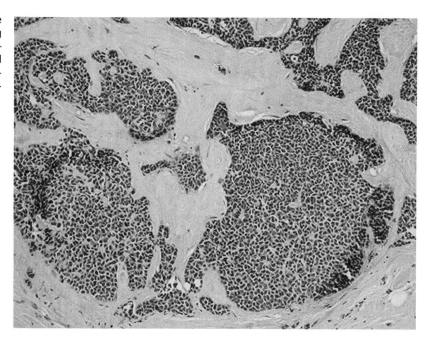

matrix-like material and globular hyaline bodies.[139] Like the salivary counterpart, ACC of breast expresses the proto-oncogene c-KIT (CD117+) and is characterized by the translocation t(6;9).[140] Insulinlike growth factor II mRNA-binding protein 3, a novel recently described biomarker of basal-like breast carcinomas, has also been shown to be overexpressed in ACC.[141]

Key Features
ADENOID CYSTIC CARCINOMA

- Subareolar in location

- Solitary or rarely multifocal

- Microscopic patterns: cribriform, trabecular/tubular, solid

- IHC: highlights dual population of epithelial and myoepithelial cells, CD117 positive

- High-grade solid basaloid variant lacks most expected markers

- Biomarkers: ER negative to weak; Her2/neu negative

- Indolent behavior but may recur locally if incompletely excised

- Delayed metastasis to lung and liver

DIAGNOSIS AND DIFFERENTIAL DIAGNOSIS

Cribriform-type invasive ductal carcinoma can closely mimic ACC (**Fig. 28**A). In one study, 7 of 27 cases of ACC were reclassified to cribriform carcinoma after review.[142] On low power, ACC looks more basaloid than cribriform carcinoma, having smaller cells with less cytoplasm, and usually lacks a DCIS component at the periphery. Cribriform carcinoma is composed of luminal epithelial cells only whereas ACC has both luminal and myoepithelial cell populations, which can be highlighted by IHC. A combined PAS/alcian blue stain may be helpful in identifying the different mucins in ACC. In addition, cribriform carcinoma is strongly and diffusely positive for ER (see **Fig. 28**B) whereas ACC usually stains weakly or lacks ER staining.[137] Cribriform DCIS can also look like ACC but immunohistochemical stains reveal myoepithelial cells confined to the periphery of the involved ducts and not surrounding the luminal spaces as in ACC (**Fig. 29**).

Other forms of invasive ductal carcinoma, in particular basal-type carcinoma, can be indistinguishable from the high-grade solid basaloid variant of ACC. The problem is compounded by the fact that both of these tumors stain, albeit variably, with myoepithelial markers and lack ER staining. Abrupt ductal differentiation of the type typically seen in ACC should be looked for carefully (**Fig. 30**), although distinguishing these two

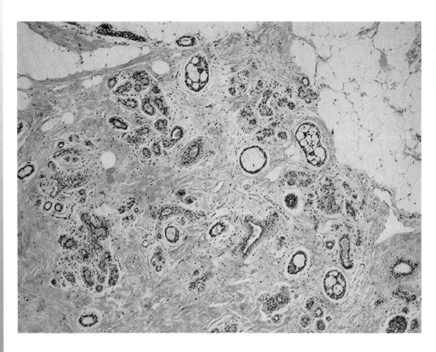

Fig. 26. ACC. Note the subtle infiltrative pattern at the periphery of the tumor where malignant tubules intermingle with normal breast lobules.

tumors may not be of clinical significance at present.

The bilayered tubular structures in AME and PA can occasionally be confused with that of ACC. These lesions, however, lack the more typical areas of ACC with well-developed cribriform structures and hyaline spherules. Besides, the myoepithelial cells of ACC tend to be smaller, more hyperchromatic, and basaloid-appearing with much less cytoplasm than those of AME and PA. Furthermore, a specific feature of ACC is that the luminal cells have eosinophilic cytoplasm and resemble eccrine ducts.

Cylindroma of the breast[143–145] is another neoplasm that closely resembles the solid variant of ACC, especially in needle biopsies. Cylindroma

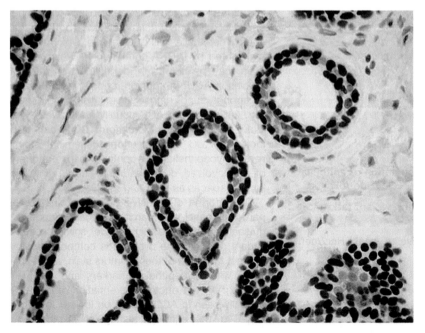

Fig. 27. ACC. p63 Immunostain shows a double layer of myoepithelial cells in the neoplastic ducts.

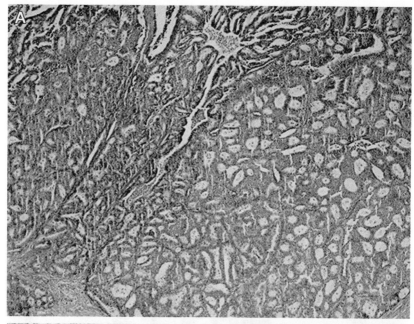

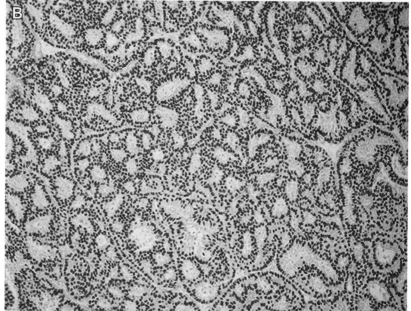

Fig. 28. Cribriform carcinoma. (*A*) Infiltrating masses of cribriform epithelium resembling ACC. (*B*) Cribriform carcinoma is strongly ER positive unlike ACC.

(Fig. 31) is distinguished from ACC by its jigsaw pattern, thick continuous basement membrane around the epithelial structures, and lack of infiltrative pattern, nuclear atypia, or mitotic figures.

The cribriform pattern and hyaline spherules of ACC can produce an appearance resembling CS, particularly in FNA.[25–30] Unlike CS, however, ACC presents as a palpable mass, shows overt stromal invasion in histologic sections, and more often expresses CD117 in the ductal epithelial component.[32] Furthermore, the epithelium in the FNAs from CS appears benign, forming cohesive

△△ **Differential Diagnosis**
ADENOID CYSTIC CARCINOMA

- Cribriform invasive ductal carcinoma
- Other forms of invasive carcinoma—basal-type carcinoma
- Cribriform DCIS
- AME
- PA
- Cylindroma
- CS

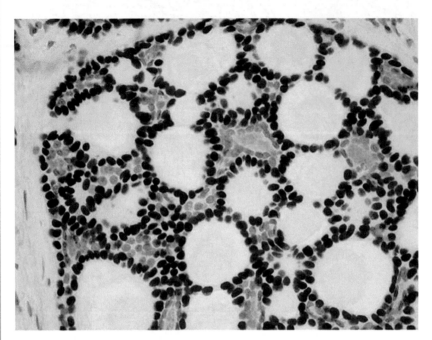

Fig. 29. ACC. The myoepithelial cells in ACC surround the luminal spaces, highlighted by p63 immunostain in this case.

groups of ductal cells with interspersed myoepithelial cells rather than the poorly cohesive pattern of ACC, and the collagenous spherules are smaller and more irregular in outline than those of ACC (**Fig. 32**; compare with **Fig. 5**).

PROGNOSIS

ACC has a good prognosis. Most tumors are cured by complete excision.[146,147] Local recurrence occurs if the tumor is incompletely excised. Axillary node metastases are uncommon. Therefore,

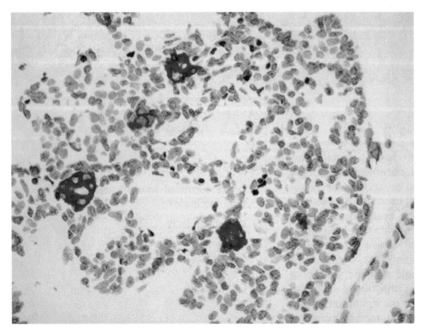

Fig. 30. ACC, high-grade solid variant. CAM 5.2 immunostain highlights the ductal differentiation.

Fig. 31. Cylindroma of the breast closely resembles the solid variant of ACC.

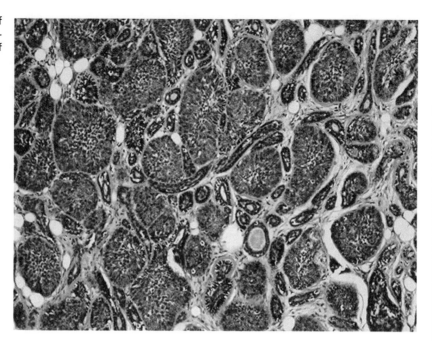

axillary lymph node dissection is contraindicated unless abnormal nodes are noted on clinical examination or imaging studies.[138,148] Hematogenous metastases to lung and liver occur in 10% of cases. These can be delayed for many years after surgical excision. Rarely, metastases occur to bone and kidney.[149] The role of chemotherapy for ACC is uncertain but breast-conserving surgery combined with radiation and chemotherapy has some proponents.[150,151]

Fig. 32. ACC. On FNA, ACC has a poorly cohesive pattern and larger spherules than those of CS.

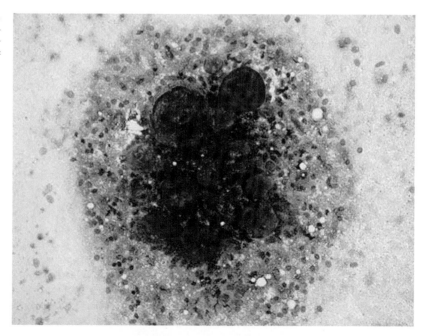

Pitfalls
EPITHELIAL-MYOEPITHELIAL LESIONS OF BREAST

! AME and PA may be mistaken for invasive ductal carcinoma in core biopsies.

! Papillomas, fibroadenomas, and phyllodes tumor may show focal myoepithelial hyperplasia resembling AME.

! AME, PA, and basaloid ACC may all be confused with metaplastic matrix-producing carcinoma.

! AME, PA, and ACC may show progression to high-grade malignancy, masking the true nature of the underlying neoplasm.

! CS may resemble ACC especially in core biopsies and FNAs.

! ACC cribriform variant may resemble cribriform DCIS or invasive cribriform carcinoma especially in core biopsies.

! The infiltrative border of tubular ACC can merge insusceptibly with normal breast tissue making margin assessment difficult.

! Cutaneous-type adnexal tumors occurring in the breast (clear cell hidradenoma and cylindroma) may be misinterpreted as AME and solid variant of ACC, respectively.

ACKNOWLEDGMENTS

The authors thank Professor V. Eusebi for his assistance with the section on AMEA.

REFERENCES

1. Lakhani SR, Ellis IO, Schnitt SJ, et al. World Health Organization Classification of tumours of the breast. 4th Edition. Lyon: IARC Press; 2012.
2. Ahmed AA, Heller DS. Malignant adenomyoepithelioma of the breast with malignant proliferation of epithelial and myoepithelial elements: a case report and review of the literature. Arch Pathol Lab Med 2000;124(4):632–6.
3. Young RH, Clement PB. Adenomyoepithelioma of the breast. A report of three cases and review of the literature. Am J Clin Pathol 1988;89(3):308–14.
4. Eusebi V, Casadei GP, Bussolati G, et al. Adenomyoepithelioma of the breast with a distinctive type of apocrine adenosis. Histopathology 1987; 11(3):305–15.
5. Kiaer H, Nielsen B, Paulsen S, et al. Adenomyoepithelial adenosis and low-grade malignant adenomyoepithelioma of the breast. Virchows Arch A Pathol Anat Histopathol 1984;405(1):55–67.
6. Eusebi V, Foschini MP, Betts CM, et al. Microglandular adenosis, apocrine adenosis, and tubular carcinoma of the breast. An immunohistochemical comparison. Am J Surg Pathol 1993; 17(2):99–109.
7. Erel S, Tuncbilek I, Kismet K, et al. Adenomyoepithelial adenosis of the breast: clinical, radiological,

and pathological findings for differential diagnosis. Breast Care (Basel) 2008;3(6):427–30.
8. Tsuda H, Mukai K, Fukutomi T, et al. Malignant progression of adenomyoepithelial adenosis of the breast. Pathol Int 1994;44(6):475–9.
9. Günhan-Bilgen I, Memiş A, Ustün EE, et al. Sclerosing adenosis: mammographic and ultrasonographic findings with clinical and histopathological correlation. Eur J Radiol 2002;44(3):232–8.
10. Nielsen BB. Adenosis tumour of the breast—a clinicopathological investigation of 27 cases. Histopathology 1987;11(12):1259–75.
11. Oztekin PS, Tuncbilek I, Kosar P, et al. Nodular sclerosing adenosis mimicking malignancy in the breast: magnetic resonance imaging findings. Breast J 2011;17(1):95–7.
12. Di Tommaso L, Pasquinelli G, Damiani S. Smooth muscle differentiation in mammary stromo-epithelial lesions with evidence of a dual origin: stromal myofibroblasts and myoepithelial cells. Histopathology 2003;42(5):448–56.
13. Clement PB, Young RH, Azzopardi JG. Collagenous spherulosis of the breast. Am J Surg Pathol 1987;11(6):411–7.
14. Hill P, Cawson J. Collagenous spherulosis presenting as a mass lesion on imaging. Breast J 2008; 14(3):301–3.
15. Resetkova E, Albarracin C, Sneige N. Collagenous spherulosis of breast: morphologic study of 59 cases and review of the literature. Am J Surg Pathol 2006;30(1):20–7.
16. Divaris DX, Smith S, Leask D, et al. Complex collagenous spherulosis of the breast presenting as a palpable

mass: a case report with immunohistochemical and ultrastructural studies. Breast J 2000;6(3):199–203.

17. Hill P, Cawson J. Collagenous spherulosis with lobular carcinoma in situ: a potential diagnostic pitfall. Pathology 2007;39(3):361–3.

18. Wells CA, Wells CW, Yeomans P, et al. Spherical connective tissue inclusions in epithelial hyperplasia of the breast ("collagenous spherulosis"). J Clin Pathol 1990;43(11):905–8.

19. Mooney EE, Kayani N, Tavassoli FA. Spherulosis of the breast. A spectrum of mucinous and collagenous lesions. Arch Pathol Lab Med 1999;123(7): 626–30.

20. Ogata K, Sakamoto G, Sakurai T. Adenoid cystic carcinoma with collagenous spherulosis-like structures in the breast: report of a case. Pathol Int 2004;54(5):332–6.

21. Stephenson TJ, Hird PM, Laing RW, et al. Nodular basement membrane deposits in breast carcinoma and atypical ductal hyperplasia: mimics of collagenous spherulosis. Pathologica 1994;86(3):234–9.

22. Grignon DJ, Ro JY, Mackay BN, et al. Collagenous spherulosis of the breast. Immunohistochemical and ultrastructural studies. Am J Clin Pathol 1989; 91(4):386–92.

23. Maluf HM, Koerner FC, Dickersin GR. Collagenous spherulosis: an ultrastructural study. Ultrastruct Pathol 1998;22(3):239–48.

24. Sgroi D, Koerner FC. Involvement of collagenous spherulosis by lobular carcinoma in situ: potential confusion with cribriform ductal carcinoma in situ. Am J Surg Pathol 1995;19(12):1366–70.

25. Jain S, Kumar N, Sodhani P, et al. Cytology of collagenous spherulosis of the breast: a diagnostic dilemma - report of three cases. Cytopathology 2002;13(2):116–20.

26. Rey A, Redondo E, Servent R. Collagenous spherulosis of the breast diagnosed by fine needle aspiration biopsy. Acta Cytol 1995;39(5):1071–3.

27. Highland KE, Finley JL, Neill JS, et al. Collagenous spherulosis. Report of a case with diagnosis by fine needle aspiration biopsy with immunocytochemical and ultrastructural observations. Acta Cytol 1993; 37(1):3–9.

28. Sola Perez J, Perez-Guillermo M, Bas Bernal A, et al. Diagnosis of collagenous spherulosis of the breast by fine needle aspiration cytology. A report of two cases. Acta Cytol 1993;37(5):725–8.

29. Johnson TL, Kini SR. Cytologic features of collagenous spherulosis of the breast. Diagn Cytopathol 1991;7(4):417–9.

30. Tyler X, Coghill SB. Fine needle aspiration cytology of collagenous spherulosis of the breast. Cytopathology 1991;2(3):159–62.

31. Azzopardi JG, Smith OD. Salivary gland tumours and their mucins. J Pathol Bacteriol 1959;77(1): 131–40.

32. Rabban JT, Swain RS, Zaloudek CJ, et al. Immunophenotypic overlap between adenoid cystic carcinoma and collagenous spherulosis of the breast: potential diagnostic pitfalls using myoepithelial markers. Mod Pathol 2006;19(10):1351–7.

33. Hamperl H. The myothelia (myoepithelial cells). Normal state; regressive changes; hyperplasia; tumors. Curr Top Pathol 1970;53:161–220.

34. Seifert G. Are adenomyoepithelioma of the breast and epithelial-myoepithelial carcinoma of the salivary glands identical tumours? [comment]. Virchows Arch 1998;433(3):285–8.

35. Foschini MP, Reis-Filho JS, Eusebi V, et al. Salivary gland-like tumours of the breast: surgical and molecular pathology. J Clin Pathol 2003;56(7):497–506.

36. Accurso A, Donofrio V, Insabato L, et al. Adenomyoepithelioma of the breast. A case report. Tumori 1990;76(6):606–10.

37. Rosen PP. Adenomyoepithelioma of the breast. Hum Pathol 1987;18(12):1232–7.

38. Howlett DC, Mason CH, Biswas S, et al. Adenomyoepithelioma of the breast: spectrum of disease with associated imaging and pathology. Am J Roentgenol 2003;180(3):799–803.

39. Huang CY, Sheen-Chen SM, Eng HL, et al. Adenomyoepithelioma of the breast. Tumori 2007;93(5): 493–5.

40. Ruiz-Delgado ML, Lopez-Ruiz JA, Eizaguirre B, et al. Benign adenomyoepithelioma of the breast: imaging findings mimicking malignancy and histopathological features. Acta Radiol 2007;48(1):27–9.

41. Buch A, Rout P, Makhija P. Adenomyoepithelioma with phyllodes tumor—a rare combination in a solitary breast lump. Indian J Pathol Microbiol 2006; 49(2):259–61.

42. Tamura G, Monma N, Suzuki Y, et al. Adenomyoepithelioma (myoepithelioma) of the breast in a male. Hum Pathol 1993;24(6):678–81.

43. Azzopardi JG, Salm R. Ductal adenoma of the breast: a lesion which can mimic carcinoma. J Pathol 1984;144(1):15–23.

44. Gusterson BA, Sloane JP, Middwood C, et al. Ductal adenoma of the breast—a lesion exhibiting a myoepithelial/epithelial phenotype. Histopathology 1987;11(1):103–10.

45. Okada K, Suzuki Y, Saito Y, et al. Two cases of ductal adenoma of the breast. Breast Cancer 2006;13(4): 354–9.

46. Kato N, Ohe S, Motoyama T. Ductal adenoma of the breast with chondromyxoid change. Pathol Int 2002;52(3):239–43.

47. Guarino M, Reale D, Squillaci S, et al. Ductal adenoma of the breast. An immunohistochemical study of five cases. Pathol Res Pract 1993;189(5):515–20.

48. Lammie GA, Millis RR. Ductal adenoma of the breast—a review of fifteen cases. Hum Pathol 1989;20(9):903–8.

49. Hikino H, Kodama K, Yasui K, et al. Intracystic adenomyoepithelioma of the breast—case report and review. Breast Cancer 2007;14(4):429–33.

50. Papaevangelou A, Pougouras I, Liapi G, et al. Cystic adenomyoepithelioma of the breast. Breast 2004;13(4):356–8.

51. Laforga JB, Aranda FI, Sevilla F. Adenomyoepithelioma of the breast: report of two cases with prominent cystic changes and intranuclear inclusions. Diagn Cytopathol 1998;19(1):55–8.

52. McLaren BK, Smith J, Schuyler PA, et al. Adenomyoepithelioma: clinical, histologic, and immunohistologic evaluation of a series of related lesions. Am J Surg Pathol 2005;29(10):1294–9.

53. Tavassoli FA. Myoepithelial lesions of the breast. Myoepitheliosis, adenomyoepithelioma, and myoepithelial carcinoma. Am J Surg Pathol 1991;15(6):554–68.

54. Fukuoka K, Kanahara T, Tamura M, et al. Basement membrane substance in adenomyoepithelioma of the breast. Acta Cytol 2001;45(2):282–3.

55. Weidner N, Levine JD. Spindle-cell adenomyoepithelioma of the breast. A microscopic, ultrastructural, and immunocytochemical study. Cancer 1988;62(8):1561–7.

56. Cai RZ, Tan PH. Adenomyoepithelioma of the breast with squamous and sebaceous metaplasia. Pathology 2005;37(6):557–9.

57. Reis-Filho JS, Fulford LG, Crebassa B, et al. Collagenous spherulosis in an adenomyoepithelioma of the breast. J Clin Pathol 2004;57(1):83–6.

58. Ohta M, Mori M, Kawada T, et al. Collagenous spherulosis associated with adenomyoepithelioma of the breast: a case report. Acta Cytol 2010;54(3):314–8.

59. Nga ME, Lim KH, Tan EY, et al. Malignant adenomyoepithelial tumor of the breast: multi-immunolabeling technique and detailed immunophenotypic study. Appl Immunohistochem Mol Morphol 2008;16(1):100–4.

60. Tamura S, Enjoji M, Toyoshima S, et al. Adenomyoepithelioma of the breast. A case report with an immunohistochemical study. Acta Pathol Jpn 1988;38(5):659–65.

61. Koyama M, Kurotaki H, Yagihashi N, et al. Immunohistochemical assessment of proliferative activity in mammary adenomyoepithelioma. Histopathology 1997;31(2):134–9.

62. Barbareschi M, Pecciarini L, Cangi MG, et al. p63, a p53 homologue, is a selective nuclear marker of myoepithelial cells of the human breast. Am J Surg Pathol 2001;25(8):1054–60.

63. Clarke C, Sandle J, Lakhani SR. Myoepithelial cells: pathology, cell separation and markers of myoepithelial differentiation. J Mammary Gland Biol Neoplasia 2005;10(3):273–80.

64. Reis-Filho JS, Milanezi F, Silva P, et al. Maspin expression in myoepithelial tumors of the breast. Pathol Res Pract 2001;197(12):817–21.

65. Simpson PT, Gale T, Reis-Filho JS, et al. Distribution and significance of 14-3-3σ, a novel myoepithelial marker, in normal, benign, and malignant breast tissue. J Pathol 2004;202(3):274–85.

66. Rosen PP. Rosen's breast pathology. 2nd edition. Philadelphia: Lippincott Williams & Wilkins; 2001. p. 130–2 & 167.

67. Knoedler D, Susnik B, Gonyo MB, et al. Giant apocrine hidradenoma of the breast. Breast J 2007;13(1):91–3.

68. Kumar N, Verma K. Clear cell hidradenoma simulating breast carcinoma: a diagnostic pitfall in fine-needle aspiration of breast. Diagn Cytopathol 1996;15(1):70–2.

69. Ohi Y, Umekita Y, Rai Y, et al. Clear cell hidradenoma of the breast: a case report with review of the literature. Breast Cancer 2007;14(3):307–11.

70. Kazakov DV, Vanecek T, Belousova IE, et al. Skin-type hidradenoma of the breast with t(11;19) translocation: hidradenoma of the breast. Am J Dermatopathol 2007;29(5):457–61.

71. Nadelman CM, Leslie KO, Fishbein MC. "Benign, " metastasizing adenomyoepithelioma of the breast: a report of 2 cases. Arch Pathol Lab Med 2006;130(9):1349–53.

72. Loose JH, Patchefsky AS, Hollander IJ, et al. Adenomyoepithelioma of the breast. A spectrum of biologic behavior. Am J Surg Pathol 1992;16(9):868–76.

73. Hayes MM. Adenomyoepithelioma of the breast: a review stressing its propensity for malignant transformation. J Clin Pathol 2011;64(6):477–84.

74. Noël JC, Simon P, Aguilar SF. Malignant myoepithelioma arising in cystic adenomyoepithelioma. Breast J 2006;12(4):386.

75. Hegyi L, Thway K, Newton R, et al. Malignant myoepithelioma arising in adenomyoepithelioma of the breast and coincident multiple gastrointestinal stromal tumours in a patient with neurofibromatosis type 1. J Clin Pathol 2009;62(7):653–5.

76. Chen PC, Chen CK, Nicastri AD, et al. Myoepithelial carcinoma of the breast with distant metastasis and accompanied by adenomyoepitheliomas. Histopathology 1994;24(6):543–8.

77. Fan F, Smith W, Wang X, et al. Myoepithelial carcinoma of the breast arising in an adenomyoepithelioma: mammographic, ultrasound and histologic features. Breast J 2007;13(2):203–4.

78. Hungermann D, Buerger H, Oehlschlegel C, et al. Adenomyoepithelial tumours and myoepithelial carcinomas of the breast–a spectrum of monophasic and biphasic tumours dominated by immature myoepithelial cells. BMC Cancer 2005;5:92.

79. Michal M, Baumruk L, Burger J, et al. Adenomyoepithelioma of the breast with undifferentiated carcinoma component. Histopathology 1994;24(3):274–6.

80. Rasbridge SA, Millis RR. Adenomyoepithelioma of the breast with malignant features. Virchows Arch 1998;432(2):123–30.

81. Han B, Mori I, Nakamura M, et al. Myoepithelial carcinoma arising in an adenomyoepithelioma of the breast: case report with immunohistochemical and mutational analysis. Pathol Int 2006;56(4):211–6.

82. Mandal S, Dhingra K, Roy S, et al. Clear cell malignant myoepithelioma—breast presenting as a fungating mass. Breast J 2007;13(6):618–20.

83. Van Dorpe J, De Pauw A, Moerman P. Adenoid cystic carcinoma arising in an adenomyoepithelioma of the breast. Virchows Arch 1998;432(2):119–22.

84. Foschini MP, Pizzicannella G, Peterse JL, et al. Adenomyoepithelioma of the breast associated with low-grade adenosquamous and sarcomatoid carcinomas. Virchows Arch 1995;427(3):243–50.

85. Van Hoeven KH, Drudis T, Cranor ML, et al. Low-grade adenosquamous carcinoma of the breast. A clinocopathologic study of 32 cases with ultrastructural analysis. Am J Surg Pathol 1993;17(3):248–58.

86. Buza N, Zekry N, Charpin C, et al. Myoepithelial carcinoma of the breast: a clinicopathological and immunohistochemical study of 15 diagnostically challenging cases. Virchows Arch 2010;457(3):337–45.

87. Oka K, Sando N, Moriya T, et al. Malignant adenomyoepithelioma of the breast with matrix production may be compatible with one variant form of matrix-producing carcinoma: a case report. Pathol Res Pract 2007;203(8):599–604.

88. Sugano I, Nagao T, Tajima Y, et al. Malignant adenomyoepithelioma of the breast: a non-tubular and matrix-producing variant. Pathol Int 2001;51(3):193–9.

89. Simpson RH, Cope N, Skálová A, et al. Malignant adenomyoepithelioma of the breast with mixed osteogenic, spindle cell, and carcinomatous differentiation. Am J Surg Pathol 1998;22(5):631–6.

90. Carter MR, Hornick JL, Lester S, et al. Spindle cell (sarcomatoid) carcinoma of the breast: a clinicopathologic and immunohistochemical analysis of 29 cases. Am J surg Pathol 2006;30(3):300–9.

91. Trojani M, Guiu M, Trouette H, et al. Malignant adenomyoepithelioma of the breast. An immunohistochemical, cytophotometric, and ultrastructural study of a case with lung metastases. Am J Clin Pathol 1992;98(6):598–602.

92. Kihara M, Yokomise H, Irie A, et al. Malignant adenomyoepithelioma of the breast with lung metastases: report of a case. Surg Today 2001;31(10):899–903.

93. Jones C, Tooze R, Lakhani SR. Malignant adenomyoepithelioma of the breast metastasizing to the liver. Virchows Arch 2003;442(5):504–6.

94. Chen KT. Pleomorphic adenoma of the breast. Am J Clin Pathol 1990;93(6):792–4.

95. Simha MR, Doctor VM, Udwadia TE. Mixed tumour of salivary gland type of the male breast. Indian J Cancer 1992;29(1):14–7.

96. van der Walt JD, Rohlova B. Pleomorphic adenoma of the human breast. A report of a benign tumour closely mimicking a carcinoma clinically. Clin Oncol 1982;8(4):361–5.

97. Sheth MT, Hathway D, Petrelli M. Pleomorphic adenoma ("mixed" tumor) of human female breast mimicking carcinoma clinico-radiologically. Cancer 1978;41(2):659–65.

98. Smith BH, Taylor HB. The occurence of bone and cartilage in mammary tumors. Am J Clin Pathol 1968;51:610–8.

99. Soreide JA, Anda O, Eriksen L, et al. Pleomorphic adenoma of the human breast with local recurrence. Cancer 1988;61(5):997–1001.

100. Moran CA, Suster S, Carter D. Benign mixed tumors (pleomorphic adenomas) of the breast. Am J Surg Pathol 1990;14(10):913–21.

101. Iyengar P, Cody HS, Brogi E. Pleomorphic adenoma of the breast: case report and review of the literature. Diagn Cytopathol 2005;33(6):416–20.

102. Reid-Nicholson M, Bleiweiss I, Pace B, et al. Pleomorphic adenoma of the breast. A case report and distinction from mucinous carcinoma. Arch Pathol Lab Med 2003;127(4):474–7.

103. Narita T, Matsuda K. Pleomorphic adenoma of the breast: case report and review of the literature. Pathol Int 1995;45(6):441–7.

104. Diaz NM, McDivitt RW, Wick MR. Pleomorphic adenoma of the breast: a clinicopathologic and immunohistochemical study of 10 cases. Hum Pathol 1991;22(12):1206–14.

105. Kumar PV, Sobhani SA, Monabati A, et al. Cytologic findings of a pleomorphic adenoma of the breast: a case report. Acta Cytol 2004;48(6):849–52.

106. Zardawi IM, Crotty A, Clark DA. Fine needle aspiration cytology of pleomorphic adenoma of the breast. Acta Cytol 2004;48(6):869–71.

107. Parham DM, Evans A. Pleomorphic adenoma of the breast; a potential for the misdiagnosis of malignancy on fine needle aspiration (FNA). Cytopathology 1998;9(5):343–8.

108. Kanter MH, Sedeghi M. Pleomorphic adenoma of the breast: cytology of fine-needle aspiration and its differential diagnosis. Diagn Cytopathol 1993;9(5):555–8.

109. Balance WA, Ro JY, el-Naggar AK, et al. Pleomorphic adenoma (benign mixed tumor) of the breast. An immunohistochemical, flow cytometric, and ultrastructural study and review of the literature. Am J Clin Pathol 1990;93(6):795–801.

110. Segen JC, Foo M, Richer S. Pleomorphic adenoma of the breast with positive estrogen receptors. N Y State J Med 1986;86(5):265–6.

111. John BJ, Griffiths C, Ebbs SR. Pleomorphic adenoma of the breast should be excised with a cuff of normal tissue. Breast J 2007;13(4):418–20.

112. Hayes MM, Lesack D, Girardet C, et al. Carcinoma ex-pleomorphic adenoma of the breast. Report of three cases suggesting a relationship to metaplastic carcinoma of matrix-producing type. Virchows Arch 2005;446(2):142–9.

113. Altemani A, Martins MT, Freitas L, et al. Carcinoma ex pleomorphic adenoma (CXPA): immunoprofile of the cells involved in carcinomatous progression. Histopathology 2005;46(6):635–41.

114. Qureshi A, Barakzai A, Sahar NU, et al. Spectrum of malignancy in mixed tumors of salivary gland: a morphological and immunohistochemical review of 23 cases. Indian J Pathol Microbiol 2009;52(2):150–4.

115. Katabi N, Gomez D, Klimstra DS, et al. Prognostic factors of recurrence in salivary carcinoma ex pleomorphic adenoma, with emphasis on the carcinoma histologic subtype: a clinicopathologic study of 43 cases. Hum Pathol 2010;41(7):927–34.

116. Olsen KD, Lewis JE. Carcinoma ex pleomorphic adenoma: a clinicopathologic review. Head Neck 2001;23(9):705–12.

117. Zaloudek C, Oertel YC, Orenstein JM. Adenoid cystic carcinoma of the breast. Am J Clin Pathol 1984;81(3):297–307.

118. Qizilbash AH, Patterson MC, Oliveira KF. Adenoid cystic carcinoma of the breast. Light and electron microscopy and a brief review of the literature. Arch Pathol Lab Med 1977;101(6):302–6.

119. Anthony PP, James PD. Adenoid cystic carcinoma of the breast: prevalence, diagnostic criteria, and histogenesis. J Clin Pathol 1975;28(8):647–55.

120. Lusted D. Structural and growth patterns of adenoid cystic carcinoma of breast. Am J Clin Pathol 1970;54(3):419–25.

121. Cavanzo FJ, Taylor HB. Adenoid cystic carcinoma of the breast. An analysis of 21 cases. Cancer 1969;24(4):740–5.

122. Foschini MP, Eusebi V. Carcinomas of the breast showing myoepithelial cell differentiation. A review of the literature. Virchows Arch 1998;432(4):303–10.

123. McCluggage WG, McManus DI, Caughley LM. Fine needle aspiration (FNA) cytology of adenoid cystic carcinoma and adenomyoepithelioma of breast: two lesions rich in myoepithelial cells. Cytopathology 1997;8(1):31–9.

124. Stahlschmidt J, Liston J, Aslam MM, et al. Educational case report. Fine needle aspiration cytology of adenoid cystic carcinoma of the breast. Cytopathology 2001;12(4):266–9.

125. Gupta RK, Green C, Naran S, et al. Fine-needle aspiration cytology of adenoid cystic carcinoma of the breast. Diagn Cytopathol 1999;20(2):82–4.

126. Ro JY, Silva EG, Gallager HS. Adenoid cystic carcinoma of the breast. Hum Pathol 1987;18(12):1276–81.

127. Kleer CG, Oberman HA. Adenoid cystic carcinoma of the breast: value of histologic grading and proliferative activity. Am J Surg Pathol 1998;22(5):569–75.

128. Cabibi D, Cipolla C, Maria Florena A, et al. Solid variant of mammary "adenoid cystic carcinoma with basaloid features" merging with "small cell carcinoma". Pathol Res Pract 2005;201(10):705–11.

129. Shin SJ, Rosen PP. Solid variant of mammary adenoid cystic carcinoma with basaloid features: a study of nine cases. Am J Surg Pathol 2002;26(4):413–20.

130. Fukuoka K, Hirokawa M, Shimizu M, et al. Basaloid type adenoid cystic carcinoma of the breast. APMIS 1999;107(8):762–6.

131. Hodgson NC, Lytwyn A, Bacopulos S, et al. Adenoid cystic breast carcinoma: high rates of margin positivity after breast conserving surgery. Am J Clin Oncol 2010;33(1):28–31.

132. Trojani M, de Mascarel I, Coindre JM. Adenoid cystic carcinoma of the breast. Value of immunohistochemical study in diagnosis. Tumori 1991;77(2):130–5.

133. Lamovec J, Us-Krasovec M, Zidar A, et al. Adenoid cystic carcinoma of the breast: a histologic, cytologic, and immunohistochemical study. Semin Diagn Pathol 1989;6(2):153–64.

134. Miettinen M, Lasota J. KIT (CD117): a review on expression in normal and neoplastic tissues, and mutations and their clinicopathologic correlation. Appl Immunohistochem Mol Morphol 2005;13(3):205–20.

135. Hill PA. c-kit expression in adenoid cystic carcinoma of the breast. Pathology 2004;36(4):362–4.

136. Trendell-Smith NJ, Peston D, Shousha S. Adenoid cystic carcinoma of the breast: a tumour commonly devoid of oestrogen receptors and related proteins. Histopathology 1999;35(3):241–8.

137. Ghabach B, Anderson WF, Curtis RE, et al. Adenoid cystic carcinoma of the breast in the United States (1977 to 2006): a population-based cohort study. Breast Cancer Res 2010;12(4):R54.

138. Vranic S, Gatalica Z, Deng H, et al. ER-α36, a novel isoform of ER-α66, is commonly over-expresed in apocrine and adenoid cystic carcinomas of the breast. J Clin Pathol 2011;64(1):54–7.

139. d'Ardenne AJ, Kirkpatrick P, Wells CA, et al. Laminin and fibronectin in adenoid cystic carcinoma. J Clin Pathol 1986;39(2):138–44.

140. Marchio C, Weigelt B, Reis-Filho JS. Adenoid cystic carcinomas of the breast and salivary glands (or 'The strange case of Dr Jekyll and Mr Hyde' of exocrine gland carcinomas). J Clin Pathol 2010;63(3):220–8.

141. Vranic S, Gurjeva O, Frkovic-Grazio S, et al. IMP3, a proposed novel basal phenotype marker, is commonly overexpressed in adenoid cystic carcinomas

but not in apocrine carcinomas of the breast. Appl Immunohistochem Mol Morphol 2011;19(5):413–6 [Epub ahead of print].

142. Sumpio BE, Jennings TA, Merino MJ, et al. Adenoid cystic carcinoma of the breast. Data from the Connecticut tumor registry and a review of the literature. Ann Surg 1987;205(3):295–301.

143. Albores-Saavedra J, Heard SC, McLaren B, et al. Cylindroma (dermal analog tumor) of the breast: a comparison with cylindroma of the skin and adenoid cystic carcinoma of the breast. Am J Clin Pathol 2005;123(6):866–73.

144. Nonaka D, Rosai J, Spagnolo D, et al. Cylindroma of the breast of skin adnexal type: a study of 4 cases. Am J Surg Pathol 2004;28(8):1070–5.

145. Mahmoud A, Hill DH, O'Sullivan MJ, et al. Cylindroma of the breast: a case report and review of the literature. Diagn Pathol 2009;4:30.

146. Page DL. Adenoid cystic carcinoma of breast, a special histopathologic type with excellent prognosis. Breast Cancer Res Treat 2005;93(3):189–90.

147. Arpino G, Clark GM, Mohsin S, et al. Adenoid cystic carcinoma of the breast: molecular markers, treatment, and clinical outcome. Cancer 2002; 94(8):2119–27.

148. Wells CA, Nicoll S, Ferguson DJ. Adenoid cystic carcinoma of the breast: a case with axillary lymph node metastasis. Histopathology 1986;10(4): 415–24.

149. Vranić S, Bilalović N, Lee LM, et al. PIK3CA and PTEN mutations in adenoid cystic carcinoma of the breast metastatic to kidney. Hum Pathol 2007; 38(9):1425–31.

150. Haddad RI, Posner MR, Busse PM, et al. Chemoradiotherapy for adenoid cystic carcinoma: preliminary results of an organ sparing approach. Am J Clin Oncol 2006;29(2):153–7.

151. Millar BA, Kerba M, Youngson B, et al. The potential role of breast conservation surgery and adjuvant breast radiation for adenoid cystic carcinoma of the breast. Breast Cancer Res Treat 2004;87(3): 225–32.

MOLECULAR CLASSIFICATION OF BREAST CANCER

Robin L. Jones, BSc, MB, MRCP[a],
Anastasia Constantinidou, MD, MSc, MRCP[b],
Jorge S. Reis-Filho, MD, PhD, FRCPath[c],*

KEYWORDS

• Molecular pathology • Breast cancer • Prognostic markers • Luminal types • Basal-like
• Normal breast–like • HER2-enriched • Claudin-low

ABSTRACT

This article reviews the conceptual and practical implications of the intrinsic subtype classification of breast cancers and the limitations of this approach. It presents the most extensively validated gene expression assays proposed as predictors of clinical outcome and discusses their potential clinical utility and limitations.

OVERVIEW

Breast cancer is a heterogeneous disease encompassing many distinct entities with variable biologic and clinical behavior and response to treatment. The management of breast cancer has been largely guided by a combination of clinical parameters (tumor size and nodal status) and pathologic features, including histologic type, grade, presence/absence of lymphovascular invasion, hormonal status, and human epidermal growth factor receptor 2 (HER2) status.[1,2] In recent years, advances in systemic treatment, including the refinement of chemotherapy regimens, the establishment of endocrine therapy in hormone receptor–positive cancers, and the addition of trastuzumab to the treatment of tumors with HER2 overexpression, have led to significant improvement in survival.[1,2] At the same time, the histopathologic classification of breast cancer has evolved with the latest World Health Organization classification (2003)[3] recognizing the existence of at least 18 distinct histologic subtypes, 17 of which are classified as "special subtypes" and account for 25% of all breast cancers.[4–6]

Over the past decade, the use of high-throughput microarray-based gene expression technology has shed light onto the biologic diversity of breast cancer and has led to a new classification through the identification of breast cancer subtypes with discrete gene expression patterns.[7–11] Five subtypes have been recognized[8–11]:

• Two of the 5 subtypes are derived largely from estrogen receptor (ER)-positive tumors: luminal A and luminal B subtypes.
• Three of the 5 subtypes are derived largely from ER-negative cancers: normal breast–like, basal-like, and HER2-enriched subtypes'.

The subtypes intrinsic biologic differences seem to be associated with both the clinical outcome and the response to treatment. The luminal A group is reported to carry the best prognosis whereas the HER2-enriched and the basal-like groups carry the worst prognosis despite better response to chemotherapy.[12] The impact of this taxonomy on

---

Disclosure: None declared.
[a] Division of Medical Oncology, Fred Hutchinson Cancer Research Center, University of Washington, 825 Eastlake Avenue East, G3630, Seattle, WA 98109-1023, USA
[b] Division of Molecular Pathology, Institute of Cancer Research, 15 Cotswold Road, Sutton SM2 5NG, United Kingdom
[c] Department of Pathology, Memorial Sloan-Kettering Cancer Center, 1275 York Ave, New York, NY 10065, United States
* Corresponding author.
E-mail address: jsreis@hotmail.com

Surgical Pathology 5 (2012) 701–717
http://dx.doi.org/10.1016/j.path.2012.06.008
1875-9181/12/$ – see front matter © 2012 Published by Elsevier Inc.

patients treated with current systemic therapy approaches, including trastuzumab for patients with HER2-positive disease, is yet to be determined.

In parallel with the class discovery studies, which unraveled the heterogeneity of breast cancers, several groups endeavored to identify multi-gene predictors (ie, gene signatures) that could predict the outcome of breast cancer patients. These supervised studies aimed to identify a group of breast cancer patients with such a good outcome that would allow oncologists to withhold chemotherapy. Despite the great initial expectations, the incorporation of microarrays into routine clinical practice has proved challenging, and validation of prognostic gene signatures in prospective clinical trials is ongoing.[1,13–18]

MOLECULAR SUBTYPES OF BREAST CANCER

In the original classification by Perou and colleagues,[7] 4 distinct subtypes were described:

1. Luminal
2. Basal-like
3. Normal breast–like
4. HER2-positive

In this seminal study of class discovery gene expression profiling, complementary DNA microarrays were used to identify gene expression patterns in 65 samples from 42 individuals, 38 of whom had primary invasive breast tumors (36 ductal and 2 lobular). The investigators selected 456 genes, called the "intrinsic gene list," all of which had a significantly higher variation between tumors from different patients than between samples from the same tumor or patient.[7] Using this intrinsic gene list, these investigators applied hierarchical cluster analysis, a technique that groups genes and samples according to similarities in their expression patterns, which revealed at least 4 molecular subtypes (luminal, basal-like, normal breast–like, and HER2-positive). The main contribution of this study and of the intrinsic gene classification was to bring to the forefront of cancer research the concepts that breast cancers are heterogeneous at the molecular level and that the transcriptomes of ER-positive and ER-negative breast cancers are fundamentally different.[1,16,17,19] Subsequent analysis divided the luminal group into subgroups (eg, luminal A and B or luminal A, B, and C), based on the expression of proliferation-related genes[8–11] (**Table 1**).

Apart from their differences at a molecular level, these groups also have differing epidemiologic, pathologic, and clinical features.[1,5,14,16,17,19] These descriptions, however, have largely been based on analysis of retrospective data sets, and advances in the therapy for some of these subgroups, such as the availability of tailored therapies for HER2 cancers (ie, addition of trastuzumab or lapatinib to chemotherapy), may significantly change their clinical outcome. Despite their distinct characteristics, the molecularly classified subtypes can be categorized into 2 large groups based on their ER expression status (ie, ER-positive and ER-negative groups), given the overwhelming transcriptomic differences between ER-positive and ER-negative disease.[13,14,16–18]

ER-POSITIVE GROUP: LUMINAL A AND B SUBTYPES

The luminal group is divided into 2 subtypes[8–11]:

1. Luminal A, a group corresponding mostly to ER-positive tumors of low histologic grade
2. Luminal B, also consisting of ER-positive tumors (although often expressing lower levels of hormone receptors), usually of high histologic grade, and consistently displaying high levels of expression of proliferation-related genes.[1,10,11,17,20,21]

The separation of the luminal group into 2 subgroups carries a prognostic significance with luminal A tumors associated with a good prognosis and luminal B tumors exhibiting more aggressive behavior compared with luminal A.[1,11,17,21] Another area of discrimination between 2 subtypes is their response to chemotherapy; although generally poor for both luminal subtypes, clinical and pathologic response to chemotherapy seems higher in luminal B cancers.[1] Despite this evidence supporting the distinct behavior of these 2 subtypes, there are several lines of evidence to demonstrate that luminal A and luminal B tumors constitute a continuum, given that their separation is primarily based on the levels of expression of proliferation-related genes, and that these genes display a normal rather than a bimodal distribution (ie, no natural cutoffs for the identification of luminal B cancers emerge).[16,19,21–23]

Despite the identification of subgroups of luminal cancers, there is no internationally accepted definition for these cancers, given that the assignment of tumors into luminal A or luminal B subgroups is strongly dependent on the methodology used.[23,24] In addition, microarrays not able to be readily applied to the analysis of formalin-fixed, paraffin-embedded samples have led several groups to devise their own surrogate markers for luminal A and luminal B cancers. None of the immunohistochemical surrogates put forward to date shows optimal concordance with the microarray definitions of luminal A and luminal B cancers.

ER-NEGATIVE GROUP: BASAL-LIKE, HER2-ENRICHED, AND NORMAL BREAST–LIKE SUBTYPES

Basal-Like

Breast cancers lacking HR receptors and expressing high molecular weight (basal) cytokeratins have long been identified by pathologists[5,25]; however, interest in these tumors re-emerged with the identification of the basal-like intrinsic subgroup.[7,26] Basal-like cancers comprise a heterogeneous group of tumors, which are more prevalent in young women and those of African American and Hispanic descent.[26–28] As a group, the clinical behavior of basal-like cancers is more aggressive than that of ER-positive cancers and comparable to that of HER2-positive cancers; however, there are special histologic types of breast cancer that consistently display a basal-like phenotype (eg, adenoid cystic carcinomas and secretory carcinomas), which have a remarkably indolent clinical course.[4,5] Basal-like cancers have a higher propensity for visceral metastases[29,30] and they carry a poor prognosis despite sensitivity to chemotherapy.[31–33]

Some of the known prognostic markers for breast cancers in general seem to have distinct impact on the outcome of patients with basal-like disease. For instance, it has been reported that even small, node-negative, basal-like tumors have poor survival.[26,34,35] Furthermore, neither an association between tumor size and lymph node metastasis nor an association between tumor size and outcome is found in patients with basal-like cancers.[26,34,35]

On histologic examination, these tumors have a pushing margin, lymphocytic infiltrate, and central necrotic zones.[36–38] They are associated with high mitotic rate and high levels of expression of proliferation-related genes[21,22] and, in more than 90%, they have high grade.[26,28] They are characterized by a specific gene expression profile of high molecular weight cytokeratins, including CK5/6 and CK17 but they may also express genes characteristic of luminal epithelia, such as CK8/18, although at lower levels than the luminal subtypes. They may also express high levels of other markers usually found in normal basal/myoepithelial cells,[26,28] including caveolins 1 and 2,[39,40] vimentin,[37] nestin,[41] CD44,[42] and fascin.[43] More than 60% of basal-like tumors show high expression levels of epidermal growth factor receptor[39,44] and more than 90% of cases harbor TP53 gene mutations.[26,28,45]

The morphologic and immunohistochemical features of basal-like tumors are similar to tumors arising in BRCA1 mutation carriers, and the prevalence of TP53 mutations observed in basal-like tumors is similar to that found in breast cancers from BRCA1 mutation carriers.[45] Two independent conditional mouse models have demonstrated that inactivation of Trp53 and Brca1 in either luminal progenitor cells[46] or basal cells[47] of the mouse mammary gland led to the development of cancers with basal-like phenotype. Taken together, there are several lines of evidence that are consistent with the hypothesis that nonhereditary basal-like cancers may constitute phenocopies of tumors arising in BRCA1 mutation carriers.[48]

HER2-Enriched Subtype

The HER2 gene is overexpressed in approximately 15% of invasive breast tumors. More than 80% are characterized by HER2 3+ expression at immunohistochemical analysis or display HER2 gene amplification. It should be emphasized, however, that the microarray-defined HER2-enriched subtype is not equivalent to the group of tumors identified as HER2-positive by Food and Drug Administration (FDA)-approved methods following the American Society of Clinical Oncology/College of American Pathologists guidelines[49] for HER2 assessment.[11,23,50] Parker and colleagues[11] showed that there is discrepancy between the clinical and the molecular classification of these tumors. Of 33 HER2 tumors, only 64% were classified as HER2-enriched by gene expression and 6% were classified as basal-like. In addition, 9% of the HER2-negative tumors were classified as HER2-enriched. de Ronde and colleagues[50] subjected a series of tumors from 195 patients treated with neoadjuvant chemotherapy to microarray-based gene expression profiling; immunohistochemistry analysis of ER, progesterone receptor (PR), and HER2; and assessment of HER2 gene amplification using in situ methods. These investigators observed that most but not all cases classified as of HER2-enriched subtype by microarray analysis were HER2-positive by immunohistochemistry and in situ hybridization. It was also observed that the majority of tumors classified by FDA-approved methods as HER2-positive were classified by microarrays as of an intrinsic subtype other than HER2 enriched.

Taken together, although HER2-enriched tumors have been shown to have a worse outcome than ER-positive cancers,[11] its predictive significance is not clear. At this stage, there are no data to support the use of trastuzumab for patients with tumors classified as HER2-enriched but

Table 1
Molecular and histopathological features of the breast cancer subtypes defined by expression profiling

Molecular Subtype	ER/PR/HER2/ MIB1[a]	Histologic Grade	Basal Markers [b]	Other Markers	Proliferation Cluster	TP53 Mutations	Outcome[c]	Special Points
Luminal A	ER+ PR+ HER2− MIB1 low	Low	−		Low	Low	Good	Distinction from the luminal B subtype is strongly dependent on the microarray definition used.
Luminal B	ER± [a] PR± HER2−/+ MIB1 high	Intermediate/ high	−		High	Intermediate	Intermediate	Distinction from the luminal A subtype is strongly dependent on the microarray definition used.
Basal-like	ER− PR− HER2− MIB1 high	High	+		High	High	Poor	A minority of tumors may express low levels of ER or harbor HER2 amplification.
HER2+/ER−	ER− PR−/+ HER2−/+ MIB1 high	High	±		High	High	Poor	This subtype does not equate with the clinically defined HER2−amplified subtype.
Molecular apocrine	ER− PR− HER2± MIB1 high[c]	Intermediate/ high	±	AR+	High	Intermediate/ high[c]	Poor	These tumors have apocrine features on histologic examination but do not meet the strict histologic criteria for apocrine cancers; therefore, the term, *molecular apocrine*.

Claudin-low	ER− PR− HER2− MIB1 intermediate	High	±	*CDH1* low/− *CLDN* low/−	High	High[c]	Intermediate	At the transcriptomic level, these tumors lack expression of E-cadherin + claudins. However, 55% and 41% of these tumors display moderate to strong protein expression of E-cadherin and/or claudins, respectively. This subtype is reported to be enriched for cells with a cancer stem cell–like phenotype and cells displaying features of epithelial to mesenchymal transition.
Normal breast-like	ER−/+ PR unknown HER2− MIB1 low	Low	+		Low	Low	Intermediate	This subtype may be an artifact due procurement of tissue samples with disproportionately high stromal content.

Abbreviations: AR, androgen receptor; CDH1, E-cadherin; CLDN, claudin; −, negative; +, positive; ±, predominantly positive; −/+, predominantly negative.

[a] Considering the majority of tumors.
[b] Basal markers: CK5, CK6, and epidermal growth factor receptor.
[c] Hypothetical.

Modified from Weigelt B, Baehner FL, Reis-Filho JS. The contribution of gene expression profiling to breast cancer classification, prognostication and prediction: a retrospective of the last decade. J Pathol 2010;220:263–80.

lacking *HER2* gene amplification/protein overexpression nor are there data to support withholding trastuzumab in patients with tumors displaying *HER2* gene amplification/protein overexpression but classified as of a molecular subtype other than HER2-enriched by microarray gene expression profiling.

Normal Breast–Like

The normal breast–like tumors are yet to be fully characterized and their clinical importance remains unclear. There are several lines of evidence to demonstrate that most if not all normal breast–like cancers constitute artifacts of tissue procurement, namely, samples with a disproportionately high content of stromal and normal breast epithelial cells.[11,16,17,20]

Molecular Apocrine, Claudin-Low, and Interferon-Rich Subtypes

In the past 5 years, additional subtypes of ER-negative cancers have emerged from subsequent microarray-based class discovery studies, namely, molecular apocrine, claudin-low, and interferon-rich (see **Table 1**).

The molecular apocrine subtype was first described by Farmer and colleagues[51] in a study of 49 tumor samples, which were divided into basal, luminal, and molecular apocrine groups based on microarray analysis and hierarchical clustering. Molecular apocrine tumors are androgen receptor–positive and display *HER2* amplification more commonly than the luminal and basal-like subtypes.[52] An independent study identified a subgroup of breast cancers with transcriptomic characteristics remarkably similar to those of molecular aprocrine tumors.[52] Although they have strong apocrine features on histologic examination (including abundant eosinophilic cytoplasm and prominent nucleoli), they do not meet the strict histopathologic criteria for apocrine carcinomas, hence, the term, *molecular apocrine tumors*.[51] These tumors seem to harbor an active androgen receptor pathway and recent data have suggested that these cancers are likely sensitive to androgen receptor targeting.[53]

The claudin-low subtype constitutes a recently identified group of ER-negative tumors characterized by high levels of expression of genes involved in epithelial-to-mesenchymal transition, including vimentin, Snail-1, Snail-2, TWIST1, TWIST2, ZEB1, and ZEB2, and down-regulation of genes involved in cell adhesion (eg, E-cadherin and claudins 3, 4, and 7).[54] These tumors were also shown to display stem cell–like features (such as high

expression of CD44/CD24 and CD2/CD24). These observations have led to the suggestion that claudin-low tumors may originate from more primitive precursor cells than the basal-like and luminal subtypes.[54,55] Some questions, however, in regards to the identification of these tumors, remain controversial, given that a substantial proportion of tumors classified as of claudin-low phenotype were formally classified as of normal breast–like phenotype using previous algorithms to classify breast cancers into the intrinsic subtypes[54]; hence, it remains to be determined whether these samples were not classified into the claudin-low subtype due to the contamination with stromal cells, which also express mesenchymal genes and usually display low levels of expression of claudins. Furthermore, at the transcriptomic level, claudin-low tumors are reported to lack or display low levels of expression of E-cadherin and claudins; surprisingly, however, 55% and 41% of tumors classified as of claudin-low phenotype by microarrays displayed moderate-to-strong expression of E-cadherin and claudin 3, respectively, at the protein level.

The interferon-rich subtype was identified in 2006 during a validation study of a breast cancer gene intrinsic classification by Hu and colleagues.[10] This subtype is characterized by high expression of interferon-regulated genes, including *STAT1*, a transcription factor responsible for mediating interferon regulation of gene expression. No further descriptions of this molecular subtype have been made since the original report. A subgroup of ER-positive tumors, however, characterized by high levels of expression of immune response-related genes, has been identified by independent groups.[19,22,56,57] These tumors, in a way akin to interferon-rich cancers, have been shown to have an outcome better than that of basal-like cancers.

The impact of the identification of these 3 subtypes (and perhaps the characterization of other, rare, yet unknown subtypes) on clinical management and decision making is yet be defined. At present, the identification of these molecular subtypes in pathology reports is not recommended.[57,58]

LIMITATIONS OF THE INTRINSIC SUBTYPE CLASSIFICATION

In the past few years, several experts in the field of microarrays have suggested that the current classification of breast cancers based on clinicopathologic features and immunohistochemical markers should be replaced by the intrinsic molecular taxonomy.[20,59]

The development of a microarray-based, gene expression–defined, molecular classification in breast cancer constituted a paradigm shift in the way breast cancer is perceived as a disease.[1,17,19,57,58] It has been revealed that breast cancer is not a single disease with subgroups but rather a collection of different diseases that affect the same anatomic site and originate in the same microanatomic structure and that ER-positive and ER-negative diseases are fundamentally different. These conceptual changes have contributed to unraveling the underlying biology of breast cancer and have the potential of revolutionizing the way breast cancer is managed in the future.

The classification of tumors into intrinsic subtypes has, however, important limitations.[16,19,23,58]

INTRINSIC CLASSIFICATION MAY NOT INCLUDE ALL BREAST CANCERS

One of the most important issues relates to molecular subtypes included in the intrinsic classification that may not include all breast cancers.[17,19,51,52,57] The majority of microarray-based gene expression profiling studies have used invasive ductal or lobular carcinoma samples.[7,8] The so-called special histologic breast types (which, among others, include tubular, medullary, mucinous, apocrine, metaplastic, and adenoid cystic carcinomas) have not been assessed and, therefore, are not sufficiently represented in this classification.[4,5,17] More recent studies, however, have demonstrated that this classification can be applied to special histopathologic subtypes, and most of these types consistently display one molecular phenotype. For example, metaplastic and medullary carcinomas display a basal-like group phenotype and tubular and mucinous carcinomas a luminal phenotype.[60]

INTRINSIC CLASSIFICATION CANNOT CLASSIFY INDIVIDUAL SAMPLES

The intrinsic subtype classification system was devised based on the identification of the molecular subtypes using hierarchic clustering analysis. This approach requires large data sets, is to some extent subjective, and cannot be used for the classification of individual samples prospectively.[14,61] To allow for the classification of individual tumors into the intrinsic subtypes, microarray single sample predictors (SSPs) were developed.[9–11] These single sample predictors are based on the correlation between the expression profile of a given sample with the centroids for each molecular subtype (ie, average expression profile of each molecular subtype). From 2003 to 2009, 3 distinct SSPs were developed.[9–11] One of these single sample predictors[11] was the basis for the development of a quantitative reverse transcriptase–polymerase chain reaction (qRT-PCR)-based or NanoString-based method (PAM50) that can be used to classify formalin-fixed, paraffin-embedded samples into the molecular subtypes.

The authors[23] and other investigators[24,62] have demonstrated that variations in the methodology for data normalization and centering, as well as in the proportion of samples from each of the subtypes, lead to changes in the classification of samples using SSPs. Independent groups have demonstrated that the classification of tumors into the molecular subtypes other than basal-like breast cancers is dependent on the SSP used.[23,24] When Sorlie's group[63] and Perou's group[64] independently classified the samples from a cohort of 295 breast cancers using the SSPs from Sorlie and colleagues[9] and Hu and colleagues,[10] the agreement was modest (ie, only 64% of the samples were classified in the same fashion; κ statistic = 0.527).[23]

Although there is a great enthusiasm with the use of this molecular taxonomy for clinical trial design and routine oncology practice,[20,59] several issues need to be taken into consideration. First, the subclassification of luminal tumors into A and B is strongly dependent on the SSP used[23] and is mainly based on the expression of proliferation-related genes,[21] which are distributed in a continuum rather than in a bimodal pattern.[16,21,23,58,65] The subclassification of ER-positive breast cancers into subtypes with distinct clinical behavior is not only a challenge for the intrinsic subtype classification. Because proliferation is distributed in a continuum in ER-positive cancers and that proliferation is a strong determinant of outcome in this group of tumors,[22] consequently the assignment of ER-positive breast cancers into good or poor prognosis using first-generation signatures (eg, MammaPrint and 76-gene assay; discussed later) or into low, intermediate, or high histologic grade is to some extent arbitrary.[16,19,57] Second, normal breast–like cancers are likely to constitute artifacts of frozen tissue procurement (ie, samples with a disproportionately high content of normal breast and stromal cells).[16,17,19,57] Third, the HER2-enriched subtype, as defined by microarrays, does not encompasses all cases classified as HER2-positive with FDA-approved methods, and not all HER2-positive cancers by clinical methods are classified as HER2-enriched subtype by microarrays.[11,50]

From a conceptual standpoint, the histogenetic implications of the intrinsic molecular subtypes put forward (ie, basal-like cancers stem from basal/progenitor cells and luminal cancers originate from luminal or luminal progenitor cells) have been called into question.[46,66] The assumption that different subtypes of breast cancer originate from different cell types is not supported by recent studies,[46,66,67] which have demonstrated that the likeliest cell of origin of basal-like breast cancers pertains to the luminal progenitor population rather than the basal or stem cell population of the normal breast. In addition, the reported enrichment for the so-called cancer stem cells in claudin-low tumors should be interpreted with caution, given the lack of standardization of the markers for the identification of breast cancer stem cells.

These observations do not invalidate the existence of the intrinsic subtypes. The authors agree with Perou and colleagues[68] and Ellis and colleagues[69] that the intrinsic subtype classification is an evolving system and that PAM50 rather the microarray-derived SSPs should be used for the identification of the intrinsic subtypes. Retrospective testing of this assay in material from prospective clinical studies has demonstrated that it is prognostic[59,69]; however, its predictive power remains to be defined.

GENE EXPRESSION PROFILING PROGNOSTIC ASSAYS

Traditionally, clinicopathologic parameters, such as tumor size, lymph node burden, tumor grade, HR, and HER2 status, have determined prognostic predictions and adjuvant therapy for patients with breast cancer.[1,2,5,16,17] Adjuvant! Online is a popular computerized tool, developed a decade ago,[70] to aid clinical decision making by using such parameters. This system has proved a valuable asset to clinicians managing early breast cancer worldwide, providing easily applicable markers of outcome for the majority of patients. Its prognostic power has been validated by independent groups.[71,72] At present, however, a large proportion of patients are treated with adjuvant chemotherapy and consequently exposed to the related cost and toxicity, yet may not benefit from this therapy. The role of Adjuvant! Online is limited by several factors, including the overestimation of overall survival for patients aged younger than 35[73] and the inability to incorporate some parameters, such as the HER2 status or the presence/absence of lymphovascular invasion, to its current form. Adjuvant! Online only provides prognostic information for an "average patient" with a given constellation of clinicopathologic features, which

may not necessarily be applicable to a given individual patient.

Over the past decade, several gene expression profiling assays have been developed in an attempt to predict the outcome of breast cancer patients more accurately and to guide individualization of therapy.[1,16,17,57,74–77] The development of these techniques has been based on the identification of prognostic gene signatures using microarrays. Two different strategies have been used to derive these signatures: the top-down (also known as supervised or empiric) approach, where the clinical outcome is already known and, therefore, incorporated in the development of the predictor or gene signature, and the bottom-up (also known as hypothesis-driven) approach, where the predictor or gene signature is defined by in vitro or in vivo experiments and is subsequently tested in the clinical setting for its predictive or prognostic role.

In most of these approaches, the heterogeneity of breast cancer at the molecular level was not taken into account. Given that the expression of genes related to proliferation and ER signaling, and to a lesser extent, immune response have been shown to be associated with the outcome of breast cancer patients, it is not surprising that this first generation of prognostic signatures resulted in algorithms that classify ER-negative cancers and highly proliferative ER-positive cancers as of poor prognosis.[1,16,17,21,22,57] Despite these caveats, some prognostic gene signatures have been shown to constitute independent predictors of outcome in multiple studies. Contrary to initial claims, which envisaged that prognostic signatures would replace prognostic algorithms based on clinicopathologic parameters,[75,78] several studies have shown that these prognostic signatures are complementary to important clinicopathologic parameters, such as tumor size and presence of lymph node metastasis.[1,16,17,21,22,57]

The first-generation prognostic signatures that have been subjected to the most extensive validation are discussed. Table 2 summarizes the characteristics of first-generation prognostic signatures.[74–77,79–82]

70-GENE ASSAY (MAMMAPRINT)

The 70-gene assay (MammaPrint) was the first breast cancer prognostic signature described[75] by researchers in the Netherlands Cancer Institute in 2002 using the top-down approach. Fresh frozen tissue was obtained from a selected group of 78 patients younger than 55 years old with node-negative disease and tumor sizes less than or equal to 5 cm. A 70-gene prognostic assay

Table 2
Breast cancer prognostic multigene signatures that are commercially available or in commercial development

Signature	Oncotype DX	MammaPrint	Veridex 76-Gene	Theros/MGI	Gemomic Grade Index
Study population	ER+, N0, and up to 3 N+, TAM or AI treated	ER+ and ER−, N0, <5-cm diameter, age <55 years	ER+ and ER−	ER+, N0	ER+ and ER−, N0 and N+
Assay	21-Gene RS	70-Gene signature	76-Gene signature	2-Gene HOXB13:IL17R/ MGI	97-Gene signature/ 8-gene PCR
Platform	RT-PCR	Microarray (Agilent)	Microarray (Affymetrix)	RT-PCR	Microarray (Affymetrix)/ RT-PCR
Tissue type	FFPE	Frozen or stabilized mRNA	Frozen	FFPE	Frozen/FFPE
Prognostic value in other populations	ER+ and 1–3 N+, ER+ postmenopausal receiving AI	Age 55–70 years, 1–3 N+, N0, and N+, HER2+	—	—	ER+ receiving aromatase inhibitors
Predictive value	Neoadjuvant and adjuvant CT[90] (high RS), response to TAM (low RS)	Neoadjuvant and adjuvant CT (poor signature)	Response to TAM (high-risk patients)	Resistance to TAM (high ratio)	Response to neoadjuvant CT (high risk)
Indication	Prediction of recurrence risk in ER+ and N0 BC treated with TAM	Prognostic in N0, <5-cm diameter, stage I/II BC, age <61 years	Prognostic in ER+ BC	Prognostic in ER+ BC, prediction of response to TAM	Molecular grading, for ER+, histologic grade II BC
Level of evidence	II	III	III	III	III
FDA approval	No	Yes	No	No	No
Randomized trial	TAILORx	MINDACT	—	—	—
Commercially available/ provider	Yes/Genomic Health	Yes/Agendia BV	No/Johnson & Johnson	Yes/bioTheranostic	Yes/Ipsogen
Availability	Europe and USA	Europe and USA	—	USA	Europe

For the description and reviews of Theros and Gemomic grade index, please see references.[79–82]

Abbreviations: AI, aromatase inhibitor; BC, breast cancer; CT, chemotherapy; FFPE, formalin-fixed, paraffin-embedded; MGI, molecular grade index; N, lymph nodes (0 or +); TAM, tamoxifen.

Adapted from Colombo PE, Milanezi F, Weigelt B, et al. Microarrays in the 2010s: the contribution of microarray-based gene expression profiling to breast cancer classification, prognostication and prediction. Breast Cancer Res 2011;13:212.

was defined by comparing the gene expression profiling of tumors from patients who relapsed within 5 years (poor prognosis group) and those who did not (good prognosis group).[75] This profile was validated in a subsequent study by the same group of researchers, where the gene signatures of 295 patients younger than 53 years old, with either node-positive disease (144 patients) or node-negative disease (151 patients), were included.[74] On multivariate analysis, this study confirmed that the 70-gene signature was a strong independent predictor of the likelihood of distant metastases (hazard ratio [HR] 4.6; 95% CI, 2.3–9.2, $P<.001$). These results, however, may constitute an overestimation of the prognostic power of the signature, given 64 patients from the original study were included in the validation study. A further validation study, however, including 307 patients aged 60 years or less, with node-negative disease, who did not receive adjuvant therapy, also confirmed this gene signature as a reliable predictor of recurrence and survival[83]; however, it did demonstrate the time dependency of this gene signature (ie, the ability of the 70-gene signature to identify patients who will develop distant relapse is greatest within 5 years of diagnosis and is somewhat reduced after 5 years). A comparison between the 70-gene signature and Adjuvant! Online revealed discordant results in 87 out of 302 cases (29%). In 68% of the discordant cases, patients were classified as high risk according to the Adjuvant! Online program and low risk according to the gene signature profile whereas 32% where classified as low risk on clinical grounds but high risk on gene signature grounds. Of the 2 methods, the gene signature profile was the one to predict the outcome more accurately.

After the publication of the previously discussed and subsequent studies, the 70-gene prognostic assay became the first microarray-based assay to be approved by the FDA to help define the prognosis and individualize therapy for patients aged younger than 61 years, with node-negative disease, tumor size of less than 5 cm, and stage I or II. The prognostic power of the 70-gene signature was only demonstrated in retrospective analyses of retrospectively accrued cohorts of breast cancer patients (ie, level III evidence). To address this issue, this assay is being assessed in a prospective study of 6000 patients, the Microarray in Node-Negative 1 to 3 Positive Lymph Node Disease May Avoid Chemotherapy (MINDACT) trial, in which 6000 patients will be tested with the 70-gene signature assay.[18] The expression profile results will be compared with the clinicopathologic characteristics and patients with concordant results will be treated according to their risk status (good prognosis vs poor prognosis) whereas patients with discordant results will be randomized to treatment according to either the gene signature or the clinicopathologic features. Patient accrual has taken longer than originally anticipated, but it is approaching completion.

The contribution of this 70-gene assay in predicting the clinical benefit from adjuvant chemotherapy has been shown in several studies, including a meta-analysis of 1637 patients where 47% of patients were categorized as high risk for recurrence and 53% as low risk. Patients with poor prognosis according to the 70-gene classifier seemed to benefit significantly from treatment with chemotherapy whereas patients with good prognosis did not.[84]

Limitations to the clinical application of the 70-gene assay are mainly associated with the requirement of fresh frozen tissue samples, the level of evidence available to support its prognostic impact (level III), and the difficulty of incorporating some of its results in clinical practice at present.[16,17,57,58] With regards to the accuracy, it seems that this may be time dependent and it should be used as a predictor of early rather than late relapse.[83] Furthermore, this signature has negligible discriminatory power in patients with ER-negative disease (ie, only 0%–4% of patients with ER-negative tumors are classified as of good prognosis[71,83,85,86]) and the best therapeutic options for patients with HER2-positive breast cancers classified as of good prognosis have yet to be defined.[85–87]

76-GENE ASSAY

This is another top-down approach also developed in 2005 in the Netherlands[76]: seventy-six genes were identified (60 from ER-positive patients and 16 from ER-negative patients) in a microarray analysis of 115 tumors. An independent test set of 171 patients with node-negative disease showed this gene assay is a strong prognostic factor for the development of distant metastasis within 5 years. Subsequent validating studies, however, showed that a major limitation of this assay is that it is time dependent.[18,22] Furthermore, when the 16-gene set of this assay was applied to 71 ER-negative patients in a study by Krieke and colleagues,[88] there was no correlation between gene expression and outcome, suggesting that the predicting ability of the 16 gene set may be limited.

Akin to the 70-gene signature, the 76-gene signature requires fresh frozen samples and has negligible discriminatory power in patients with ER-negative disease, and its prognostic value is strongly time dependent and only supported by level III evidence.[16,17,57,58]

21-GENE ASSAY (ONCOTYPE DX)

Concurrently with the development of microarray-based prognostic signatures, Paik and colleagues[89] developed Oncotype DX (Genomic Health, Redwood City, California), a qRT-PCR–based analysis of 21 genes (16 cancer-related and 5 reference genes) that can be performed with RNA extracted from formalin-fixed, paraffin-embedded tissue samples. The expression of these genes is presented as a single recurrence score (RS) (continuous variable, with score 0–100), which is a measure of the risk of distant relapse within 10 years and can be used for risk stratification of ER-positive, node-negative breast cancers from patients treated with adjuvant tamoxifen. This score divides patients in 3 categories according to their risk of recurrence: low risk (RS <18), intermediate risk (RS 18–31), and high risk (RS ≥31). A retrospective analysis of 668 tumor blocks from node-negative patients treated with tamoxifen within the National Surgical Adjuvant Breast and Bowel Project B-14 trial, demonstrated an association between the RS and distant relapse with low-risk, intermediate-risk, and high-risk groups presenting 10-year relapse rates of 7%, 14%, and 30%, respectively. In addition, the RS seems to correlate with response to adjuvant chemotherapy: patients with ER-positive disease and low RS have low risk of recurrence and limited benefit from adjuvant chemotherapy whereas patients with ER-positive disease and high RS have high risk of recurrence and greater benefit from chemotherapy.[90] The management of the intermediate-risk group remains an issue of debate and it is currently addressed in the Trial Assigning Individualized Options for Treatment (TAILORx). In this trial, patients with ER-positive, node-negative breast cancer are assessed for risk of relapse after surgery and assigned to low-risk (RS <11), intermediate-risk (RS 11–25), and high-risk groups (RS >25). Patients with intermediate risk are then offered either hormonal therapy alone or in combination with chemotherapy.

Subsequent retrospective analyses of material from prospective clinical trials have validated the prognostic power of OncotypeDx for patients with ER-positive disease treated with aromatase inhibitors[91] and for patients with ER-positive breast cancers with up to 3 positive lymph nodes[92] (reviewed by Kim and Paik[93]).

When the prognostic utility of Oncotype DX is compared with that of the clinicopathologic parameters in ER-positive node-negative breast cancer, it becomes clear that although the accuracy of the RS of Oncotype DX in predicting relapse seems higher than the associated clinicopathologic parameters, the information it provides cannot replace these parameters entirely.[58,94,95]

Given that Oncotype Dx can be applied to formalin-fixed, paraffin-embedded tissue samples, level I evidence for its prognostic and predictive power has been accrued through retrospective analyses of the samples from multiple prospective clinical trials. Therefore, it should not come as a surprise that the National Comprehensive Cancer Network has included Oncotype DX in its guidelines not only as a predictor of recurrence but also as a useful guide for treatment decision making in early ER-positive, node-negative breast cancer. Oncotype DX assay is also included in the American Society of Clinical Oncology guidelines as a tumor marker of recurrence.[1,17] The St Gallen International Expert Consensus on the Primary Therapy of Early Breast Cancer recommends that a validated assay (such as Oncotype DX) should be considered as an adjunct to high-quality pathology phenotyping if there is doubt about the indication of chemotherapy after consideration of other factors.[96]

FIRST-GENERATION PROGNOSTIC GENE SIGNATURES: ARE THEY READY FOR CLINICAL PRACTICE?

First-generation signatures undoubtedly provide powerful information for outcome prediction; however, with the exception of OncotypeDx, they are yet to be incorporated into clinical practice. At present, there is no first-generation microarray-based prognostic signature supported by level I evidence for its prognostic power.[1,17,57] Although the MINDACT trial may provide the required level of evidence for MammaPrint, its use in clinical practice is likely to prove challenging given the fresh frozen tissue requirement.

Several studies have demonstrated that the lists of genes comparing the first generation signatures are unstable and that multiple signatures with equivalent prognostic power can be identified in a given data set.[97,98] Meta-analyses have demonstrated that despite the negligible overlap in their constituent genes, first-generation signatures have similar performance and show a good concordance in their prognostic classification, identifying similar but not identical subgroups of patients with poor prognosis.[21,64,99]

The prognostic power of first-generation prognostic signatures to determine prognosis seems primarily related to the assessment of proliferation-related/cell-cycle–related genes.[16,21,22,57] Some investigators have argued that these first-generation signatures are nothing but mere surrogates of proliferation.[16,21,58] This observation provides a rationale for several of the limitations of prognostic signatures.

1. First, proliferation has been shown prognostic only in ER-positive disease and not in ER-negative cancers; hence, it is not surprising that the discriminatory power of first-generation signatures is almost restricted to patients with ER-positive and HER2-negative breast cancers.[1,16,17,19,57]

2. Second, given that the expression level of proliferation-related genes in ER-positive cancers has been demonstrated to constitute a continuum rather than a bimodal distribution, the subdivision of ER-positive cancers into good and poor prognosis groups is artificial.[16,21,22,57,58] The only first-generation prognostic signature to take this finding into account was Oncotype Dx; the continuous nature of the RS derived from this signature is more representative of the ranges of prognosis of patients with ER-positive disease.

3. Third, as discussed previously, the prognostic power of first-generation prognostic signatures seems to be time dependent (ie, optimal predictions at approximately 5 years of follow-up), with a reduced prognostic value after 5 to 10 years.[65,83] Therefore, these signatures may represent early distant recurrence surrogates, which are unable to predict late relapses with the same accuracy. Thus, an unmet clinical need is present in that there are no gene signatures that can identify patients with a higher risk of late relapse after 10 years of follow-up. This is particularly relevant given after 8 years of follow-up; the risk of distant relapse of patients with ER-positive disease is higher than that of patients with ER-negative breast cancers.[100]

4. Finally, first-generation signatures do not constitute a replacement for current clinicopathologic parameters for the management of breast cancer patients. Clinicopathologic variables have been shown to add prognostic information independent of that offered by first-generation signatures.[1,16,57,58] Therefore, these gene signatures are perhaps best perceived as ancillary tools that complement current methods based on the clinicopathologic features of the tumors rather than a replacement for them.[1,16,58]

The prognostic information provided by first-generation signatures in addition to that provided by current clinicopathologic parameters and immunohistochemical markers seems limited, given that when clinicopathologic parameters are analyzed in a centralized fashion with standardized methods (ie, central and standardized reassessment of histologic grade, ER, PR, HER2, and proliferation rate as defined by Ki67 immunohistochemical analysis),[94] first-generation prognostic signatures provide minimal additional prognostic information. Therefore, the contribution of first-generation signatures beyond histologic and immunohistochemical assessment of tumors remains to be determined.[58]

Recently, second-generation signatures, specific for the distinct subtypes of breast cancers, have been reported studying breast cancer microenvironment or host immune response.[56,101,102] Immune response–related signatures have been shown to be potential prognosticators in ER-negative breast cancers or triple-negative breast cancers.[56,103,104] Although promising, because they are able to identify a group of ER-negative or ER-negative/HER2-negative breast cancer patients with good prognosis, it is unclear whether the risk of distant relapses in the good prognosis group would be sufficiently low for patients classified as good prognosis to forgo adjuvant chemotherapy.[19,57] Additional evidence in support of the use of these signatures as potential predictors of outcome is still required.

PREDICTIVE SIGNATURES

The issue of multigene classifiers predictive of response to specific therapeutic agents is beyond the scope of this review and is discussed elsewhere.[57,105] Several signatures designed to predict response to specific chemotherapy agents or regimens have been developed, mainly through supervised microarray analyses of cohorts of breast cancer treated in the neoadjuvant and/or metastatic setting. These signatures, however, have not been translated into diagnostic tests for several reasons, including heterogeneous patient populations and therapies as well as small sample sizes with inadequate validation (reviewed by Borst and Wessels[105]). Articles describing some of the most promising predictive signatures derived from the analysis of cancer cell lines have recently been withdrawn.[105] Despite the limited success of first-generation predictive signatures, more recent studies have demonstrated that by combining predictive gene signatures, prediction of response to anthracycline-based chemotherapy[106] and anthracycline-taxane–based regimens[107] may be possible.

SUMMARY

The past decade has resulted in a dramatic change in the perception and understating of breast cancer. The seminal gene expression studies by the Stanford group[7-11] confirmed that breast cancer is a collection of different diseases. These findings have had far-reaching effects with substantial alteration in the design and implementation of breast cancer research. As with other malignancies, identifying the molecular drivers of these diseases will lead not only to a better understating of the biology but also potentially to improved therapies. The unraveling of the biologic diversity of breast cancer has not only provided insight into the molecular mechanisms of disease but has also had practical consequences. Clinical trials should be conducted with greater precision and less cost rather than applying the one-size-fits-all approach of the past. Despite these conceptual advancements, microarray-based gene expression profiling only provided incremental improvements in the ability to predict the outcome and response to specific therapies. It could be argued that first-generation prognostic signatures only constitute a reproducible and quantitative analysis of tumor cell proliferation. Furthermore, it has become clear that the first-generation prognostic gene signatures provide information that is complementary to and not a replacement for that provided by current prognostic algorithms based on clinicopathologic features. The enthusiasm for the use of microarrays in clinical practice has waned somewhat; however, the breast cancer research community ought to learn from the lessons from microarray studies in the past decade in terms of disease heterogeneity, study design, and validation of molecular classifiers.

With the advent of next-generation sequencing and the ability to characterize the entire repertoire of mutations, gene copy number aberrations, and somatic rearrangements of a cancer in a single experiment,[108,109] the opportunities for the development of more accurate prognostic and predictive tests for each subgroup/subtype of breast cancers are unprecedented; however, the challenges that will have to be faced are also formidable. It is anticipated that this time, the information provided by pathology will be taken into account in the design of studies aiming to unravel the drivers of this complex and heterogeneous group of diseases.

REFERENCES

1. Sotiriou C, Pusztai L. Gene-expression signatures in breast cancer. N Engl J Med 2009;360:790–800.

2. Weigel MT, Dowsett M. Current and emerging biomarkers in breast cancer: prognosis and prediction. Endocr Relat Cancer 2010;17:R245–62.

3. Tumours of the Breast and Female Genital Organs. Oxford [Oxfordshire]: Oxford University Press 2003.

4. Weigelt B, Geyer FC, Reis-Filho JS. Histological types of breast cancer: how special are they? Mol Oncol 2010;4:192–208.

5. Weigelt B, Reis-Filho JS. Histological and molecular types of breast cancer: is there a unifying taxonomy? Nat Rev Clin Oncol 2009;6:718–30.

6. Bombonati A, Sgroi DC. The molecular pathology of breast cancer progression. J Pathol 2011;223: 307–17.

7. Perou CM, Sorlie T, Eisen MB, et al. Molecular portraits of human breast tumours. Nature 2000; 406:747–52.

8. Sorlie T, Perou CM, Tibshirani R, et al. Gene expression patterns of breast carcinomas distinguish tumor subclasses with clinical implications. Proc Natl Acad Sci U S A 2001;98:10869–74.

9. Sorlie T, Tibshirani R, Parker J, et al. Repeated observation of breast tumor subtypes in independent gene expression data sets. Proc Natl Acad Sci U S A 2003;100:8418–23.

10. Hu Z, Fan C, Oh DS, et al. The molecular portraits of breast tumors are conserved across microarray platforms. BMC Genomics 2006;7:96.

11. Parker JS, Mullins M, Cheang MC, et al. Supervised risk predictor of breast cancer based on intrinsic subtypes. J Clin Oncol 2009;27:1160–7.

12. Rouzier R, Perou CM, Symmans WF, et al. Breast cancer molecular subtypes respond differently to preoperative chemotherapy. Clin Cancer Res 2005;11:5678–85.

13. Pusztai L. Current status of prognostic profiling in breast cancer. Oncologist 2008;13:350–60.

14. Pusztai L, Mazouni C, Anderson K, et al. Molecular classification of breast cancer: limitations and potential. Oncologist 2006;11:868–77.

15. Pusztai L, Cristofanilli M, Paik S. New generation of molecular prognostic and predictive tests for breast cancer. Semin Oncol 2007;34:S10–6.

16. Reis-Filho JS, Weigelt B, Fumagalli D, et al. Molecular profiling: moving away from tumor philately. Sci Transl Med 2010;2:47ps43.

17. Weigelt B, Baehner FL, Reis-Filho JS. The contribution of gene expression profiling to breast cancer classification, prognostication and prediction: a retrospective of the last decade. J Pathol 2010; 220:263–80.

18. Cardoso F, Van't Veer L, Rutgers E, et al. Clinical application of the 70-gene profile: the MINDACT trial. J Clin Oncol 2008;26:729–35.

19. Iwamoto T, Pusztai L. Predicting prognosis of breast cancer with gene signatures: are we lost in a sea of data? Genome Med 2010;2:81.

20. Peppercorn J, Perou CM, Carey LA. Molecular subtypes in breast cancer evaluation and management: divide and conquer. Cancer Invest 2008;26:1–10.

21. Wirapati P, Sotiriou C, Kunkel S, et al. Meta-analysis of gene expression profiles in breast cancer: toward a unified understanding of breast cancer subtyping and prognosis signatures. Breast Cancer Res 2008;10:R65.

22. Desmedt C, Haibe-Kains B, Wirapati P, et al. Biological processes associated with breast cancer clinical outcome depend on the molecular subtypes. Clin Cancer Res 2008;14:5158–65.

23. Weigelt B, Mackay A, A'Hern R, et al. Breast cancer molecular profiling with single sample predictors: a retrospective analysis. Lancet Oncol 2010;11:339–49.

24. Haibe-Kains B, Culhane A, Desmedt C, et al. Robustness of breast cancer molecular subtypes identification. Ann Oncol 2010;21:iv49–59.

25. Santini D, Ceccarelli C, Taffurelli M, et al. Differentiation pathways in primary invasive breast carcinoma as suggested by intermediate filament and biopathological marker expression. J Pathol 1996;179:386–91.

26. Foulkes WD, Smith IE, Reis-Filho JS. Triple-negative breast cancer. N Engl J Med 2010;363:1938–48.

27. Bauer KR, Brown M, Cress RD, et al. Descriptive analysis of estrogen receptor (ER)-negative, progesterone receptor (PR)-negative, and HER2-negative invasive breast cancer, the so-called triple-negative phenotype: a population-based study from the California cancer Registry. Cancer 2007;109:1721–8.

28. Rakha EA, Reis-Filho JS, Ellis IO. Basal-like breast cancer: a critical review. J Clin Oncol 2008;26:2568–81.

29. Fulford LG, Reis-Filho JS, Ryder K, et al. Basal-like grade III invasive ductal carcinoma of the breast: patterns of metastasis and long-term survival. Breast Cancer Res 2007;9:R4.

30. Smid M, Wang Y, Zhang Y, et al. Subtypes of breast cancer show preferential site of relapse. Cancer Res 2008;68:3108–14.

31. Liedtke C, Mazouni C, Hess KR, et al. Response to neoadjuvant therapy and long-term survival in patients with triple-negative breast cancer. J Clin Oncol 2008;26:1275–81.

32. Dent R, Trudeau M, Pritchard KI, et al. Triple-negative breast cancer: clinical features and patterns of recurrence. Clin Cancer Res 2007;13:4429–34.

33. Carey LA, Dees EC, Sawyer L, et al. The triple negative paradox: primary tumor chemosensitivity of breast cancer subtypes. Clin Cancer Res 2007;13:2329–34.

34. Foulkes WD, Reis-Filho JS, Narod SA. Tumor size and survival in breast cancer–a reappraisal. Nat Rev Clin Oncol 2010;7:348–53.

35. Dent R, Hanna WM, Trudeau M, et al. Time to disease recurrence in basal-type breast cancers: effects of tumor size and lymph node status. Cancer 2009;115:4917–23.

36. Fulford LG, Easton DF, Reis-Filho JS, et al. Specific morphological features predictive for the basal phenotype in grade 3 invasive ductal carcinoma of breast. Histopathology 2006;49:22–34.

37. Livasy CA, Karaca G, Nanda R, et al. Phenotypic evaluation of the basal-like subtype of invasive breast carcinoma. Mod Pathol 2006;19:264–71.

38. Turner NC, Reis-Filho JS, Russell AM, et al. BRCA1 dysfunction in sporadic basal-like breast cancer. Oncogene 2007;26:2126–32.

39. Tan DS, Marchio C, Jones RL, et al. Triple negative breast cancer: molecular profiling and prognostic impact in adjuvant anthracycline-treated patients. Breast Cancer Res Treat 2008;111:27–44.

40. Savage K, Leung S, Todd SK, et al. Distribution and significance of caveolin 2 expression in normal breast and invasive breast cancer: an immunofluorescence and immunohistochemical analysis. Breast Cancer Res Treat 2008;110:245–56.

41. Parry S, Savage K, Marchio C, et al. Nestin is expressed in basal-like and triple negative breast cancers. J Clin Pathol 2008;61:1045–50.

42. Klingbeil P, Natrajan R, Everitt G, et al. CD44 is overexpressed in basal-like breast cancers but is not a driver of 11p13 amplification. Breast Cancer Res Treat 2010;120:95–109.

43. Rodriguez-Pinilla SM, Sarrio D, Honrado E, et al. Prognostic significance of basal-like phenotype and fascin expression in node-negative invasive breast carcinomas. Clin Cancer Res 2006;12:1533–9.

44. Nielsen TO, Hsu FD, Jensen K, et al. Immunohistochemical and clinical characterization of the basal-like subtype of invasive breast carcinoma. Clin Cancer Res 2004;10:5367–74.

45. Manie E, Vincent-Salomon A, Lehmann-Che J, et al. High frequency of TP53 mutation in BRCA1 and sporadic basal-like carcinomas but not in BRCA1 luminal breast tumors. Cancer Res 2009;69:663–71.

46. Molyneux G, Geyer FC, Magnay FA, et al. BRCA1 basal-like breast cancers originate from luminal epithelial progenitors and not from basal stem cells. Cell Stem Cell 2010;7:403–17.

47. Liu X, Holstege H, van der Gulden H, et al. Somatic loss of BRCA1 and p53 in mice induces mammary tumors with features of human BRCA1-mutated basal-like breast cancer. Proc Natl Acad Sci U S A 2007;104:12111–6.

48. Turner NC, Reis-Filho JS. Basal-like breast cancer and the BRCA1 phenotype. Oncogene 2006;25:5846–53.

49. Wolff AC, Hammond ME, Schwartz JN, et al. American Society of Clinical Oncology/College of

American Pathologists guideline recommendations for human epidermal growth factor receptor 2 testing in breast cancer. J Clin Oncol 2007;25: 118–45.

50. de Ronde JJ, Hannemann J, Halfwerk H, et al. Concordance of clinical and molecular breast cancer subtyping in the context of preoperative chemotherapy response. Breast Cancer Res Treat 2010;119:119–26.

51. Farmer P, Bonnefoi H, Becette V, et al. Identification of molecular apocrine breast tumours by microarray analysis. Oncogene 2005;24:4660–71.

52. Doane AS, Danso M, Lal P, et al. An estrogen receptor-negative breast cancer subset characterized by a hormonally regulated transcriptional program and response to androgen. Oncogene 2006;25:3994–4008.

53. Robinson JL, Macarthur S, Ross-Innes CS, et al. Androgen receptor driven transcription in molecular apocrine breast cancer is mediated by FoxA1. EMBO J 2011;30(15):3019–27.

54. Prat A, Parker JS, Karginova O, et al. Phenotypic and molecular characterization of the claudin-low intrinsic subtype of breast cancer. Breast Cancer Res 2010;12:R68.

55. Hennessy BT, Gonzalez-Angulo AM, Stemke-Hale K, et al. Characterization of a naturally occurring breast cancer subset enriched in epithelial-to-mesenchymal transition and stem cell characteristics. Cancer Res 2009;69:4116–24.

56. Teschendorff AE, Caldas C. A robust classifier of high predictive value to identify good prognosis patients in ER-negative breast cancer. Breast Cancer Res 2008;10:R73.

57. Colombo PE, Milanezi F, Weigelt B, et al. Microarrays in the 2010s: the contribution of microarray-based gene expression profiling to breast cancer classification, prognostication and prediction. Breast Cancer Res 2011;13:212.

58. Weigelt B, Reis-Filho JS. Molecular profiling currently offers no more than tumour morphology and basic immunohistochemistry. Breast Cancer Res 2010;12(Suppl 4):S5.

59. Nielsen TO, Parker JS, Leung S, et al. A comparison of PAM50 intrinsic subtyping with immunohistochemistry and clinical prognostic factors in tamoxifen-treated estrogen receptor-positive breast cancer. Clin Cancer Res 2010;16: 5222–32.

60. Weigelt B, Horlings HM, Kreike B, et al. Refinement of breast cancer classification by molecular characterization of histological special types. J Pathol 2008;216:141–50.

61. Mackay A, Weigelt B, Grigoriadis A, et al. Microarray-based class discovery for molecular classification of breast cancer: analysis of interobserver agreement. J Natl Cancer Inst 2011;103:662–73.

62. Lusa L, McShane LM, Reid JF, et al. Challenges in projecting clustering results across gene expression-profiling datasets. J Natl Cancer Inst 2007;99:1715–23.

63. Chang HY, Nuyten DS, Sneddon JB, et al. Robustness, scalability, and integration of a wound-response gene expression signature in predicting breast cancer survival. Proc Natl Acad Sci U S A 2005;102:3738–43.

64. Fan C, Oh DS, Wessels L, et al. Concordance among gene-expression-based predictors for breast cancer. N Engl J Med 2006;355:560–9.

65. Desmedt C, Piette F, Loi S, et al. Strong time dependence of the 76-gene prognostic signature for node-negative breast cancer patients in the TRANSBIG multicenter independent validation series. Clin Cancer Res 2007;13:3207–14.

66. Molyneux G, Smalley MJ. The cell of origin of BRCA1 mutation-associated breast cancer: a cautionary tale of gene expression profiling. J Mammary Gland Biol Neoplasia 2011;16: 51–5.

67. Lim E, Vaillant F, Wu D, et al. Aberrant luminal progenitors as the candidate target population for basal tumor development in BRCA1 mutation carriers. Nat Med 2009;15:907–13.

68. Perou CM, Parker JS, Prat A, et al. Clinical implementation of the intrinsic subtypes of breast cancer. Lancet Oncol 2010;11:718–9.

69. Ellis MJ, Suman VJ, Hoog J, et al. Randomized phase II neoadjuvant comparison between letrozole, anastrozole, and exemestane for postmenopausal women with estrogen receptor-rich stage 2 to 3 breast cancer: clinical and biomarker outcomes and predictive value of the baseline PAM50-based intrinsic subtype—ACOSOG Z1031. J Clin Oncol 2011;29:2342–9.

70. Ravdin PM, Siminoff LA, Davis GJ, et al. Computer program to assist in making decisions about adjuvant therapy for women with early breast cancer. J Clin Oncol 2001;19:980–91.

71. Mook S, Schmidt MK, Viale G, et al. The 70-gene prognosis-signature predicts disease outcome in breast cancer patients with 1-3 positive lymph nodes in an independent validation study. Breast Cancer Res Treat 2009;116:295–302.

72. Campbell HE, Taylor MA, Harris AL, et al. An investigation into the performance of the Adjuvant! Online prognostic programme in early breast cancer for a cohort of patients in the United Kingdom. Br J Cancer 2009;101:1074–84.

73. Olivotto IA, Bajdik CD, Ravdin PM, et al. Population-based validation of the prognostic model ADJUVANT! for early breast cancer. J Clin Oncol 2005;23:2716–25.

74. van de Vijver MJ, He YD, van't Veer LJ, et al. A gene-expression signature as a predictor of

survival in breast cancer. N Engl J Med 2002;347: 1999–2009.

75. van 't Veer LJ, Dai H, van de Vijver MJ, et al. Gene expression profiling predicts clinical outcome of breast cancer. Nature 2002;415:530–6.

76. Wang Y, Klijn JG, Zhang Y, et al. Gene-expression profiles to predict distant metastasis of lymph-node-negative primary breast cancer. Lancet 2005;365:671–9.

77. Sotiriou C, Wirapati P, Loi S, et al. Gene expression profiling in breast cancer: understanding the molecular basis of histologic grade to improve prognosis. J Natl Cancer Inst 2006;98:262–72.

78. van't Veer LJ, Bernards R. Enabling personalized cancer medicine through analysis of gene-expression patterns. Nature 2008;452:564–70.

79. Filho OM, Ignatiadis M, Sotiriou C. Genomic grade index: an important tool for assessing breast cancer tumor grade and prognosis. Crit Rev Oncol Hematol 2011;77:20–9.

80. Toussaint J, Sieuwerts AM, Haibe-Kains B, et al. Improvement of the clinical applicability of the Genomic Grade Index through a qRT-PCR test performed on frozen and formalin-fixed paraffin-embedded tissues. BMC Genomics 2009;10:424.

81. Ma XJ, Wang Z, Ryan PD, et al. A two-gene expression ratio predicts clinical outcome in breast cancer patients treated with tamoxifen. Cancer Cell 2004;5:607–16.

82. Sgroi DC. The HOXB13:IL17BR gene-expression ratio: a biomarker providing information above and beyond tumor grade. Biomark Med 2009;3:99–102.

83. Buyse M, Loi S, van't Veer L, et al. Validation and clinical utility of a 70-gene prognostic signature for women with node-negative breast cancer. J Natl Cancer Inst 2006;98:1183–92.

84. Knauer M, Mook S, Rutgers EJ, et al. The predictive value of the 70-gene signature for adjuvant chemotherapy in early breast cancer. Breast Cancer Res Treat 2010;120:655–61.

85. Bueno-de-Mesquita JM, van Harten WH, Retel VP, et al. Use of 70-gene signature to predict prognosis of patients with node-negative breast cancer: a prospective community-based feasibility study (RASTER). Lancet Oncol 2007;8:1079–87.

86. Straver ME, Glas AM, Hannemann J, et al. The 70-gene signature as a response predictor for neoadjuvant chemotherapy in breast cancer. Breast Cancer Res Treat 2010;119:551–8.

87. Knauer M, Cardoso F, Wesseling J, et al. Identification of a low-risk subgroup of HER-2-positive breast cancer by the 70-gene prognosis signature. Br J Cancer 2010;103:1788–93.

88. Kreike B, van Kouwenhove M, Horlings H, et al. Gene expression profiling and histopathological characterization of triple-negative/basal-like breast carcinomas. Breast Cancer Res 2007;9:R65.

89. Paik S, Shak S, Tang G, et al. A multigene assay to predict recurrence of tamoxifen-treated, node-negative breast cancer. N Engl J Med 2004;351:2817–26.

90. Paik S, Tang G, Shak S, et al. Gene expression and benefit of chemotherapy in women with node-negative, estrogen receptor-positive breast cancer. J Clin Oncol 2006;24:3726–34.

91. Dowsett M, Cuzick J, Wale C, et al. Prediction of risk of distant recurrence using the 21-gene recurrence score in node-negative and node-positive postmenopausal patients with breast cancer treated with anastrozole or tamoxifen: a TransATAC study. J Clin Oncol 2010;28:1829–34.

92. Albain KS, Barlow WE, Shak S, et al. Prognostic and predictive value of the 21-gene recurrence score assay in postmenopausal women with node-positive, oestrogen-receptor-positive breast cancer on chemotherapy: a retrospective analysis of a randomised trial. Lancet Oncol 2010;11:55–65.

93. Kim C, Paik S. Gene-expression-based prognostic assays for breast cancer. Nat Rev Clin Oncol 2010; 7:340–7.

94. Cuzick J, Dowsett M, Wale C, et al. Prognostic value of a combined ER, PgR, Ki67, HER2 immuno-histochemical (IHC4) score and comparison with the GHI recurrence score - results from TransATAC [abstract]. Cancer Res 2009;69:503S.

95. Goldstein LJ, Gray R, Badve S, et al. Prognostic utility of the 21-gene assay in hormone receptor-positive operable breast cancer compared with classical clinicopathologic features. J Clin Oncol 2008;26:4063–71.

96. Goldhirsch A, Ingle JN, Gelber RD, et al. Thresholds for therapies: highlights of the St Gallen International Expert Consensus on the primary therapy of early breast cancer 2009. Ann Oncol 2009;20:1319–29.

97. Michiels S, Koscielny S, Hill C. Prediction of cancer outcome with microarrays: a multiple random validation strategy. Lancet 2005;365:488–92.

98. Ein-Dor L, Kela I, Getz G, et al. Outcome signature genes in breast cancer: is there a unique set? Bioinformatics 2005;21:171–8.

99. Haibe-Kains B, Desmedt C, Piette F, et al. Comparison of prognostic gene expression signatures for breast cancer. BMC Genomics 2008;9:394.

100. Blows FM, Driver KE, Schmidt MK, et al. Subtyping of breast cancer by immunohistochemistry to investigate a relationship between subtype and short and long term survival: a collaborative analysis of data for 10,159 cases from 12 studies. PLoS Med 2010;7:e1000279.

101. Bergamaschi A, Tagliabue E, Sorlie T, et al. Extracellular matrix signature identifies breast cancer subgroups with different clinical outcome. J Pathol 2008;214:357–67.

102. Finak G, Bertos N, Pepin F, et al. Stromal gene expression predicts clinical outcome in breast cancer. Nat Med 2008;14:518–27.

103. Rody A, Holtrich U, Pusztai L, et al. T-cell metagene predicts a favorable prognosis in estrogen receptor-negative and HER2-positive breast cancers. Breast Cancer Res 2009;11:R15.

104. Yau C, Esserman L, Moore DH, et al. A multigene predictor of metastatic outcome in early stage hormone receptor-negative and triple-negative breast cancer. Breast Cancer Res 2010;12:R85.

105. Borst P, Wessels L. Do predictive signatures really predict response to cancer chemotherapy? Cell Cycle 2010;9:4836–40.

106. Desmedt C, Di Leo A, de Azambuja E, et al. Multi-factorial approach to predicting resistance to an-thracyclines. J Clin Oncol 2011;29:1578–86.

107. Hatzis C, Pusztai L, Valero V, et al. A genomic predictor of response and survival following taxane-anthracycline chemotherapy for invasive breast cancer. JAMA 2011;305:1873–81.

108. Aparicio SA, Huntsman DG. Does massively parallel DNA resequencing signify the end of histo-pathology as we know it? J Pathol 2010;220:307–15.

109. Natrajan R, Reis-Filho JS. Next-generation se-quencing applied to molecular diagnostics. Expert Rev Mol Diagn 2011;11:425–44.

METASTASES TO AND FROM THE BREAST

Alessandro Bombonati, MD[a], Melinda F. Lerwill, MD[b,c],*

KEYWORDS

• Breast • Carcinoma • Metastasis • Immunohistochemistry

ABSTRACT

Breast cancer is a common source of systemic metastatic disease. Distinguishing metastatic breast cancer from other types of malignancies can be diagnostically challenging but is important for correct treatment and prognosis. Nonmammary tumors can also metastasize to the breast, although this is a rare phenomenon. Differentiating a metastasis to the breast from a primary breast cancer can likewise be difficult. Knowledge of the clinical history and careful morphologic evaluation are the cornerstones of diagnosis. A panel of immunohistochemical stains tailored to the differential diagnosis at hand can provide helpful information in ambiguous cases.

OVERVIEW

Breast cancer is a strikingly common disease. It is the most common type of cancer affecting women worldwide (excluding nonmelanoma skin cancers), representing 23% of all cancers in women and 1.38 million new cases per year.[1] In the United States, it accounts for 26% of all cancers in women, with an annual incidence of approximately 182,500.[1] As of 2008, slightly more than 2.63 million women diagnosed with breast cancer were alive in the United States.[2] Distant metastatic disease ultimately develops in 20% to 30% of patients with invasive breast cancer. Given that breast cancer and, consequently, its metastases affect a large number of patients, it is no surprise that spread of breast cancer is a frequent diagnostic consideration in routine pathology practice.

Key Features
DIFFERENTIATION OF BREAST CARCINOMA FROM OTHER MALIGNANCIES

1. A combination of morphology and clinical history is often sufficient to differentiate breast carcinoma from other types of tumors.

2. Comparison of the histologic features of the current tumor with those of any prior malignancy is often the single most informative test a pathologist performs when trying to differentiate a new primary tumor from a metastasis.

3. Tumors often demonstrate variable morphologic patterns, and occasionally a minor pattern in the main tumor dominates in the metastasis.

4. Although most cases of metastatic breast cancer maintain the same estrogen receptor (ER)/progesterone receptor (PR)/Her-2 profile as the primary tumor, changes in hormone receptor or Her-2 status are seen in minority of cases.

5. Immunohistochemical (IHC) markers for site of origin can be useful for differentiating adenocarcinomas of breast origin from those arising from other sites; however, the specificity and sensitivity of the individual markers vary depending on the particular subtypes of carcinoma under consideration.

6. IHC panels for site of origin should be tailored to the differential diagnosis at hand; broad, nonspecific panels often yield misleading results.

7. IHC studies should always be interpreted in the context of the morphologic findings and clinical history.

[a] Department of Pathology, Thomas Jefferson University Hospitals, Methodist Division, 2301 South Broad Street, Philadelphia, PA 19148, USA
[b] James Homer Wright Pathology Laboratories of the Massachusetts General Hospital, 55 Fruit Street, Boston, MA 02114, USA
[c] Department of Pathology, Harvard Medical School, 25 Shattuck street, Boston, MA 02115, USA
* Corresponding author. James Homer Wright Pathology Laboratories, Massachusetts General Hospital, 55 Fruit Street, Boston, MA 02114.
E-mail address: mlerwill@partners.org

Surgical Pathology 5 (2012) 719–747
http://dx.doi.org/10.1016/j.path.2012.06.004
1875-9181/12/$ - see front matter © 2012 Elsevier Inc. All rights reserved.

surgpath.theclinics.com

The need to distinguish breast carcinoma from nonmammary malignancies can arise in a variety of clinical settings. A patient with a history of breast cancer may develop a new lesion in a different organ, such as lung or ovary; is the new finding a metastasis or a separate primary tumor? Or perhaps a patient has a history of more than one type of malignancy, including breast cancer, and develops distant metastatic disease; correct identification of the source of the metastasis is important for clinical management. In other instances, a patient may present with widely metastatic disease originating from an unknown primary. And rarely, nonmammary malignancies may metastasize to the breast and should not be confused with breast cancer. In all such scenarios, proper differentiation of breast cancer from other types of malignancies has important therapeutic and prognostic implications.

Correct identification of the tumor type can often be made by careful evaluation of the morphology but, in some cases, the histologic features are ambiguous. Comparison with slides of any prior cancers can prove invaluable, as can the clinical history. Unfortunately, prior slides and history are not always available. In difficult cases, the use of IHC markers can be helpful for determining a tumor's site of origin. No individual marker is entirely specific or sensitive in this regard, but a panel of selected IHC markers in conjunction with the histology and available clinical history should enable a pathologist to arrive at a definitive diagnosis or, at a minimum, to direct the clinical investigation to a few likely candidates of origin.

This review discusses the spread of breast cancer to distant sites, the secondary involvement of the breast by other malignancies, and the use of IHC markers to differentiate breast carcinoma from nonmammary malignancies.

METASTATIC BREAST CANCER

Breast cancer is not fastidious in terms of its metastatic targets and shows frequent involvement of diverse sites. In an autopsy study of 3827 patients that examined the frequency and distribution of metastases from a broad range of cancers, breast cancer was the leading contributor of metastases and accounted for 24% of all metastatic lesions.[3] Averaging 5.2 metastases per primary lesion, it contributed the largest proportion of metastases to the broadest range of sites. Lung, liver, and bone represent the most common sites of distant metastasis.

Patterns of Spread by Histologic Subtype

The pattern of metastatic disease shows some differences according to histologic subtype: ductal carcinomas more frequently involve the lung and pleura, whereas lobular carcinomas more frequently involve the bone marrow, gastrointestinal tract, gynecologic organs, peritoneum, and retroperitoneum.[4-8] Widespread serosal involvement, consisting of numerous tiny tumor nodules, is particularly characteristic of the peritoneal spread of lobular carcinoma.[4]

Patterns of Spread by Molecular Subtype

Differences in metastatic pattern have also been described among more recently defined molecular subtypes of breast cancer (luminal A, luminal B, Her-2+, and basal-like):

- Her-2+ and basal-like carcinomas are associated with increased rates of brain metastases.[9-14]
- Basal-like carcinomas show more frequent lung metastases and fewer bone metastases than nonbasal or luminal subtypes of breast cancer.[9,11,13,14]
- Some studies demonstrate lower rates of liver metastases in the basal-like subgroup.[13,14]
- Triple-negative breast cancers, which lack expression of ER, PR, and Her-2 and overlap in large part with the group of basal-like cancers, show similar patterns of metastatic spread as the latter.[15,16]
- ER− tumors have higher rates of first relapse in viscera and soft tissue, whereas ER+ breast cancers have higher rates of first relapse in bone.[16,17]

Comparison of Primary and Metastatic Breast Cancer

Metastatic lesions generally retain the histologic features of the primary breast tumor (Fig. 1). Occasionally, a minor pattern of growth in the primary tumor predominates in the metastasis. The metastatic tumor sometimes demonstrates more confluent growth than the primary tumor, because the degree of stromal reaction may be less than that encountered in the breast parenchyma. Nevertheless, the cytomorphologic features of the metastatic and primary lesions are usually sufficiently similar to permit a diagnosis of metastatic breast cancer on the basis of histologic comparison alone.

Although the majority of primary tumors and their distant metastases have parallel hormone receptor profiles, loss or gain of ER or PR expression in the metastases has been documented.[18-22] Reported rates of ER discordance between primary and metastatic tumors range from 7.5% to as high as 30% (Table 1). The frequency of positive-to-negative conversions and negative-to-positive

Fig. 1. Metastatic breast carcinoma to the lung. The (*A*) lung metastasis and the (*B*) primary breast carcinoma have identical histologic features.

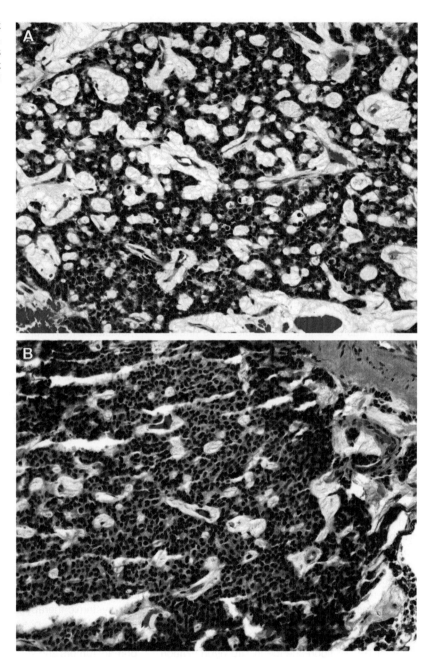

conversions are similar. PR expression shows more frequent and consistent discordance: more than one-third of cases demonstrate a change of PR status in the metastatic lesion (see **Table 1**), and loss of PR expression in the metastasis is particularly frequent. Such positive-to-negative conversions account for 78% to 100% of discordant cases in some studies.[18–22] There seems to

be no significant effect of metastatic site, time interval between diagnosis of the primary tumor and development of metastases, use of chemotherapy, use of endocrine therapy, primary tumor grade, Her-2 status, or method of sampling on the rate of hormone receptor discordance.[18–20,22] Gong and colleagues[22] noted that among their cases with discordant ER results, variability in

Table 1
Hormone receptor discordance rates between primary and metastatic tumors

Study	N	ER Discordance	PR Discordance
Lower et al,[18] 2005	ER = 200 PR = 173	30%	39.3%
Guarneri et al,[19] 2008	ER = 75 PR = 75	22%	36%
Broom et al,[20] 2009	ER = 62 PR = 59	17.7%	37.3%
Liedtke et al,[21] 2009	ER = 228 PR = 216	18.4%	40.3%
Gong et al,[22] 2011	ER = 227	7.5%	—

testing methods (eg, the primary and metastatic tumors were evaluated at different institutions) and marginal scores were common. Because the conventional 10% or greater cutoff for ER and PR positivity was used in these studies, it is unclear how many discordant cases had low-positive scores or results in the 1% to 9% range of expression that were classified as negative. In such instances, changes in hormone receptor status classification between primary and metastatic lesions are not surprising.

Her-2 status can also vary between primary tumors and their metastases (**Table 2**). Some studies demonstrate low rates of Her-2 discordance between primary and metastatic tumors, ranging from 0% to 7%; others show intermediate levels of discordance, approximately 14% to 16%; and yet others find that up to 33% of cases have discordant Her-2 results.[19–21,23–28] The study reporting the highest rate of discordance, one-third of cases, was based on IHC analysis for Her-2 expression.[28] Both 2+ and 3+ scores were considered positive. When cases with 2+ scores were reclassified as negative, the rate of discordance was lower but still notable at 22%. Discordant results are encountered regardless of whether IHC or fluorescence in situ hybridization (FISH) is used for analysis. Aggregate data from studies based on IHC alone show an 18% rate of Her-2 discordance between primary and metastatic tumors (**Table 3**). Aggregate data from studies in which FISH or chromogenic in situ hybridization (CISH) was performed in all cases, or in which FISH was used at a minimum to evaluate all 2+ IHC scores, demonstrate a 10% rate of discordance (**Table 4**).

The Her-2 status can change from positive in the primary tumor to negative in the metastases or vice versa (see **Table 2**).[19–21,23–28] There does not seem to be a distinct predilection for either positive-to-negative conversion or negative-to-positive conversion. Variation in Her-2 status among different metastatic lesions in the same patient can also occur. In one study, 17 patients had distant metastases from more than 1 site available for analysis.[24] Her-2 discordance between different metastatic lesions was 18% by IHC and 19% by FISH. Curiously, the IHC-discordant cases were concordant by FISH, and the FISH-discordant cases were concordant by IHC.

Whether the use of systemic therapy, in particular targeted therapy with trastuzumab, is associated with changes in Her-2 status in subsequent metastases is not well studied. Loss of Her-2 amplification in primary tumors after treatment with trastuzumab-containing neoadjuvant chemotherapy regimens has been observed.[29] Such alterations may reflect biologic changes in the tumor or preferential survival of nonamplified clones in tumors with heterogeneous Her-2 status. Extrapolation to the metastatic setting suggests that similar mechanisms could potentially be at play in cases with discordant Her-2 results, but so far, the limited data do not indicate that systemic therapy is a significant factor. Gong and colleagues[26] observed no effect of interval chemotherapy on Her-2 concordance between primary tumors and subsequent metastases. Guarneri and colleagues[19] found no differences in metastatic site, time interval between diagnosis of the primary tumor and development of metastases, and prior therapies between patients who did or did not experience a change in Her-2 status. Furthermore, loss of Her-2 expression in metastatic lesions can occur even in patients who do not receive trastuzumab.[25,28]

ER, PR, and Her-2 analyses are all subject to a variety of preanalytical and analytical variables that may have an impact on discordance rates.[30,31] Borderline or equivocal scores may also contribute to inconsistent results between primary and

Table 2
Her-2 discordance rates between primary and metastatic tumors

Study	N	LR vs Distant Metastases N	Method of Assessment[a]	Her-2 Discordance	Primary +/ Metastasis −	Primary −/ Metastasis +
Tanner et al,[23] 2001	46	LR = 33 Distant = 12	IHC and CISH	0%	0%	0%
Gancberg et al,[24] 2002	100 68	Distant = 100 Distant = 68	IHC FISH	6% 7%	0% 3%	6% 4%
Regitnig et al,[25] 2004	31 17 10	Distant = 31 Distant = 17 Regional LN = 10	IHC FISH IHC and FISH	16% 24% 0%	3% 0% 0%	13% 24% 0%
Gong et al,[26] 2005	60	LR = 43 Distant = 17	FISH	3%	3%	0%
Zidan et al,[27] 2005	58	Not specified	IHC[b] and FISH	14%	2%	12%
Guarneri et al,[19] 2008	75	LR soft tissue = 30 Distant = 45	IHC[b] and/or FISH	16%	3%	13%
Lower et al,[28] 2009	382	Not specified	IHC (2+ or 3+ = positive)	33%	24%	9%
	—	—	IHC (3+ = positive)	22%	NA	NA
Broom et al,[20] 2009	18	Not specified[c]	IHC[d] and/or FISH	5.5%	5.5%	0%
Liedtke et al,[21] 2009	528	Not specified	IHC and/or FISH	13.6%	NA	NA

Abbreviations: LN, lymph node; LR, locoregional; NA, not available.
[a] Unless otherwise noted, IHC scores of 3+ were considered positive.
[b] Cases with IHC scores of 2+ were also evaluated by FISH.
[c] Axillary lymph node metastases excluded.
[d] IHC threshold for positivity not stated.

metastatic lesions, even though the quantitative difference between positive and negative scores in such examples may be slight. The presence of multiple primary tumor nodules could potentially be a confounding factor in a small subset of cases, if the nodules were characterized by different receptor profiles but only one was tested. Although such technical and sampling issues might explain discordant results between primary and metastatic tumors in a percentage of cases, there seems to be true discordance in some instances. Therefore, repeat receptor testing of the metastasis is suggested if the metastatic lesion is readily accessible to biopsy, because the findings may alter the course of treatment. It is prudent to remember, however, that heterogeneity among metastases

Table 3
Her-2 discordance between primary and metastatic tumors by IHC analysis alone

Study	Discordant Cases (N)	Total Cases (N)	Her-2 Discordance Rate
Gancberg et al,[24] 2002	6	100	6%
Regitnig et al,[25] 2004	5	31	16%
Lower et al,[28] 2009	83[a]	382	22%
Total	94	513	18%

[a] Extrapolated results when only IHC scores of 3+ were considered positive.

Table 4
Her-2 discordance between primary and metastatic tumors in studies with comprehensive FISH/CISH evaluation or FISH validation of 2+ IHC scores

Study	Discordant Cases (N)	Total Cases (N)	Her-2 Discordance Rate
Tanner et al,[23] 2001	0	46	0%
Gancberg et al,[24] 2002	5	68	7%
Regitnig et al,[25] 2004	4	17	24%
Gong et al,[26] 2005	2	60	3%
Zidan et al,[27] 2005	8	58	14%
Guarneri et al,[19] 2008	12	75	16%
Total	31	324	10%

exists in some cases, and the presence of a certain receptor profile in one metastasis may not be reflective of the entirety of a patient's metastatic disease.

METASTASES TO THE BREAST

The breast is a remarkably uncommon site of secondary tumor involvement. Less than 1% of metastatic lesions are found in the breast.[3] Melanomas, carcinomas from a wide variety of sites, sarcomas, lymphomas, leukemias, mesotheliomas, and germ cell tumors have all been reported to spread to the breast (Figs. 2–6). The most common source of metastatic disease is actually the contralateral breast (Figs. 7 and 8; Table 5); lymphatic spread of breast cancer from the opposite breast across the anterior chest wall accounts for this phenomenon.[3,32–35] When tumors of mammary origin are excluded, metastatic solid tumors account for 0.2% to 1.1% of all breast malignancies (see Table 5).[32,34,36–40] The most common solid extramammary tumor to spread to the breast is melanoma, followed by pulmonary, gynecologic, renal, and gastrointestinal carcinomas.[33,34,36–38,40–46] In men, prostate cancer is a frequent culprit.[37,43,47] In countries with different disease prevalences, other types of malignancies are more common; for example, in a report from South Korea, gastric carcinomas were the leading source of metastases to the breast.[39]

Secondary hematologic tumors account for 0.02% to 0.4% of all breast malignancies (see Table 5).[32,34,36,39,40] These include both neoplasms that relapse in the breast and those that involve the breast as part of widespread disease. B-cell lymphomas are the most common, but other types of lymphoma, leukemia, and myeloma can be seen (Fig. 9).[34,48,49]

Postmortem studies examining the rate of secondary breast involvement in consecutive patients with malignant tumors have found that 3.6% to 5.9% of patients harbor breast metastases from contralateral breast carcinomas, 3.9% show secondary involvement of the breast by hematologic malignancies, and 1.4% have metastases from extramammary solid tumors.[32,35]

Metastases to the breast occur over a wide age range, from 12 to 90 years; the mean, however, is between the fifth and sixth decades.[34,36–42,44–46,50,51] The majority of patients have a known history of extramammary malignancy, but in 21%, the breast tumor represents the initial presentation of disease.[32,34,36,38,39,41,44–46,49,51,52] The most common clinical manifestation is that of a solitary discrete mass. Multiple nodules are seen in 28% of patients, and bilateral tumors are present in 17%.[36–40,42,45,46,49–53] The upper outer quadrant is the most frequent site of involvement.[36] The tumors are often superficially located and may be adherent to skin.[36,38] They tend to be round or oval with well-defined to slightly irregular margins on mammography; occasional tumors may be less well-circumscribed.[40,50,53] Only rare tumors demonstrate a stellate configuration akin to that of primary breast carcinoma.[52,54] Calcifications are distinctly unusual, but when seen, they are most often encountered in the setting of metastatic serous carcinoma from the female genital tract.[33,39] A minority of patients present with skin thickening or edema of the breast rather than a mass lesion, and occasionally a clinical picture of inflammatory carcinoma is observed.[33,40,49,53,55–60] A few patients have normal findings on mammography.[40]

Most metastases from extramammary tumors demonstrate unusual histologic features that are not typical of primary breast carcinoma (see Figs. 3A, 4, and 5). For example, the hierarchical branching of serous carcinoma, the mucinous glands of colonic carcinoma, and the pigmented cells of melanoma all represent findings that are uncharacteristic of breast carcinoma. Extensive lymphatic

Fig. 2. (*A*) Metastasis to the breast from a pulmonary adenocarcinoma. (*B*) The majority of the primary lung tumor had micropapillary and acinar features and did not resemble the metastasis. (*C*) Only a small portion of the primary tumor demonstrated a solid nesting pattern, which was the component that metastasized to the breast.

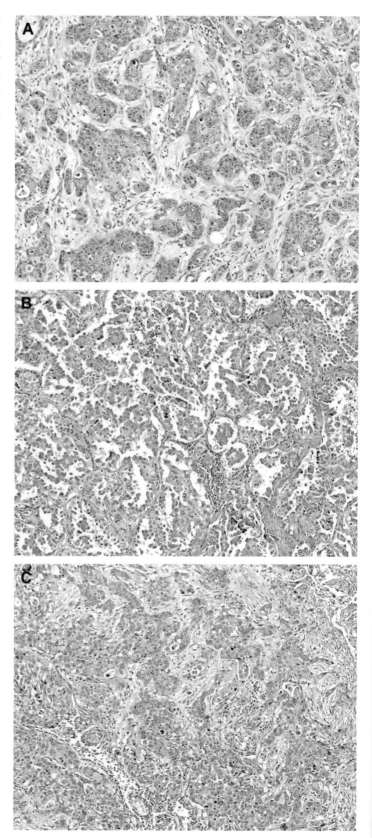

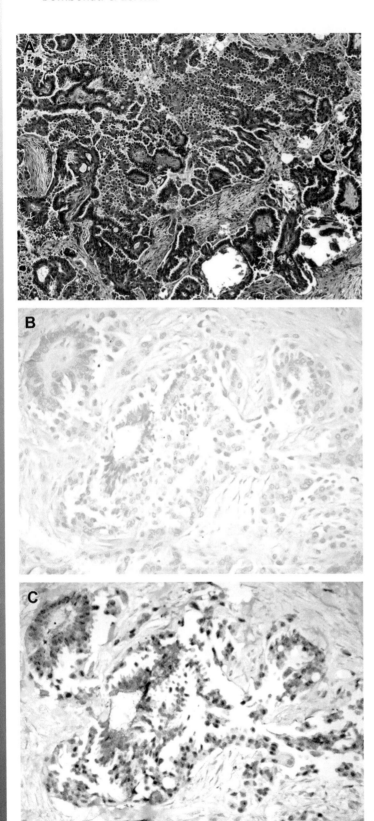

Fig. 3. (*A*) Metastatic ovarian serous papillary carcinoma to the breast. The tumor cells are (*B*) negative for GCDFP-15 and (*C*) positive for WT-1, supporting the diagnosis.

Fig. 4. Metastasis to the breast from a parotid acinic cell carcinoma. The cytoplasmic features are unusual for a primary breast carcinoma and should raise consideration of a non-mammary neoplasm.

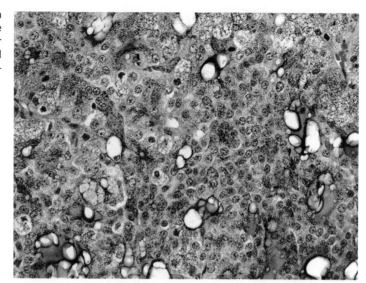

Fig. 5. Metastatic melanoma involving the breast with spindle cell morphology and focal pigment.

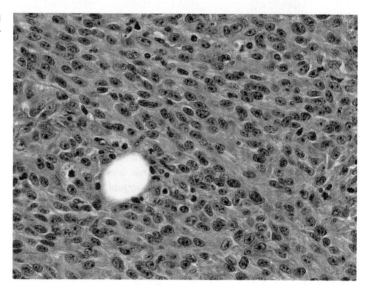

Fig. 6. Metastatic melanoma involving the breast with epithelioid aggregates that mimic carcinoma.

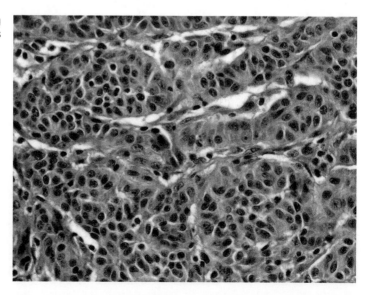

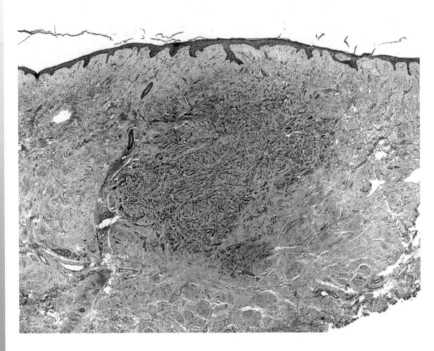

Fig. 7. Metastasis to breast skin from a contralateral invasive ductal carcinoma.

invasion, disproportionate to the size of the tumor, is sometimes seen. In some patients, the clinically detected mass may be caused by extensive vascular space invasion rather than by stromal infiltration.[36,61] The finding of a well-circumscribed tumor with multiple satellite nodules also suggests secondary tumor involvement.[52] The presence of any unusual morphologic findings, such as these, can be an important clue to the metastatic nature of a breast tumor.

Unfortunately, some metastatic tumors show histologic features that overlap significantly with those of primary breast carcinoma. This is particularly true of high-grade neoplasms with nonspecific solid or nested growth patterns, such as those that may be seen in poorly differentiated

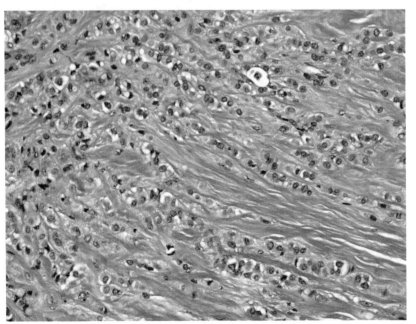

Fig. 8. Metastasis to breast parenchyma from a contralateral invasive lobular carcinoma. The patient had a contralateral 16 cm invasive lobular carcinoma with 23 positive axillary lymph nodes that was resected 2 years earlier. A few widely scattered foci of invasive lobular carcinoma only a few millimeters in size were identified in the nonindex breast with no associated in situ lobular neoplasia. The clinical history, pattern of disease, and lack of in situ component suggested metastatic rather than primary disease.

Table 5
Frequency of different types of metastases to the breast

Source of Metastases	Percentage of All Breast Malignancies (Rates Reported in Individual Studies)	Percentage of All Breast Malignancies (Aggregate Data from Multiple Studies)
All sources (contralateral breast cancers, hematologic malignancies, and solid tumors)	1.3%–3%	2.8%
Contralateral breast cancers	0.1%–2.8%	2.4%
Hematologic malignancies	0.02%–0.4%	0.2%
Solid tumors	0.2%–1.1%	0.4%

Data from Refs.[32,34,36–40,53]

adenocarcinomas and melanomas. Additionally, signet ring cell carcinomas of the stomach and breast may be indistinguishable by morphology alone. Review of the clinical history and of slides from any prior malignancies is critical for correct diagnosis. If the breast tumor and the extramammary primary are morphologically similar, this is generally sufficient evidence to recognize the breast tumor as a metastasis. When comparing histologic features, attention should be paid to even small areas of morphologic heterogeneity: a minor histologic component in the primary tumor may become the dominant or sole component in the breast metastasis (see **Fig. 2**).

The presence or absence of an in situ component is also helpful for differentiating primary from secondary tumors of the breast. Identification of

in situ carcinoma in the vicinity of, and with similar cytologic features to, the invasive tumor supports a diagnosis of primary breast carcinoma. In contrast, metastatic lesions lack a corresponding in situ component. Some primary breast carcinomas, however, do not have a demonstrable in situ component, so the lack thereof is not sufficient, by itself, to identify a tumor as metastatic in nature.

Additionally, 2 patterns of metastatic disease can mimic in situ carcinoma:

1. Metastatic tumor can occlude and distend lymphatic vessels and thereby resemble ducts involved by in situ carcinoma.[61] Attention to the configuration and distribution of the carcinoma and evaluation for contiguous areas of more overt vascular space invasion are helpful

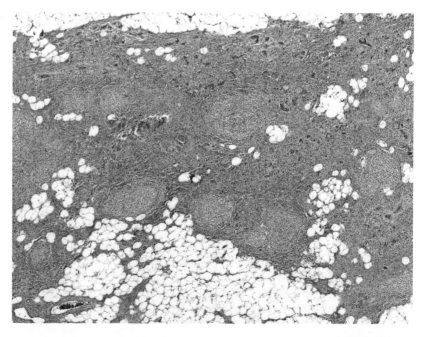

Fig. 9. Hairy cell leukemia involving the breast.

for recognizing this phenomenon. IHC staining for D2-40, a lymphatic endothelial cell marker, and comparison with a myoepithelial cell marker, such as p63, can be useful for differentiating occlusive lymphatic tumor emboli from in situ carcinoma.[62]

2. Hajdu and Urban[36] report but do not illustrate a second pattern of metastatic tumor that can mimic in situ carcinoma wherein secondary colonization of existing ducts and lobules results in an in situ carcinoma-like picture.

Finally, given that breast cancer is a common disease, it is possible for invasive or in situ breast carcinoma to coexist with a secondary tumor in rare instances.[63]

It is easy to appreciate how a metastasis from a contralateral breast carcinoma could be readily mistaken for a new primary cancer. A few findings can be helpful in this distinction, however. Involvement of the skin and/or lymphatics without evidence of parenchymal tumor is consistent with metastatic disease (see **Fig. 7**). Lack of an in situ component corroborates interpretation as a metastasis, but as discussed previously, is not independently diagnostic of such. Conversely, the presence of an in situ component supports a diagnosis of a second primary tumor. If 2 tumors are morphologically distinct, that indicates dual primaries rather than metastatic disease.

Review of the clinicopathologic features of the prior tumor can be helpful in assessing the likelihood of spread to the opposite breast. For example, it would not be surprising for an inflammatory carcinoma or a large, node-positive carcinoma to metastasize (see **Fig. 8**), but it would be quite unlikely for a subcentimeter low-grade tumor to do so. Overall, dual primaries are more common than breast-to-breast metastases.[41]

Because secondary tumors of the breast are rare and therefore not a common diagnostic consideration, they can be easily misdiagnosed as primary breast carcinomas. A low threshold of

suspicion is appropriate when there are features that seem unusual for a primary breast tumor, and these should prompt a pathologist to explore the clinical history in greater detail. Comparison with the morphology of any prior tumors is perhaps the single most valuable diagnostic tool that can be employed. Correct identification of a metastatic tumor by core needle biopsy or fine-needle aspiration can spare a patient unnecessary surgery, but in cases with ambiguous histologic features, excisional biopsy may be required to fully evaluate the morphology. Metastases to the breast most often occur in the setting of widely disseminated disease, and consequently, prognosis is generally poor.[36–38,41] Isolated metastatic disease in the breast is rare.

DIAGNOSTIC IMMUNOHISTOCHEMISTRY FOR BREAST CARCINOMA

IHC can provide invaluable information regarding the site of origin of a malignancy, but the findings must always be integrated with the morphology and clinical history. Too heavy a reliance on IHC findings can be misleading, because no site-specific marker is 100% specific or sensitive. The best approach is to develop a specific differential diagnosis based on the histologic and clinical findings and then to tailor the IHC work-up accordingly. Use of broad, non-specific panels of antibodies without regard to the particular considerations at hand often leads to aberrant findings, which can result in diagnostic confusion and even misdiagnosis.

This section reviews the IHC profile of breast carcinoma and then discusses the use of IHC within the context of specific differential diagnoses (**Table 6**).

Breast Carcinoma

Carcinomas of breast origin are usually positive for cytokeratin 7 and negative for cytokeratin 20 (CK7+/CK20–).[64,65] This profile overlaps with

Table 6	
Useful immunohistochemical markers for differentiating breast carcinoma from other malignancies	
Differential Diagnosis	**Helpful Antibodies**
Pulmonary carcinoma	TTF-1/napsin A/GCDFP-15/mammaglobin
Ovarian carcinoma	WT-1/PAX8/GCDFP-15/mammaglobin
Endometrial carcinoma	PAX8/GCDFP-15
Gastric carcinoma	CK20/CDX-2/GCDFP-15/mammaglobin/ER
Melanoma	HMB-45/MART-1/cytokeratin
Sweat gland carcinoma	p63/D2-40/high molecular weight cytokeratins

that of many other common adenocarcinomas, such as those arising from the lung or the gynecologic tract, diminishing the utility of the CK7/CK20 expression pattern for identifying breast carcinoma. Additionally, up to 11% of breast carcinomas are negative for CK7, so the absence of CK7 expression does not exclude the breast as a site of origin.[66] CK7 expression can be patchy, and sampling issues may potentially affect interpretation. Variance from the classical CK7+/CK20− profile occurs with CK20 as well. Approximately 7% of breast carcinomas are positive for CK20, and its expression can be either diffuse or focal.[66,67] Mucinous and lobular carcinomas seem to have a slightly greater propensity for CK20 expression than other subtypes of breast cancer.[67] Most often these CK20+ tumors coexpress CK7 (CK7+/CK20+); only rare breast cancers demonstrate a CK7−/CK20+ colonic-type profile.[66,67]

One useful marker for breast origin is gross cystic disease fluid protein-15 (GCDFP-15). GCDFP-15 is 1 of 4 major constituent proteins found in breast cyst fluid.[68] It is strongly expressed in the cytoplasm of cells demonstrating apocrine differentiation and is found in normal breast epithelium.[69,70] IHC expression of GCDFP-15 is seen in 62% to 74% of primary breast carcinomas.[70–73] In locally recurrent or metastatic breast cancer, the reported rates of expression range from 11% to 71% (Fig. 10).[70,74–79] Staining is typically heterogeneous and commonly focal,

which may affect detection in small biopsies and tissue microarray-based studies. Data from some studies suggest that lobular carcinomas show more frequent and more extensive staining for GCDFP-15 than ductal carcinomas.[75,77] Although the sensitivity of GCDFP-15 is only moderate, its specificity is excellent at 95%.[71] It is only uncommonly expressed in tumors from other sites, including[71,72,75,76,78,80,81]

- Lung (3%–15%)
- Prostate (10%)
- Ovary (4%)
- Stomach (3%)
- Kidney (3%)
- Bladder (2%)

Higher rates of expression are seen in salivary gland carcinomas (41% to 76%) and apocrine sweat gland tumors of the skin (100%), but these tumors typically have a clinical picture that is distinct from that of breast carcinoma.[82,83] In general, a positive result for GCDFP-15 is highly suggestive of breast origin, but a negative result does not exclude the possibility, because a significant proportion of breast carcinomas do not express this marker.

Another IHC marker for breast origin is mammaglobin. Mammaglobin is a small secretory protein that was initially identified based on its overexpression in human primary breast carcinoma.[84] IHC reactivity for mammaglobin can be observed in benign breast tissue, where its expression is

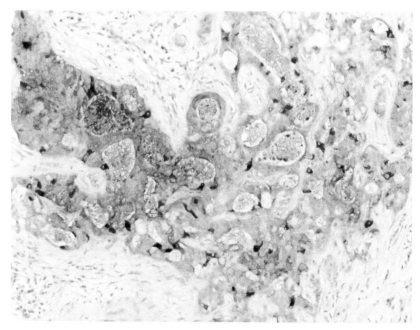

Fig. 10. GCDFP-15 positivity in metastatic breast cancer involving a mediastinal lymph node.

typically focal, and in breast carcinomas.[70,85] 48% to 72% of primary breast carcinomas show cytoplasmic positivity for mammaglobin as do 48% to 87% of locally recurrent and metastatic breast carcinomas (Fig. 11).[70,72–74,76–78,85–88] Like GCDFP-15, its expression is often heterogeneous, but it tends to be positive in a higher percentage of tumor cells than GCDFP-15.[74,77] In studies that have compared the 2 markers, the sensitivity of mammaglobin is similar or superior to that of GCDFP-15.[70,72–74,76–78,87,89] It is, however, a less specific marker of breast origin. Mammaglobin expression has been reported in 11% to 58% of endometrial adenocarcinomas, including 77% of endometrioid-type carcinomas in one study, and in 31% of endocervical adenocarcinomas.[77,85,86,90] Expression is also seen in up to 40% of tumors from the cutaneous sweat glands; 20% from the salivary gland, thyroid, and bladder; 17% from the lung; 13% from the stomach; 12% from the colorectum; 10% from the hepatobiliary tract; 3% from the ovary (serous carcinoma); and 1% from the pancreas.[76,77,91] Positivity for mammaglobin has even been reported in 6% of melanomas.[77]

Combined use of GCDFP-15 and mammaglobin results in increased sensitivity for the detection of breast origin. In one study of 165 primary breast carcinomas, GCDFP-15 was positive in 73.3% of cases and mammaglobin in 72.1%[70]; 91.8% of the cases, however, expressed at least 1 of the 2 markers. The specificity of dual positivity for GCDFP-15 and mammaglobin is not well studied.

Both GCDFP-15 and mammaglobin are more frequently expressed in luminal A, luminal B, and Her-2–overexpressing tumors than in basal-like and unclassified triple-negative carcinomas.[89] Infrequent expression of GCDFP-15 and mammaglobin in the latter 2 groups adds to the difficulty in distinguishing these often poorly differentiated tumors from other high-grade neoplasms arising from nonbreast sites.

Breast Versus Lung

Distinguishing breast carcinoma from lung carcinoma is a common diagnostic problem. Breast and lung cancers are both common malignancies, and patients not infrequently have primary tumors at both sites. The lung is also a major site of metastasis for breast cancer (see Fig. 1). A new lung nodule in a patient with a history of breast cancer, therefore, has a reasonable likelihood of representing either a new primary tumor or a metastasis, and there are major differences in clinical management depending on which of the 2 it is. Additionally, both lung and breast carcinomas are important considerations in the differential diagnosis of carcinomas of unknown primary, and although metastases to the breast are rare, lung carcinoma is one of the more common solid tumors to secondarily involve the breast (see Fig. 2).

For tumors involving the lung, a combination of clinical, radiographic, and histologic features usually enables appropriate classification. Knowledge of any prior history of malignancy is

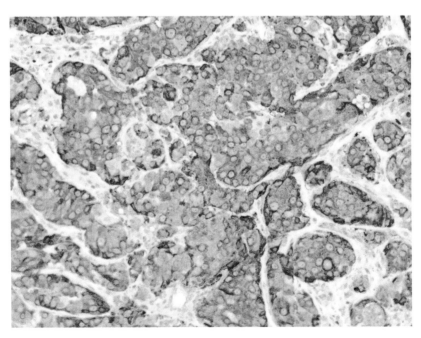

Fig. 11. Mammaglobin positivity in primary breast cancer.

invaluable, although this information is not always conveyed to the pathologist. The imaging characteristics of the tumor are helpful: primary lung cancers are typically spiculated, whereas metastases tend to have more rounded contours. The presence of multiple lung nodules favors metastasis. Histologic examination of primary lung adenocarcinomas often reveals central scarring as well as lepidic growth at the periphery; metastases usually lack these features. A lymphangitic pattern and multifocal pleural involvement may be seen in metastases. Comparison with slides of any prior malignancy is, as always, prudent.

IHC stains that are useful in the differentiation of lung adenocarcinoma from breast carcinoma include thyroid transcription factor-1 (TTF-1) and napsin A for lung origin (**Fig. 12**) and GCDFP-15 and mammaglobin for breast origin. The CK 7/20 profile of lung and breast adenocarcinomas is similar and, therefore, not discriminatory.

TTF-1 is a member of the NKX2 family of homeodomain transcription factors. Nuclear TTF-1 expression is highly specific for carcinomas of lung and thyroid origin. TTF-1 is probably the most widely used marker for confirming pulmonary origin. It is positive in 72% to 88% of primary lung adenocarcinomas; mucinous and poorly differentiated adenocarcinomas are less likely to stain.[72,92–96] TTF-1 is infrequently expressed in pulmonary squamous cell carcinomas (<10%). Most small cell carcinomas of the lung are positive; however, TTF-1 is also often expressed in extrapulmonary small cell carcinomas, including 20% of those that arise in the breast.[97–101]

The 2 most commonly used antibody clones for the detection of TTF-1 are 8G7G3/1 (DakoCytomation) and SPT24 (Novocastra, Leica Microsystems). The Leica/Novocastra SPT24 clone is generally considered more sensitive but less specific than the Dako 8G7G3/1 clone for lung adenocarcinoma.[102] Nearly all reported examples of breast adenocarcinoma, either primary or metastatic, have been negative for TTF-1 when stained with either clone. Exceptions are reported in only one systematic study. Robens and colleagues[103] found that 13 of 546 (2.4%) breast carcinomas were positive for TTF-1 using the SPT24 clone. The positive cases consisted of 12 invasive ductal carcinomas and 1 invasive lobular carcinoma. Staining was most often focal and weak, but a few cases showed diffuse and strong positivity. Overall, TTF-1 is a highly specific marker for lung origin when attempting to discriminate adenocarcinoma of the lung from that of the breast, but reactivity may be encountered in rare breast carcinomas, particularly when using the SPT24 clone.[104]

Napsin A is a more recently described IHC marker of lung adenocarcinoma. It is an aspartic proteinase that is expressed in type II pneumocytes and is involved in the processing of prosurfactant protein B.[105,106] It is also expressed in the proximal and convoluted tubules of the kidney and the exocrine glands and ducts of the pancreas.[105] Between 80% and 90% of primary

Fig. 12. TTF-1 (brown nuclear staining) and napsin A (red cytoplasmic staining) positivity in primary lung adenocarcinoma.

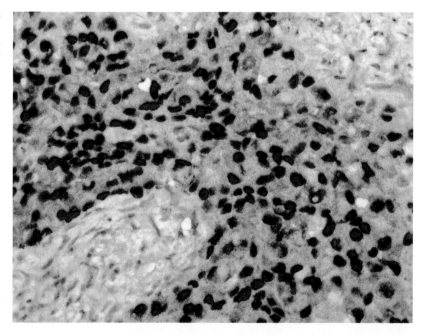

lung adenocarcinomas are positive for napsin A, which demonstrates a granular cytoplasmic staining pattern.[72,105,107–110] Pulmonary squamous cell, large cell, and small cell carcinomas are usually negative. Among nonpulmonary malignancies, napsin A is frequently expressed in renal cell carcinomas: 80% of papillary renal cell carcinomas and 34% of clear cell renal cell carcinomas are positive for this marker.[108,110] Expression has also been reported in 5% of papillary thyroid carcinomas.[108] Although data are relatively limited, other carcinomas from various nonpulmonary sites, including the breast, are largely negative for napsin A.[107,108,110] Napsin A expression has been described in breast carcinoma in only 2 reports. One of the early studies on napsin A documents a few cases of adenocarcinoma from the pancreas, breast, colon, and ovary with weak napsin A expression, a pattern that differs from the strong granular staining seen in lung adenocarcinoma.[105] A more recent abstract report describes napsin A expression in 4 out of 30 triple-negative breast carcinomas, but staining was focal and seen in only 5% to 10% of tumor cells.[111] Altogether, combined use of napsin A and TTF-1 leads to increased sensitivity for identification of pulmonary origin, and dual positivity for both napsin A and TTF-1 seems highly specific for primary lung adenocarcinoma.[108,110]

Several studies have documented positivity for GCDFP-15 in 2.5% to 5% of lung carcinomas.[72,76,80,81] A single study identified positivity in 15% of primary lung adenocarcinomas, but this result seems aberrantly high.[78] When seen, GCDFP-15 expression is typically focal. Most studies show no expression of mammaglobin in primary lung adenocarcinoma (>350 cases tested),[72,78,86] although 1 study of only 30 lung cancers had a 17% rate of positivity.[76] The rate of ER positivity in lung carcinoma varies from less than 1% to upward of 30% of cases and depends on the antibody clone that is used; expression is usually focal if present.[72,112]

A panel of antibodies incorporating TTF-1, napsin A, GCDFP-15, and mammaglobin is most informative for differentiating lung from breast adenocarcinoma. Positivity for TTF-1 or napsin A strongly suggests lung origin, especially if there is dual positivity for both markers. Rare breast cancers may stain for either of these pulmonary markers, however, so awareness of the antibody clone used and attention to the extent and pattern of staining are important. Positivity for GCDFP-15 or mammaglobin is most suggestive of breast origin, but a small percentage of primary lung carcinomas are reactive. Lack of immunoreactivity for GCDFP-15 and mammaglobin also does not exclude

a diagnosis of breast carcinoma because neither marker is wholly sensitive. ER may be helpful in certain cases, but there is a degree of overlap between breast and lung carcinomas from this standpoint, and technical considerations, such as the choice of antibody clone, can influence the results.

Breast Versus Ovary

Breast and ovarian cancers are common in the same patient population, particularly in women with germline mutations in BRCA1 or BRCA2. The need to distinguish between the 2 types of malignancies therefore arises not infrequently. Fortunately, the morphologic features are sufficiently distinctive in many cases. For example, the hierarchical branching and occasional fibrovascular cores of papillary serous carcinoma of the ovary (see Fig. 3A) are not typical features of micropapillary carcinoma of the breast, and the tall columnar cells and elongated glands of endometrioid carcinoma are not usually seen in invasive ductal carcinoma. Poorly differentiated tumors arising from either site, however, can be more difficult to distinguish from one another. Careful examination for focal areas with more distinctive patterns can be invaluable (Figs. 13 and 14). Additionally, when evaluating neoplasms in the ovary, identification of background endometriosis or an underlying adenofibroma helps support a diagnosis of primary ovarian carcinoma (see Fig. 14C), whereas bilaterality, surface involvement, multinodular growth (Fig. 15), and prominent lymphatic invasion are features more common to tumors metastatic to the ovary.

IHC can be of great utility in difficult cases. The most useful markers are Wilms tumor 1 (WT-1) and paired box gene 8 (PAX8) for ovarian origin and GCDFP-15 and mammaglobin for breast origin. The applicability of these different immunostains, however, depends on the particular subtypes of carcinoma in the differential diagnosis.

WT-1 is expressed in the nuclei of 82% to 100% of ovarian, tubal, and peritoneal serous carcinomas and transitional cell carcinomas (see Figs. 3C and 13E).[79,113–124] Expression is typically diffuse and strong in these tumors. WT-1 is uncommonly expressed in endometrioid (6%), clear cell (4%), and mucinous (0%) carcinomas arising from these sites.[79,114,116–121,124–126] In unselected breast carcinomas, nuclear WT-1 expression is seen in only 3% of tumors.[79,113,116,118,120,127,128] Subtype analysis, however, reveals that WT-1 expression is present in almost half of pure and mixed mucinous carcinomas of the breast.[126,128] Most show only weak to moderate positivity for

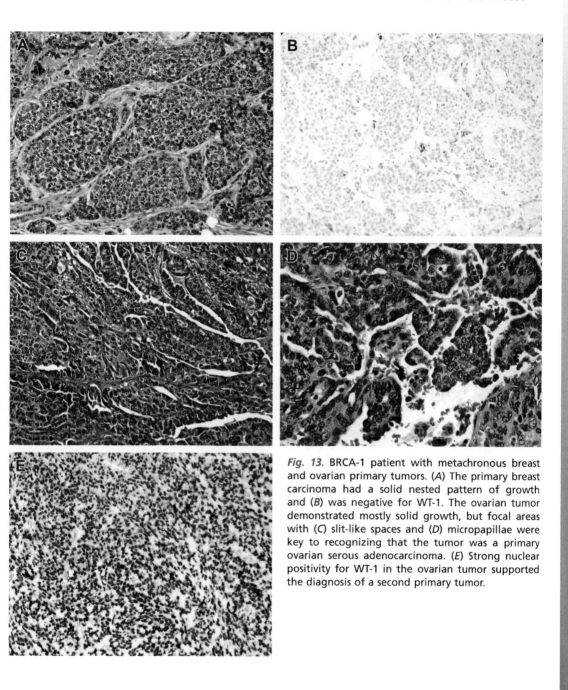

Fig. 13. BRCA-1 patient with metachronous breast and ovarian primary tumors. (*A*) The primary breast carcinoma had a solid nested pattern of growth and (*B*) was negative for WT-1. The ovarian tumor demonstrated mostly solid growth, but focal areas with (*C*) slit-like spaces and (*D*) micropapillae were key to recognizing that the tumor was a primary ovarian serous adenocarcinoma. (*E*) Strong nuclear positivity for WT-1 in the ovarian tumor supported the diagnosis of a second primary tumor.

WT-1, but occasional tumors demonstrate strong and diffuse reactivity (**Fig. 16**). A minority (11%) of micropapillary carcinomas of the breast, in particular those with mixed mucinous differentiation, may also show reactivity for WT-1; however, in those examples without a mucinous component, expression is usually limited (≤10% of cells) and only of weak to moderate intensity.[122,128–130]

Overall, WT-1 is useful for distinguishing ovarian serous or transitional cell carcinomas from breast carcinomas. Diffuse strong positivity favors an ovarian primary whereas a negative reaction favors a breast primary. WT-1 expression may be seen in certain subtypes of breast carcinoma, but reactivity is typically focal and only of weak to moderate intensity. WT-1 is generally not useful for distinguishing ovarian endometrioid, clear cell, or mucinous carcinomas from breast carcinoma, because all are usually negative for this antigen. Additionally, it is important to remember that other

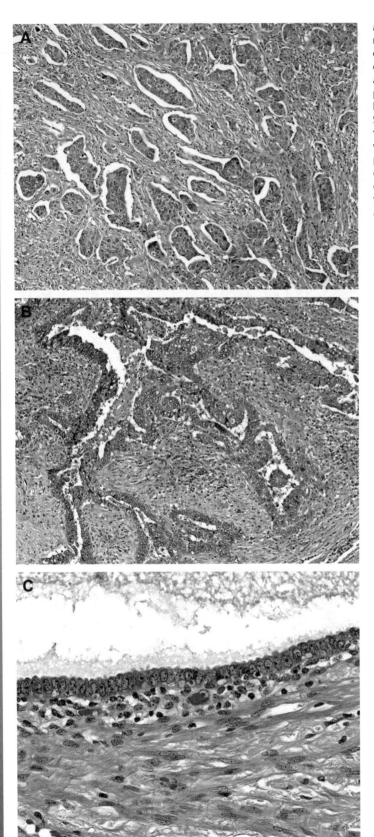

Fig. 14. Primary ovarian carcinoma mimicking a metastasis. (*A*) The pattern of irregular nests was unusual for an ovarian surface epithelial carcinoma and suggested a metastasis. The patient had a history of node-positive breast carcinoma 17 years prior. (*B*) Submission of additional sections from the ovarian tumor revealed focal areas with more typical endometrioid morphology and (*C*) associated atypical endometriosis, supporting a diagnosis of a poorly differentiated endometrioid adenocarcinoma rather than a metastasis.

Fig. 15. Multinodular growth pattern of a metastatic breast cancer involving the ovary.

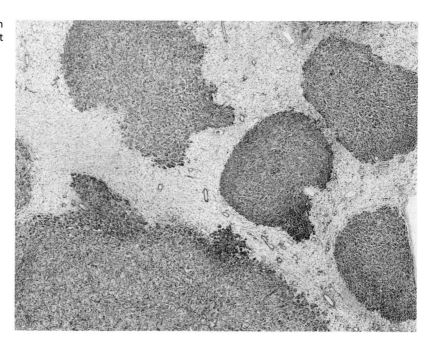

tumors, such as mesothelioma and desmoplastic small round cell tumor, also express WT-1, so a WT-1–positive tumor in the abdomen is not necessarily of mullerian derivation.[131]

PAX8 is a paired box transcription factor that plays an important role in the embryonic development of the mullerian system, kidneys, and thyroid.

It is expressed in solid tumors arising from those organs as well as thymic tumors.[132] Among tumors of the ovary, nuclear expression is seen in 91% of serous, 81% of clear cell, 61% of endometrioid, and 27% of mucinous carcinomas.[120–122,125,126,132–138] It is also expressed in ovarian transitional cell carcinomas, but only

Fig. 16. Mixed mucinous carcinoma of the breast demonstrating strong reactivity for WT-1.

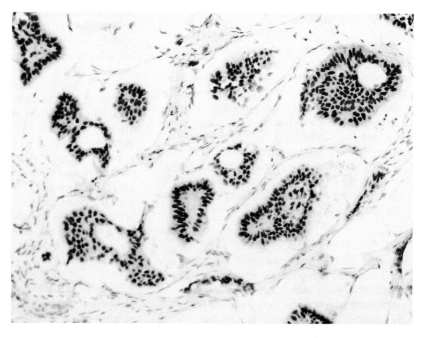

a few cases have so far been evaluated.[132] Of more than 600 breast carcinomas reported to date, none has shown positivity for PAX8.[120,122,126,132,134–137,139,140] Therefore, reactivity for PAX8 is supportive of an ovarian origin in this differential diagnosis, but the diagnostic value of a negative result depends on the particular subtype of ovarian carcinoma under consideration.

As discussed previously, a small minority (4%) of ovarian carcinomas express GCDFP-15, but in general, a positive reaction should lead to strong consideration of a breast primary. A negative result, however, is noninformative because the sensitivity of GCDFP-15 for breast carcinoma is only moderate. Mammaglobin expression has been reported in 3% of ovarian serous carcinomas but has not been extensively studied in these tumors, and there is little information regarding the rate of reactivity in other subtypes of ovarian surface epithelial carcinoma. Because mammaglobin is expressed in a high percentage of endometrioid adenocarcinomas originating from the uterus, reactivity in endometrioid adenocarcinomas of ovarian origin is likely. Therefore, a positive reaction for mammaglobin should be interpreted cautiously when an endometrioid-type tumor is a consideration based on the morphology.

Breast Versus Endometrium

As with ovarian carcinoma, morphology often provides enough clues to distinguish endometrial carcinoma from breast carcinoma, but less differentiated tumors can present diagnostic difficulty (**Fig. 17**). WT-1 is less useful in this setting because only 21% of endometrial serous carcinomas are positive.[115,117,119,124,141] WT-1 expression is also uncommon in endometrial endometrioid (13%) and clear cell (9%) carcinomas.[117,119,124,141] PAX8, however, is positive in 97% of endometrioid, 91% of serous, and up to 100% of clear cell carcinomas of the endometrium and, therefore, is useful for distinguishing these tumors from breast carcinoma (see **Fig. 17**D).[132,135,137,138] Rare endometrial carcinomas may express GCDFP-15 (see **Fig. 17**E). Mammaglobin is commonly expressed in endometrial carcinomas, in particular those of endometrioid type, and therefore is of limited utility in this differential diagnosis.

Breast Versus Stomach

Metastatic breast carcinoma can mimic a primary gastrointestinal malignancy on clinical, radiographic, and even endoscopic evaluation. Most gastrointestinal primaries, however, are histologically distinct from breast carcinoma. When diagnostic problems arise, they are often related to gastric signet ring cell carcinomas, which bear a strong resemblance to invasive lobular carcinoma of the breast. Further complicating matters is that lobular carcinoma metastasizes more frequently to the gastrointestinal tract than ductal carcinoma, and it accounts for approximately 70% of gastrointestinal metastases of breast cancer.[4,8] Additionally, some patients are at risk for both types of cancer: women with hereditary inactivating mutations in the E-cadherin gene *CDH1* are at increased risk for diffuse-type gastric cancer (approximately 70% lifetime risk) as well as lobular carcinoma (additional 20%–40% risk).[142]

By immunohistochemistry, metastatic breast carcinomas to the gastrointestinal tract are more often positive for ER (72–76%), GCDFP-15 (62–78%), and mammaglobin (52%) than primary gastric carcinomas (ER, 0–28%; GCDFP-15, 0%; mammaglobin, 13%).[76,77,86,143–147] Primary gastric carcinomas are more often positive for CK20 (50–100%) and CDX-2 (70–90%) than metastatic breast carcinomas (CK20, 0–7%; CDX-2, 0%).[65–67,143,144,148–151] Positivity for GCDFP-15 or mammaglobin, therefore, supports a mammary origin (**Fig. 18**), but negative results are noninformative. An ER+ signet ring cell carcinoma is more likely of breast origin, whereas a CK20+ or CDX-2+ tumor is more likely to be of gastrointestinal origin. Because there is some overlap in ER and CK7/CK20 profiles between breast and gastric carcinomas, and because the more site-specific markers (GCDFP-15, mammaglobin, and CDX-2) are not entirely sensitive, a panel of IHC markers provides the most information when working up this differential diagnosis.

Evaluation of mucin glycoprotein antigens can provide additional information, but the results should be integrated with the aforementioned studies.[143,144,152] Primary gastric carcinomas frequently express MUC5AC (58–85%), whereas metastatic breast cancers to the gastrointestinal tract infrequently do so (5%–6%). MUC6 is expressed in subset of gastric carcinomas (27%–39%), but is usually negative in gastric metastases of breast carcinoma. MUC6 expression, however, has been reported in up to 50% of primary mucinous breast carcinomas.[126] MUC2 is positive in approximately 50% of gastric carcinomas, but it is also expressed in 24% of breast cancer metastases and has a high rate of expression in primary mucinous carcinomas of the breast (up to 100%).[126,153]

Breast Versus Melanoma

Malignant melanoma, especially minimally pigmented or amelanotic examples, can be mistaken

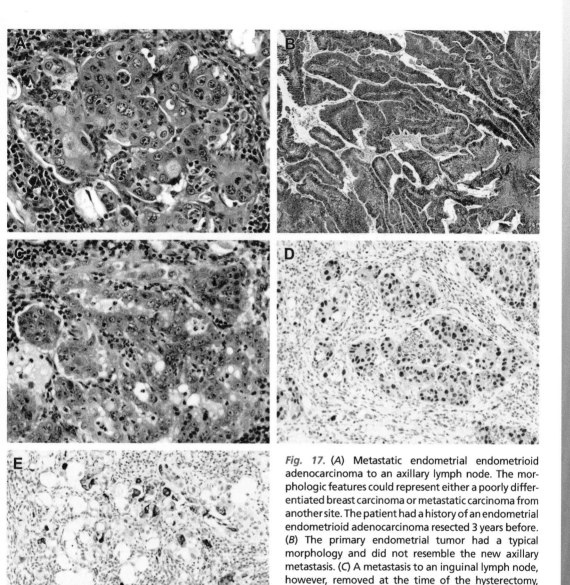

Fig. 17. (A) Metastatic endometrial endometrioid adenocarcinoma to an axillary lymph node. The morphologic features could represent either a poorly differentiated breast carcinoma or metastatic carcinoma from another site. The patient had a history of an endometrial endometrioid adenocarcinoma resected 3 years before. (B) The primary endometrial tumor had a typical morphology and did not resemble the new axillary metastasis. (C) A metastasis to an inguinal lymph node, however, removed at the time of the hysterectomy, showed morphologic similarity to the subsequent tumor in the axilla. (D) The metastatic tumor in the axilla showed strong nuclear positivity for PAX8, supportive of mullerian origin. (E) The tumor also showed focal reactivity for GCDFP-15, which could have lead to a misdiagnosis of breast carcinoma if viewed in isolation.

for high-grade breast carcinoma (see Fig. 6). A high index of suspicion in patients with a history of melanoma is important. Attention to any areas of pigmentation or unusual morphologic growth, such as spindle cell areas, can alert pathologists to the possibility of melanoma (see Fig. 5). Immunoreactivity for HMB-45 and MART-1 and lack of cytokeratin expression distinguish melanoma from breast carcinoma. S-100 is not discriminatory

because breast carcinomas can also express S-100. Rare primary breast carcinomas may contain areas with melanocytic differentiation, but these areas merge with those exhibiting the morphologic and IHC features of carcinoma.[154,155]

Breast Versus Skin Adnexa

The most common cause of cutaneous metastases in women is breast cancer.[156] Because

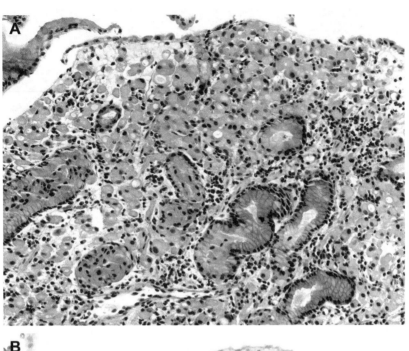

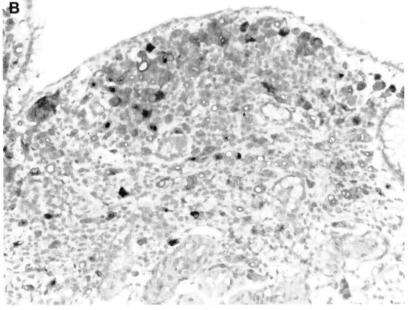

Fig. 18. (*A*) Metastatic lobular carcinoma to the stomach. (*B*) Positivity for GCDFP-15 supports the diagnosis.

breast and skin adnexal carcinomas can demonstrate morphologic overlap, IHC is occasionally needed to help differentiate them. Useful markers in this regard include p63, D2-40, and high molecular weight cytokeratins. p63 is positive in 90% to 100% and D2-40 in 44% to 100% of primary skin adnexal carcinomas.[91,157–161] Both of these markers react with the basaloid cells of primary adnexal carcinomas. High molecular weight cytokeratins, such as cytokeratins 5, 14, 15, and 17, are also expressed in 40% to 91% of skin adnexal carcinomas.[91,157,160] Reactivity for p63 and high molecular weight cytokeratins is less common in primary breast carcinoma, and reactivity for

D2-40 is generally not seen. Studies of cutaneous metastases of breast carcinoma reveal positivity for p63 in 0% to 8% of cases, high molecular weight cytokeratins in 6% to 17%, and D2-40 in only rare examples.[91,157–162] Significant overlap exists between breast and skin adnexal carcinomas in terms of their reactivity for GCDFP-15, ER, and PR, and therefore these markers have no reliable discriminatory value.[83,163–165] Mammaglobin has not been extensively studied in skin adnexal carcinomas, but its expression is reported in a minority of eccrine carcinomas.[91]

A note of caution applies to primary apocrine carcinomas of the skin. Morphologically, these tumors may be indistinguishable from metastatic apocrine carcinoma from the breast. They are largely indistinguishable by IHC means as well. Data are limited, but cutaneous apocrine carcinomas are often negative for p63, D2-40, and high molecular weight cytokeratins, similar to apocrine carcinomas of the breast.[158,160,162] They are also, like their mammary counterparts, positive for GCDFP-15. Consequently, IHC markers are of little discriminatory value. Another note of caution applies to adenocarcinomas involving the skin of the axilla in the absence of a primary neoplasm in the breast. Although superficial biopsies may raise consideration of a primary skin adnexal carcinoma, in the authors' experience, these tumors often turn out to represent mammary carcinomas arising in underlying axillary breast tissue, a fact that only becomes evident on wide local excision.

Pitfalls
IMMUNOHISTOCHEMISTRY FOR SITE OF ORIGIN

! GCDFP-15 is only moderately sensitive for breast carcinoma, and a negative result for this marker does not exclude breast origin.

! Mammaglobin seems somewhat more sensitive but less specific than GCDFP-15 for breast origin; it is often positive in endometrioid adenocarcinomas.

! TTF-1 expression is seen in 2.4% of breast adenocarcinomas, particularly when using the Leica/Novocastra SPT24 antibody clone.

! Focal or weak napsin A expression has been reported in a small number of breast cancers.

! WT-1 positivity is seen in many examples of pure or mixed mucinous carcinomas of the breast.

! PAX8 demonstrates a broader range of positivity than WT-1 among female genital tract adenocarcinomas, but it is often negative in mucinous tumors and does not discriminate between adnexal/peritoneal and uterine origin.

! Primary gastric adenocarcinomas may show variable CK7/CK20 expression patterns, and a minority are reported to be positive for ER.

! S-100 can be positive in breast adenocarcinomas and, therefore, HMB-45 and MART-1 are better markers for discriminating between breast cancer and melanoma.

! Skin adnexal tumors show notable morphologic and IHC overlap with breast carcinoma, although a panel of p63, D2-40, and high molecular weight cytokeratin can be helpful in nonapocrine tumors.

IDENTIFICATION OF METASTATIC CARCINOMA

Proper recognition of metastases to and from the breast requires careful attention to the clinical history and the morphologic findings. Judicious use of a selected panel of IHC stains, tailored to the specific differential diagnosis suggested by the morphology, can provide helpful information in difficult cases. No marker is completely specific or sensitive for site of origin, however. An awareness of the limitations of each individual IHC marker is essential for successful use of these adjunct studies. Furthermore, the IHC results cannot be interpreted in isolation, and they must be integrated with the morphologic and clinical features to arrive at the correct diagnosis.

REFERENCES

1. Ferlay J, Shin HR, Bray F, et al. GLOBOCAN 2008, Cancer Incidence and Mortality Worldwide: IARC CancerBase No. 10. Available at: http://globocan. iarc.fr. Accessed June 19, 2011.
2. Howlader N, Noone AM, Krapcho M, et al. SEER Cancer Statistics Review, 1975-2008. Available at: http://seer.cancer.gov/csr/1975_2008. Accessed June 20, 2011.
3. Disibio G, French SW. Metastatic patterns of cancers: results from a large autopsy study. Arch Pathol Lab Med 2008;132(6):931–9.
4. Harris M, Howell A, Chrissohou M, et al. A comparison of the metastatic pattern of infiltrating lobular carcinoma and infiltrating duct carcinoma of the breast. Br J Cancer 1984;50(1):23–30.
5. Dixon AR, Ellis IO, Elston CW, et al. A comparison of the clinical metastatic patterns of invasive lobular and ductal carcinomas of the breast. Br J Cancer 1991;63(4):634–5.

6. Lamovec J, Bracko M. Metastatic pattern of infiltrating lobular carcinoma of the breast: an autopsy study. J Surg Oncol 1991;48(1):28–33.

7. Jain S, Fisher C, Smith P, et al. Patterns of metastatic breast cancer in relation to histological type. Eur J Cancer 1993;29A(15):2155–7.

8. Borst MJ, Ingold JA. Metastatic patterns of invasive lobular versus invasive ductal carcinoma of the breast. Surgery 1993;114(4):637–41.

9. Tsuda H, Takarabe T, Hasegawa F, et al. Large, central acellular zones indicating myoepithelial tumor differentiation in high-grade invasive ductal carcinomas as markers of predisposition to lung and brain metastases. Am J Surg Pathol 2000; 24(2):197–202.

10. Hicks DG, Short SM, Prescott NL, et al. Breast cancers with brain metastases are more likely to be estrogen receptor negative, express the basal cytokeratin CK5/6, and overexpress HER2 or EGFR. Am J Surg Pathol 2006;30(9):1097–104.

11. Smid M, Wang Y, Zhang Y, et al. Subtypes of breast cancer show preferential site of relapse. Cancer Res 2008;68(9):3108–14.

12. Leyland-Jones B. Human epidermal growth factor receptor 2-positive breast cancer and central nervous system metastases. J Clin Oncol 2009; 27(31):5278–86.

13. Kennecke H, Yerushalmi R, Woods R, et al. Metastatic behavior of breast cancer subtypes. J Clin Oncol 2010;28(20):3271–7.

14. Fulford LG, Reis-Filho JS, Ryder K, et al. Basal-like grade III invasive ductal carcinoma of the breast: patterns of metastasis and long-term survival. Breast Cancer Res 2007;9(1):R4.

15. Lin NU, Claus E, Sohl J, et al. Sites of distant recurrence and clinical outcomes in patients with metastatic triple-negative breast cancer: high incidence of central nervous system metastases. Cancer 2008;113(10):2638–45.

16. Liedtke C, Mazouni C, Hess KR, et al. Response to neoadjuvant therapy and long-term survival in patients with triple-negative breast cancer. J Clin Oncol 2008;26(8):1275–81.

17. Hess KR, Pusztai L, Buzdar AU, et al. Estrogen receptors and distinct patterns of breast cancer relapse. Breast Cancer Res Treat 2003;78(1):105–18.

18. Lower EE, Glass EL, Bradley DA, et al. Impact of metastatic estrogen receptor and progesterone receptor status on survival. Breast Cancer Res Treat 2005;90(1):65–70.

19. Guarneri V, Giovannelli S, Ficarra G, et al. Comparison of HER-2 and hormone receptor expression in primary breast cancers and asynchronous paired metastases: impact on patient management. Oncologist 2008;13(8):838–44.

20. Broom RJ, Tang PA, Simmons C, et al. Changes in estrogen receptor, progesterone receptor and Her-2/neu status with time: discordance rates between primary and metastatic breast cancer. Anticancer Res 2009;29(5):1557–62.

21. Liedtke C, Broglio K, Moulder S, et al. Prognostic impact of discordance between triple-receptor measurements in primary and recurrent breast cancer. Ann Oncol 2009;20(12):1953–8.

22. Gong Y, Han EY, Guo M, et al. Stability of estrogen receptor status in breast carcinoma: a comparison between primary and metastatic tumors with regard to disease course and intervening systemic therapy. Cancer 2011;117(4):705–13.

23. Tanner M, Jarvinen P, Isola J. Amplification of HER-2/neu and topoisomerase IIα in primary and metastatic breast cancer. Cancer Res 2001;61(14): 5345–8.

24. Gancberg D, Di Leo A, Cardoso F, et al. Comparison of HER-2 status between primary breast cancer and corresponding distant metastatic sites. Ann Oncol 2002;13(7):1036–43.

25. Regitnig P, Schippinger W, Lindbauer M, et al. Change of HER-2/neu status in a subset of distant metastases from breast carcinomas. J Pathol 2004; 203(4):918–26.

26. Gong Y, Booser DJ, Sneige N. Comparison of HER-2 status determined by fluorescence in situ hybridization in primary and metastatic breast carcinoma. Cancer 2005;103(9):1763–9.

27. Zidan J, Dashkovsky I, Stayerman C, et al. Comparison of HER-2 overexpression in primary breast cancer and metastatic sites and its effect on biological targeting therapy of metastatic disease. Br J Cancer 2005;93(5):552–6.

28. Lower EE, Glass E, Blau R, et al. HER-2/neu expression in primary and metastatic breast cancer. Breast Cancer Res Treat 2009;113(2):301–6.

29. Mittendorf EA, Wu Y, Scaltriti M, et al. Loss of HER2 amplification following trastuzumab-based neoadjuvant systemic therapy and survival outcomes. Clin Cancer Res 2009;15(23):7381–8.

30. Hammond ME, Hayes DF, Dowsett M, et al. American Society of Clinical Oncology/College of American Pathologists guideline recommendations for immunohistochemical testing of estrogen and progesterone receptors in breast cancer (unabridged version). Arch Pathol Lab Med 2010; 134(7):e48–72.

31. Wolff AC, Hammond ME, Schwartz JN, et al. American Society of Clinical Oncology/College of American Pathologists guideline recommendations for human epidermal growth factor receptor 2 testing in breast cancer. Arch Pathol Lab Med 2007; 131(1):18–43.

32. Sandison AT. Metastatic tumours in the breast. Br J Surg 1959;47:54–8.

33. Paulus DD, Libshitz HI. Metastasis to the breast. Radiol Clin North Am 1982;20(3):561–8.

34. Georgiannos SN, Chin J, Goode AW, et al. Secondary neoplasms of the breast: a survey of the 20th Century. Cancer 2001;92(9):2259–66.

35. Abrams HL, Spiro R, Goldstein N. Metastases in carcinoma: analysis of 1000 autopsied cases. Cancer 1950;3(1):74–85.

36. Hajdu SI, Urban JA. Cancers metastatic to the breast. Cancer 1972;29(6):1691–6.

37. Toombs BD, Kalisher L. Metastatic disease to the breast: clinical, pathologic, and radiographic features. AJR Am J Roentgenol 1977;129(4):673–6.

38. Alvarado Cabrero I, Carrera Alvarez M, Perez Montiel D, et al. Metastases to the breast. Eur J Surg Oncol 2003;29(10):854–5.

39. Lee SK, Kim WW, Kim SH, et al. Characteristics of metastasis in the breast from extramammary malignancies. J Surg Oncol 2010;101(2):137–40.

40. Noguera JJ, Martinez-Miravete P, Idoate F, et al. Metastases to the breast: a review of 33 cases. Australas Radiol 2007;51(2):133–8.

41. McIntosh IH, Hooper AA, Millis RR, et al. Metastatic carcinoma within the breast. Clin Oncol 1976;2(4): 393–401.

42. Di Bonito L, Luchi M, Giarelli L, et al. Metastatic tumors to the female breast. An autopsy study of 12 cases. Pathol Res Pract 1991;187(4):432–6.

43. Alva S, Shetty-Alva N. An update of tumor metastasis to the breast data. Arch Surg 1999;134(4):450.

44. David O, Gattuso P, Razan W, et al. Unusual cases of metastases to the breast. A report of 17 cases diagnosed by fine needle aspiration. Acta Cytol 2002;46(2):377–85.

45. Williams SA, Ehlers RA 2nd, Hunt KK, et al. Metastases to the breast from nonbreast solid neoplasms: presentation and determinants of survival. Cancer 2007;110(4):731–7.

46. Wood B, Sterrett G, Frost F, et al. Diagnosis of extramammary malignancy metastatic to the breast by fine needle biopsy. Pathology 2008;40(4):345–51.

47. Salyer WR, Salyer DC. Metastases of prostatic carcinoma to the breast. J Urol 1973;109(4):671–5.

48. Ferry J. Lymphomas of the breast. In: Extranodal lymphomas. Philadelphia: Elsevier Saunders; 2011. p. 125–7.

49. McCrea ES, Johnston C, Haney PJ. Metastases to the breast. AJR Am J Roentgenol 1983;141(4):685–90.

50. Bohman LG, Bassett LW, Gold RH, et al. Breast metastases from extramammary malignancies. Radiology 1982;144(2):309–12.

51. Chaignaud B, Hall TJ, Powers C, et al. Diagnosis and natural history of extramammary tumors metastatic to the breast. J Am Coll Surg 1994;179(1): 49–53.

52. Vergier B, Trojani M, de Mascarel I, et al. Metastases to the breast: differential diagnosis from primary breast carcinoma. J Surg Oncol 1991;48(2): 112–6.

53. Chung SY, Oh KK. Imaging findings of metastatic disease to the breast. Yonsei Med J 2001;42(5): 497–502.

54. Recine MA, Deavers MT, Middleton LP, et al. Serous carcinoma of the ovary and peritoneum with metastases to the breast and axillary lymph nodes: a potential pitfall. Am J Surg Pathol 2004; 28(12):1646–51.

55. Kayikcioglu F, Boran N, Ayhan A, et al. Inflammatory breast metastases of ovarian cancer: a case report. Gynecol Oncol 2001;83(3):613–6.

56. Nebesio CL, Goulet RJ Jr, Helft PR, et al. Metastatic esophageal carcinoma masquerading as inflammatory breast carcinoma. Int J Dermatol 2007; 46(3):303–5.

57. Papakonstantinou K, Antoniou A, Palialexis K, et al. Fallopian tube cancer presenting as inflammatory breast carcinoma: report of a case and review of the literature. Eur J Gynaecol Oncol 2009;30(5):568–71.

58. Khalifeh I, Deavers MT, Cristofanilli M, et al. Primary peritoneal serous carcinoma presenting as inflammatory breast cancer. Breast J 2009;15(2):176–81.

59. Klein RL, Brown AR, Gomez-Castro CM, et al. Ovarian cancer metastatic to the breast presenting as inflammatory breast cancer: a case report and literature review. J Cancer 2010;1:27–31.

60. Mandato VD, Pirillo D, Gelli MC, et al. Gastric cancer in a pregnant woman presenting with low back pain and bilateral erythematous breast hypertrophy mimicking primary inflammatory breast carcinoma. Anticancer Res 2011;31(2):681–5.

61. Gupta D, Merino MI, Farhood A, et al. Metastases to breast simulating ductal carcinoma in situ: report of two cases and review of the literature. Ann Diagn Pathol 2001;5(1):15–20.

62. Rabban JT, Chen YY. D2-40 expression by breast myoepithelium: potential pitfalls in distinguishing intralymphatic carcinoma from in situ carcinoma. Hum Pathol 2008;39(2):175–83.

63. Farkash EA, Ferry JA, Harris NL, et al. Rare lymphoid malignancies of the breast: a report of two cases illustrating potential diagnostic pitfalls. J Hematop 2009;2(4):237–44.

64. Wang NP, Zee S, Zarbo RJ, et al. Coordinate expression of cytokeratins 7 and 20 defines unique subsets of carcinomas. Appl Immunohistochem 1995;3(2):99–107.

65. Chu P, Wu E, Weiss LM. Cytokeratin 7 and cytokeratin 20 expression in epithelial neoplasms: a survey of 435 cases. Mod Pathol 2000;13(9):962–72.

66. Tot T. Cytokeratins 20 and 7 as biomarkers: usefulness in discriminating primary from metastatic adenocarcinoma. Eur J Cancer 2002;38(6):758–63.

67. Tot T. Patterns of distribution of cytokeratins 20 and 7 in special types of invasive breast carcinoma: a study of 123 cases. Ann Diagn Pathol 1999;3(6): 350–6.

68. Haagensen DE Jr, Mazoujian G, Dilley WG, et al. Breast gross cystic disease fluid analysis. I. Isolation and radioimmunoassay for a major component protein. J Natl Cancer Inst 1979;62(2):239–47.

69. Mazoujian G, Pinkus GS, Davis S, et al. Immunohistochemistry of a gross cystic disease fluid protein (GCDFP-15) of the breast. A marker of apocrine epithelium and breast carcinomas with apocrine features. Am J Pathol 1983;110(2):105–12.

70. Fritzsche FR, Thomas A, Winzer KJ, et al. Co-expression and prognostic value of gross cystic disease fluid protein 15 and mammaglobin in primary breast cancer. Histol Histopathol 2007; 22(11):1221–30.

71. Wick MR, Lillemoe TJ, Copland GT, et al. Gross cystic disease fluid protein-15 as a marker for breast cancer: immunohistochemical analysis of 690 human neoplasms and comparison with alpha-lactalbumin. Hum Pathol 1989;20(3):281–7.

72. Yang M, Nonaka D. A study of immunohistochemical differential expression in pulmonary and mammary carcinomas. Mod Pathol 2010;23(5):654–61.

73. Yan Z, Gidley J, Horton D, et al. Diagnostic utility of mammaglobin and GCDFP-15 in the identification of metastatic breast carcinoma in fluid specimens. Diagn Cytopathol 2009;37(7):475–8.

74. Chia SY, Thike AA, Cheok PY, et al. Utility of mammaglobin and gross cystic disease fluid protein-15 (GCDFP-15) in confirming a breast origin for recurrent tumors. Breast 2010;19(5):355–9.

75. Kaufmann O, Deidesheimer T, Muehlenberg M, et al. Immunohistochemical differentiation of metastatic breast carcinomas from metastatic adenocarcinomas of other common primary sites. Histopathology 1996;29(3):233–40.

76. Han JH, Kang Y, Shin HC, et al. Mammaglobin expression in lymph nodes is an important marker of metastatic breast carcinoma. Arch Pathol Lab Med 2003;127(10):1330–4.

77. Bhargava R, Beriwal S, Dabbs DJ. Mammaglobin vs GCDFP-15: an immunohistologic validation survey for sensitivity and specificity. Am J Clin Pathol 2007;127(1):103–13.

78. Takeda Y, Tsuta K, Shibuki Y, et al. Analysis of expression patterns of breast cancer-specific markers (mammaglobin and gross cystic disease fluid protein 15) in lung and pleural tumors. Arch Pathol Lab Med 2008;132(2):239–43.

79. Tornos C, Soslow R, Chen S, et al. Expression of WT1, CA 125, and GCDFP-15 as useful markers in the differential diagnosis of primary ovarian carcinomas versus metastatic breast cancer to the ovary. Am J Surg Pathol 2005;29(11):1482–9.

80. Striebel JM, Dacic S, Yousem SA. Gross cystic disease fluid protein-(GCDFP-15): expression in primary lung adenocarcinoma. Am J Surg Pathol 2008;32(3):426–32.

81. Wang LJ, Greaves WO, Sabo E, et al. GCDFP-15 positive and TTF-1 negative primary lung neoplasms: a tissue microarray study of 381 primary lung tumors. Appl Immunohistochem Mol Morphol 2009;17(6):505–11.

82. Swanson PE, Pettinato G, Lillemoe TJ, et al. Gross cystic disease fluid protein-15 in salivary gland tumors. Arch Pathol Lab Med 1991;115(2):158–63.

83. Wick MR, Ockner DM, Mills SE, et al. Homologous carcinomas of the breasts, skin, and salivary glands. A histologic and immunohistochemical comparison of ductal mammary carcinoma, ductal sweat gland carcinoma, and salivary duct carcinoma. Am J Clin Pathol 1998;109(1):75–84.

84. Watson MA, Fleming TP. Mammaglobin, a mammary-specific member of the uteroglobin gene family, is overexpressed in human breast cancer. Cancer Res 1996;56(4):860–5.

85. Wang Z, Spaulding B, Sienko A, et al. Mammaglobin, a valuable diagnostic marker for metastatic breast carcinoma. Int J Clin Exp Pathol 2009;2(4):384–9.

86. Sasaki E, Tsunoda N, Hatanaka Y, et al. Breast-specific expression of MGB1/mammaglobin: an examination of 480 tumors from various organs and clinicopathological analysis of MGB1-positive breast cancers. Mod Pathol 2007;20(2):208–14.

87. Kanner WA, Galgano MT, Stoler MH, et al. Distinguishing breast carcinoma from Mullerian serous carcinoma with mammaglobin and mesothelin. Int J Gynecol Pathol 2008;27(4):491–5.

88. Ciampa A, Fanger G, Khan A, et al. Mammaglobin and CRxA-01 in pleural effusion cytology: potential utility of distinguishing metastatic breast carcinomas from other cytokeratin 7-positive/cytokeratin 20-negative carcinomas. Cancer 2004;102(6):368–72.

89. Lewis GH, Subhawong AP, Nassar H, et al. Relationship between molecular subtype of invasive breast carcinoma and expression of gross cystic disease fluid protein 15 and mammaglobin. Am J Clin Pathol 2011;135(4):587–91.

90. Onuma K, Dabbs DJ, Bhargava R. Mammaglobin expression in the female genital tract: immunohistochemical analysis in benign and neoplastic endocervix and endometrium. Int J Gynecol Pathol 2008;27(3):418–25.

91. Rollins-Raval M, Chivukula M, Tseng GC, et al. An immunohistochemical panel to differentiate metastatic breast carcinoma to skin from primary sweat gland carcinomas with a review of the literature. Arch Pathol Lab Med 2011;135(8):975–83.

92. Bejarano PA, Baughman RP, Biddinger PW, et al. Surfactant proteins and thyroid transcription factor-1 in pulmonary and breast carcinomas. Mod Pathol 1996;9(4):445–52.

93. Pelosi G, Fraggetta F, Pasini F, et al. Immunoreactivity for thyroid transcription factor-1 in stage I

non-small cell carcinomas of the lung. Am J Surg Pathol 2001;25(3):363–72.

94. Yatabe Y, Mitsudomi T, Takahashi T. TTF-1 expression in pulmonary adenocarcinomas. Am J Surg Pathol 2002;26(6):767–73.

95. Park SY, Kim BH, Kim JH, et al. Panels of immunohistochemical markers help determine primary sites of metastatic adenocarcinoma. Arch Pathol Lab Med 2007;131(10):1561–7.

96. Stenhouse G, Fyfe N, King G, et al. Thyroid transcription factor 1 in pulmonary adenocarcinoma. J Clin Pathol 2004;57(4):383–7.

97. Lau SK, Luthringer DJ, Eisen RN. Thyroid transcription factor-1: a review. Appl Immunohistochem Mol Morphol 2002;10(2):97–102.

98. Agoff SN, Lamps LW, Philip AT, et al. Thyroid transcription factor-1 is expressed in extrapulmonary small cell carcinomas but not in other extrapulmonary neuroendocrine tumors. Mod Pathol 2000;13(3):238–42.

99. Kaufmann O, Dietel M. Expression of thyroid transcription factor-1 in pulmonary and extrapulmonary small cell carcinomas and other neuroendocrine carcinomas of various primary sites. Histopathology 2000;36(5):415–20.

100. Shin SJ, DeLellis RA, Rosen PP. Small cell carcinoma of the breast – additional immunohistochemical studies. Am J Surg Pathol 2001;25(6):831–2.

101. Jagirdar J. Application of immunohistochemistry to the diagnosis of primary and metastatic carcinoma to the lung. Arch Pathol Lab Med 2008;132(3):384–96.

102. Matoso A, Singh K, Jacob R, et al. Comparison of thyroid transcription factor-1 expression by 2 monoclonal antibodies in pulmonary and nonpulmonary primary tumors. Appl Immunohistochem Mol Morphol 2010;18(2):142–9.

103. Robens J, Goldstein L, Gown AM, et al. Thyroid transcription factor-1 expression in breast carcinomas. Am J Surg Pathol 2010;34(12):1881–5.

104. Bisceglia M, Galliani C, Rosai J. TTF-1 expression in breast carcinoma-the chosen clone matters. Am J Surg Pathol 2011;35(7):1087–8.

105. Hirano T, Auer G, Maeda M, et al. Human tissue distribution of TA02, which is homologous with a new type of aspartic proteinase, napsin A. Jpn J Cancer Res 2000;91(10):1015–21.

106. Ueno T, Linder S, Na CL, et al. Processing of pulmonary surfactant protein B by napsin and cathepsin H. J Biol Chem 2004;279(16):16178–84.

107. Suzuki A, Shijubo N, Yamada G, et al. Napsin A is useful to distinguish primary lung adenocarcinoma from adenocarcinomas of other organs. Pathol Res Pract 2005;201(8–9):579–86.

108. Bishop JA, Sharma R, Illei PB. Napsin A and thyroid transcription factor-1 expression in carcinomas of the lung, breast, pancreas, colon, kidney, thyroid, and malignant mesothelioma. Hum Pathol 2010;41(1):20–5.

109. Ueno T, Linder S, Elmberger G. Aspartic proteinase napsin is a useful marker for diagnosis of primary lung adenocarcinoma. Br J Cancer 2003;88(8):1229–33.

110. Ye J, Findeis-Hosey JJ, Yang Q, et al. Combination of napsin A and TTF-1 immunohistochemistry helps in differentiating primary lung adenocarcinoma from metastatic carcinoma in the lung. Appl Immunohistochem Mol Morphol 2011;19(4):313–7.

111. Tanner S, Redfield S, Brown A. Immunohistochemical expression of Napsin A in triple-negative breast carcinomas. ASCP Poster Presentations. 2011. Available at: http://www.ascponline.org/ascp-static/planner_public/index.php.

112. Gomez-Fernandez C, Mejias A, Walker G, et al. Immunohistochemical expression of estrogen receptor in adenocarcinomas of the lung: the antibody factor. Appl Immunohistochem Mol Morphol 2010;18(2):137–41.

113. Kumar-Singh S, Segers K, Rodeck U, et al. WT1 mutation in malignant mesothelioma and WT1 immunoreactivity in relation to p53 and growth factor receptor expression, cell-type transition, and prognosis. J Pathol 1997;181(1):67–74.

114. Goldstein NS, Bassi D, Uzieblo A. WT1 is an integral component of an antibody panel to distinguish pancreaticobiliary and some ovarian epithelial neoplasms. Am J Clin Pathol 2001;116(2):246–52.

115. Goldstein NS, Uzieblo A. WT1 immunoreactivity in uterine papillary serous carcinomas is different from ovarian serous carcinomas. Am J Clin Pathol 2002;117(4):541–5.

116. Lee BH, Hecht JL, Pinkus JL, et al. WT1, estrogen receptor, and progesterone receptor as markers for breast or ovarian primary sites in metastatic adenocarcinoma to body fluids. Am J Clin Pathol 2002;117(5):745–50.

117. Hashi A, Yuminamochi T, Murata S, et al. Wilms tumor gene immunoreactivity in primary serous carcinomas of the fallopian tube, ovary, endometrium, and peritoneum. Int J Gynecol Pathol 2003;22(4):374–7.

118. Hwang H, Quenneville L, Yaziji H, et al. Wilms tumor gene product: sensitive and contextually specific marker of serous carcinomas of ovarian surface epithelial origin. Appl Immunohistochem Mol Morphol 2004;12(2):122–6.

119. Acs G, Pasha T, Zhang PJ. WT1 is differentially expressed in serous, endometrioid, clear cell, and mucinous carcinomas of the peritoneum, fallopian tube, ovary, and endometrium. Int J Gynecol Pathol 2004;23(2):110–8.

120. Nonaka D, Chiriboga L, Soslow RA. Expression of Pax8 as a useful marker in distinguishing ovarian carcinomas from mammary carcinomas. Am J Surg Pathol 2008;32(10):1566–71.

121. Kobel M, Kalloger SE, Boyd N, et al. Ovarian carcinoma subtypes are different diseases: implications for biomarker studies. PLoS Med 2008;5(12):e232.

122. Lotan TL, Ye H, Melamed J, et al. Immunohistochemical panel to identify the primary site of invasive micropapillary carcinoma. Am J Surg Pathol 2009;33(7):1037–41.

123. Logani S, Oliva E, Amin MB, et al. Immunoprofile of ovarian tumors with putative transitional cell (urothelial) differentiation using novel urothelial markers: histogenetic and diagnostic implications. Am J Surg Pathol 2003;27(11):1434–41.

124. Al-Hussaini M, Stockman A, Foster H, et al. WT-1 assists in distinguishing ovarian from uterine serous carcinoma and in distinguishing between serous and endometrioid ovarian carcinoma. Histopathology 2004;44:109–15.

125. Tabrizi AD, Kalloger SE, Kobel M, et al. Primary ovarian mucinous carcinoma of intestinal type: significance of pattern of invasion and immunohistochemical expression profile in a series of 31 cases. Int J Gynecol Pathol 2010;29(2):99–107.

126. Chu PG, Chung L, Weiss LM, et al. Determining the site of origin of mucinous adenocarcinoma: an immunohistochemical study of 175 cases. Am J Surg Pathol 2011;35(12):1830–6.

127. Ordonez NG. Value of thyroid transcription factor-1, E-cadherin, BG8, WT1, and CD44S immunostaining in distinguishing epithelial pleural mesothelioma from pulmonary and nonpulmonary adenocarcinoma. Am J Surg Pathol 2000;24(4):598–606.

128. Domfeh AB, Carley AL, Striebel JM, et al. WT1 immunoreactivity in breast carcinoma: selective expression in pure and mixed mucinous subtypes. Mod Pathol 2008;21(10):1217–23.

129. Lee AH, Paish EC, Marchio C, et al. The expression of Wilms' tumour-1 and Ca125 in invasive micropapillary carcinoma of the breast. Histopathology 2007;51(6):824–8.

130. Moritani S, Ichihara S, Hasegawa M, et al. Serous papillary adenocarcinoma of the female genital organs and invasive micropapillary carcinoma of the breast. Are WT1, CA125, and GCDFP-15 useful in differential diagnosis? Hum Pathol 2008;39(5):666–71.

131. Barcena C, Oliva E. WT1 expression in the female genital tract. Adv Anat Pathol 2011;18(6):454–65.

132. Laury AR, Perets R, Piao H, et al. A comprehensive analysis of PAX8 expression in human epithelial tumors. Am J Surg Pathol 2011;35(6):816–26.

133. Bowen NJ, Logani S, Dickerson EB, et al. Emerging roles for PAX8 in ovarian cancer and endosalpingeal development. Gynecol Oncol 2007;104(2):331–7.

134. Nonaka D, Tang Y, Chiriboga L, et al. Diagnostic utility of thyroid transcription factors Pax8 and TTF-2 (FoxE1) in thyroid epithelial neoplasms. Mod Pathol 2008;21(2):192–200.

135. Wiseman W, Michael CW, Roh MH. Diagnostic utility of PAX8 and PAX2 immunohistochemistry in the identification of metastatic Mullerian carcinoma in effusions. Diagn Cytopathol 2011;39(9):651–6.

136. Tacha D, Zhou D, Cheng L. Expression of PAX8 in normal and neoplastic tissues: a comprehensive immunohistochemical study. Appl Immunohistochem Mol Morphol 2011;19(4):293–9.

137. Tong GX, Devaraj K, Hamele-Bena D, et al. Pax8: a marker for carcinoma of Mullerian origin in serous effusions. Diagn Cytopathol 2011;39(8):567–74.

138. Ozcan A, Liles N, Coffey D, et al. PAX2 and PAX8 expression in primary and metastatic mullerian epithelial tumors: a comprehensive comparison. Am J Surg Pathol 2011;35(12):1837–47.

139. Fujiwara M, Taube J, Sharma M, et al. PAX8 discriminates ovarian metastases from adnexal tumors and other cutaneous metastases. J Cutan Pathol 2010;37(9):938–43.

140. Ozcan A, Shen SS, Hamilton C, et al. PAX 8 expression in non-neoplastic tissues, primary tumors, and metastatic tumors: a comprehensive immunohistochemical study. Mod Pathol 2011;24(6):751–64.

141. Dupont J, Wang X, Marshall DS, et al. Wilms Tumor Gene (WT1) and p53 expression in endometrial carcinomas: a study of 130 cases using a tissue microarray. Gynecol Oncol 2004;94(2):449–55.

142. Cisco RM, Ford JM, Norton JA. Hereditary diffuse gastric cancer: implications of genetic testing for screening and prophylactic surgery. Cancer 2008;113(Suppl 7):1850–6.

143. O'Connell FP, Wang HH, Odze RD. Utility of immunohistochemistry in distinguishing primary adenocarcinomas from metastatic breast carcinomas in the gastrointestinal tract. Arch Pathol Lab Med 2005;129(3):338–47.

144. Koyama T, Sekine S, Taniguchi H, et al. Hepatocyte nuclear factor 4A expression discriminates gastric involvement by metastatic breast carcinomas from primary gastric adenocarcinomas. Hum Pathol 2011;42(11):1777–84.

145. Yokozaki H, Takekura N, Takanashi A, et al. Estrogen receptors in gastric adenocarcinoma: a retrospective immunohistochemical analysis. Virchows Arch A Pathol Anat Histopathol 1988;413(4):297–302.

146. Kojima O, Takahashi T, Kawakami S, et al. Localization of estrogen receptors in gastric cancer using immunohistochemical staining of monoclonal antibody. Cancer 1991;67(9):2401–6.

147. Chaubert P, Bouzourene H, Saraga E. Estrogen and progesterone receptors and pS2 and ERD5 antigens in gastric carcinomas from the European population. Mod Pathol 1996;9(3):189–93.

148. Werling RW, Yaziji H, Bacchi CE, et al. CDX2, a highly sensitive and specific marker of adenocarcinomas of intestinal origin: an immunohistochemical survey

of 476 primary and metastatic carcinomas. Am J Surg Pathol 2003;27(3):303–10.

149. Chu PG, Weiss LM. Immunohistochemical characterization of signet-ring cell carcinomas of the stomach, breast, and colon. Am J Clin Pathol 2004;121(6):884–92.

150. Tot T. The role of cytokeratins 20 and 7 and estrogen receptor analysis in separation of metastatic lobular carcinoma of the breast and metastatic signet ring cell carcinoma of the gastrointestinal tract. APMIS 2000;108(6):467–72.

151. Mazziotta RM, Borczuk AC, Powell CA, et al. CDX2 immunostaining as a gastrointestinal marker: expression in lung carcinomas is a potential pitfall. Appl Immunohistochem Mol Morphol 2005;13(1):55–60.

152. Lau SK, Weiss LM, Chu PG. Differential expression of MUC1, MUC2, and MUC5AC in carcinomas of various sites: an immunohistochemical study. Am J Clin Pathol 2004;122(1):61–9.

153. Adsay NV, Merati K, Nassar H, et al. Pathogenesis of colloid (pure mucinous) carcinoma of exocrine organs: coupling of gel-forming mucin (MUC2) production with altered cell polarity and abnormal cell-stroma interaction may be the key factor in the morphogenesis and indolent behavior of colloid carcinoma in the breast and pancreas. Am J Surg Pathol 2003;27(5):571–8.

154. Ruffolo EF, Koerner FC, Maluf HM. Metaplastic carcinoma of the breast with melanocytic differentiation. Mod Pathol 1997;10(6):592–6.

155. Padmore RF, Lara JF, Ackerman DJ, et al. Primary combined malignant melanoma and ductal carcinoma of the breast. A report of two cases. Cancer 1996;78(12):2515–25.

156. Brownstein MH, Helwig EB. Patterns of cutaneous metastasis. Arch Dermatol 1972;105(6):862–8.

157. Qureshi HS, Ormsby AH, Lee MW, et al. The diagnostic utility of p63, CK5/6, CK 7, and CK 20 in distinguishing primary cutaneous adnexal neoplasms from metastatic carcinomas. J Cutan Pathol 2004;31(2):145–52.

158. Ivan D, Nash JW, Prieto VG, et al. Use of p63 expression in distinguishing primary and metastatic cutaneous adnexal neoplasms from metastatic adenocarcinoma to skin. J Cutan Pathol 2007;34(6):474–80.

159. Plaza JA, Ortega PF, Stockman DL, et al. Value of p63 and podoplanin (D2-40) immunoreactivity in the distinction between primary cutaneous tumors and adenocarcinomas metastatic to the skin: a clinicopathologic and immunohistochemical study of 79 cases. J Cutan Pathol 2010;37(4):403–10.

160. Mahalingam M, Nguyen LP, Richards JE, et al. The diagnostic utility of immunohistochemistry in distinguishing primary skin adnexal carcinomas from metastatic adenocarcinoma to skin: an immunohistochemical reappraisal using cytokeratin 15, nestin, p63, D2-40, and calretinin. Mod Pathol 2010;23(5):713–9.

161. Liang H, Wu H, Giorgadze TA, et al. Podoplanin is a highly sensitive and specific marker to distinguish primary skin adnexal carcinomas from adenocarcinomas metastatic to skin. Am J Surg Pathol 2007;31(2):304–10.

162. Fernandez-Flores A. Podoplanin immunostaining in cutaneous apocrine carcinoma and in cutaneous metastasis from the breast. Appl Immunohistochem Mol Morphol 2010;18(6):573–4.

163. Wallace ML, Longacre TA, Smoller BR. Estrogen and progesterone receptors and anti-gross cystic disease fluid protein 15 (BRST-2) fail to distinguish metastatic breast carcinoma from eccrine neoplasms. Mod Pathol 1995;8(9):897–901.

164. Busam KJ, Tan LK, Granter SR, et al. Epidermal growth factor, estrogen, and progesterone receptor expression in primary sweat gland carcinomas and primary and metastatic mammary carcinomas. Mod Pathol 1999;12(8):786–93.

165. Swanson PE, Mazoujian G, Mills SE, et al. Immunoreactivity for estrogen receptor protein in sweat gland tumors. Am J Surg Pathol 1991;15(9):835–41.

PATHOLOGY CONSIDERATIONS IN PATIENTS TREATED WITH NEOADJUVANT CHEMOTHERAPY

Sunati Sahoo, MD[a],*, Susan C. Lester, MD, PhD[b]

KEYWORDS

- Breast cancer • Neoadjuvant therapy • NAT • Preoperative therapy • Histology
- Pathologic diagnosis • Tumor markers

ABSTRACT

Neoadjuvant therapy (NAT) was first used to treat women with locally advanced disease but is currently offered to women with earlier-stage and operable breast carcinoma. NAT allows more women to be eligible for breast conservation surgery and provides an opportunity to assess the response of carcinomas to therapy. This review focuses on predictors of therapeutic response in pretreatment biopsy, evaluation of post-treatment breast and lymph node specimens, classification systems to evaluate degree of response to NAT, and reporting of post-treatment specimens.

OVERVIEW

Neoadjuvant therapy (NAT) is offered to women with locally advanced carcinomas to reduce tumor burden and make patients eligible for surgical treatment. Clinical trials have shown no difference in the locoregional control and metastasis free survival for patients who receive adjuvant chemotherapy vs NAT.[1–6] However, patients who achieve a pathologic complete response (pCR) have improved long-term survival, disease-free survival (DFS), and overall survival (OS) compared with patients who have partial or no response to NAT.[7–10] Individual patients may benefit from this information by being able to change treatment when no response is evident or receive additional treatment if response is not complete. Alternatively, patients with good responses benefit by knowing their prognosis and making decisions about types of treatment, including prophylactic

Pathologic Key Features
ANALYSIS OF BREAST CARCINOMA IN
NEOADJUVANT SETTING

- Identification, thorough sampling, and microscopic documentation of the tumor bed are essential, particularly in cases of complete or near-complete response.

- Microscopically, the tumor bed appears as a loose vascularized fibrotic area often associated with edema, myxoid change, and lymphohistiocytic infiltrate.

- The extent, largest contiguous focus, cellularity, and treatment effect of any residual tumor should be analyzed carefully to grade the extent of response in both the breast and lymph nodes.

- Tumor bed transected at the margin should be reported, particularly in specimens where residual invasive carcinoma or ductal carcinoma in situ (DCIS) is identified.

- Repeat studies on residual tumor for hormone receptors, human epidermal growth factor receptor 2 (HER2) and proliferation marker (eg, Ki-67) can provide additional prognostic and therapeutic information.

a Department of Pathology, UT Southwestern Medical Center, 5323 Harry Hines Boulevard, Dallas, TX 75390, USA
b Department of Pathology, Brigham and Women's Hospital, 75 Francis Street, Boston, MA 02115, USA
* Corresponding author.
E-mail address: sunati.sahoo@utsouthwestern.edu

Surgical Pathology 5 (2012) 749–774
http://dx.doi.org/10.1016/j.path.2012.06.005
1875-9181/12/$ – see front matter Published by Elsevier Inc

surgpath.theclinics.com

surgery. Tumor response has also been used as a short-term endpoint for clinical trials. Information about the effectiveness of a treatment is available in months to 1 to 2 years, in contrast to the endpoints of recurrence or death—events that typically do not occur for many years or even decades after adjuvant treatment. Finally, the ability to correlate pretreatment and post-treatment tumor samples directly to treatment response has provided a wealth of information about tumor biology and will hopefully yield better methods of predicting response as well as identify additional targets for treatment.

Patients undergoing NAT are diagnosed by a core needle biopsy. Pretreatment tumor size and extent are determined by imaging studies. A clip or clips must be placed at the time of diagnostic core needle biopsy and/or during the first

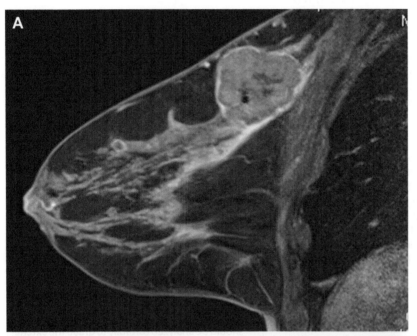

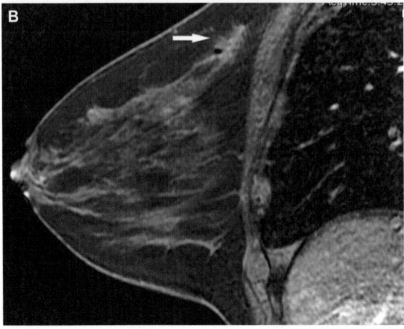

Fig. 1. Pretreatment and post-treatment contrast enhanced MRI images of breast carcinoma. (*A*) Pretreatment maximum intensity projection image of a patient presented with a large palpable breast mass that abutted but did not involve the skin or chest wall. (*B*) The postchemotherapy maximum intensity projection image shows complete resolution of the prior mass (*arrow*). Microscopic evaluation did reveal, however, scattered residual tumor in the area of prior abnormality (tumor bed).

few cycles of NAT to ensure the tumor bed can be identified, particularly for patients who become eligible for breast-conserving surgery.[11] Patients with palpable axillary lymph nodes or with abnormal node found on ultrasound may undergo fine-needle aspiration to document a positive node. If no enlarged nodes are detected and a sentinel node biopsy confirms node-negative status, no further nodal evaluation is performed. If nodes are not evaluated before treatment, it may not be possible to determine a patient's initial node status or response of metastases to therapy, and much valuable information is lost.

During therapy, patients are monitored by clinical examination and imaging studies. Clinical complete response, partial response (PR), minimal or no response, and progressive disease are defined by the change in tumor size from pretreatment clinical and/or radiologic measurements to post-treatment measurements (**Fig. 1**).

The extent of response to NAT determined by physical examination and imaging is helpful but often inaccurate. False-positive results may result from residual acellular fibrotic tumor bed mimicking residual carcinoma. Alternatively, false-negative results may occur because cancers often become softer and less dense. Recent breast imaging modalities, such as dynamic contrast-enhanced MRI and dynamic fluodeoxyglucose F 18 positron emission tomography (PET), have shown promising results in the evaluation of treatment response.[12,13] To obtain the optimal information regarding treatment effect, however, some of the systems have to be used in combination. Such combined PET/CT or PET/MRI systems are currently in technical development and yet to be used by most centers as a routine method for predicting and evaluating tumor response. Pathologic examination is currently the only method that can accurately determine the presence and the extent of residual disease.[11]

pCR rate (defined as the absence of invasive carcinoma in the breast and in the lymph nodes after completion of NAT) ranges from 15% to 30%.[2,7,8,10,14–16] Residual in situ carcinoma may be present, but this finding does not alter OS.[17,18] A pCR is a straightforward category to define and is often used to compare different treatment regimens. Although many classification systems to evaluate PR have been devised, it is difficult to consistently quantify residual carcinoma and, thus, to compare groups across studies.

Hormonal agents improve survival for hormone receptor HR-positive (HR+) patients but pCR is rarely observed with these agents. Therefore, other endpoints such as inhibition of growth more appropriate for assessment of treatment effect. A decrease in proliferation has been suggested as an alternative, but the best method for predicting prognosis after hormonal therapy has not yet been determined.

A deviation from the standard NAT by using very short-term treatment course between diagnosis and definitive surgery has been tried primarily as a research tool to look for biomarker changes. For example, the response of DCIS to hormonal treatment has been studied in this manner.[19]

EVALUATION OF PRETREATMENT CORE NEEDLE BIOPSIES

The initial diagnostic specimen must contain quantitatively sufficient core biopsies of the tumor to make a definitive diagnosis of invasive carcinoma and to determine tumor markers. There may not be another opportunity to evaluate the carcinoma if there is a complete or near-complete response. If only a small area of invasive carcinoma is present (eg, <0.5 cm), a repeat biopsy to confirm negative results for HR or HER2 should be considered.

Pathologic features of the carcinoma that are known to predict response to therapy are discussed.

HISTOLOGIC TYPE

Lobular carcinomas are less likely to respond than carcinomas of no special type.[20] These carcinomas are usually estrogen receptor (ER) positive and have a low proliferative rate. These features are also associated with a low response rate in nonlobular (ie, well-differentiated) ductal carcinomas.

HISTOLOGIC GRADE

Higher-grade carcinomas respond to a greater extent than low-grade tumors.[21] Carcinomas with high mitotic count or with high proliferative rates by Ki-67 (MIB-1) also have higher response rates.[22,23]

TUMOR NECROSIS

Areas of necrosis in the invasive carcinoma are predictive of response.[24] This feature also correlates with higher-grade and high proliferative rate tumors.

TUMOR INFILTRATING LYMPHOCYTES

High-grade HR-negative (HR−) carcinomas are often associated with a dense lymphocytic infiltrate, and this feature is frequently associated with BRCA1 mutations. Carcinomas with a lymphocytic infiltrate are more likely to respond to chemotherapy than cancers without this feature.[25]

TUMOR MARKERS

ER, progesterone receptor (PgR), and HER2 are often used to classify patients into groups for NAT clinical trials. HR− tumors achieve a higher pCR rate compared with HR+ tumors.[10,26,27] In one study, 27% of ER-/PR-/HER2- (triple-negative breast cancer [TNBC]) and 36% of ER−/HER2+ tumors achieved pCR compared with 7% of HR+ tumors (luminal subtypes).[26] Similarly, patients with HER2+ tumors who receive HER2-targeted therapy (eg, trastuzumab) as part of the NAT achieve higher breast and nodal pCR (rates up to 60%) compared with patients who do not receive targeted therapy.[15,28–30] The greatest benefit of trastuzumab in the neoadjuvant setting is seen in patients who have HR−/HER2+ tumors versus HR+/HER2+ tumors because response to treatment declines with increased tumor ER expression.[31]

TNBC and ER−/HER2+ carcinomas are more likely to achieve pCR than ER+ carcinomas; patients who fail to achieve a pCR have a worse outcome (frequent relapse and decreased OS) compared with patients who have ER+ tumors and residual disease. This phenomenon has been described as the triple-negative paradox or the HR− paradox.[26,27] This observation suggests that there are 2 types of high-grade carcinomas—one that is treatment sensitive with a good prognosis and the other that is treatment resistant with a poor prognosis. Currently, the only means to identify these 2 types of carcinoma with any degree of certainty is with NAT.

Studies using gene expression profile of tumors have reported similar factors associated with better responses to therapy.[32–35] Additionally, gene microarray studies have shown that a defective DNA repair gene expression signature in sporadic TNBC may predict tumors that are sensitive to anthracyclines and that are resistant to taxane-based chemotherapy.[36]

EVALUATION OF POST-TREATMENT SPECIMENS

GROSS EVALUATION

Breast Specimens

In order to optimally examine a post-treatment specimen, a pathologist must have information regarding the pretreatment tumor size and location, the presence of clips or radiologic calcifications marking the tumor, the presence or absence of multiple tumors, and possible pretreatment involvement of skin, nipple, and chest wall. Carcinomas with a minimal response generally remain palpable and are easily identified in the specimen. Finding the tumor bed can be challenging, however, if there has been a marked or

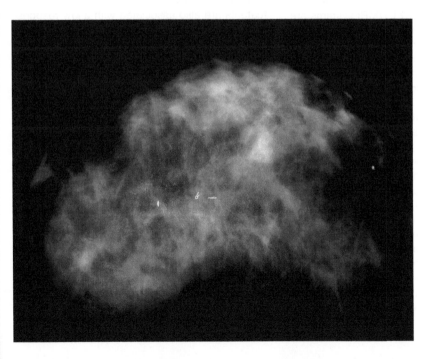

Fig. 2. Post-treatment excisional biopsy specimen radiograph shows 3 clips left after the original diagnostic needle biopsy and subsequent needle biopsies as part of research protocol.

Fig. 3. Pathologic minimal response. Post-treatment mastectomy specimen shows still a large somewhat fibrotic tumor bed after chemotherapy. Microscopic examination of this tumor showed minimal response to therapy.

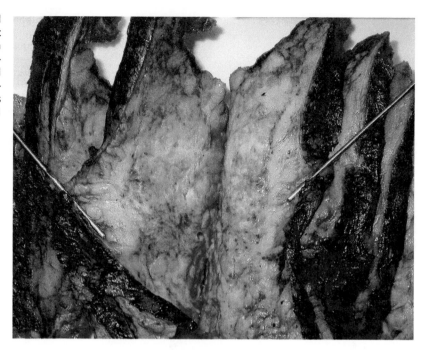

complete clinical response. It is essential to obtain a specimen radiograph in wire-localized biopsies demonstrating the clip or density corresponding to the tumor bed (**Fig. 2**). Mastectomies without an easily identifiable palpable mass should undergo radiography before processing. If no clip was placed, calcifications if present in the carcinoma can be used to identify the tumor bed. In the absence of radiologic guidance, a detailed description of the pretreatment tumor location (eg, quadrant and distance from nipple) or sutures placed by a surgeon at the site of the previous mass may help find the tumor bed.

The gross appearance of residual carcinoma in cases with minimal response is similar to that of untreated carcinoma (**Fig. 3**). In cases with a complete or near-complete response to NAT, the tumor bed may appear as a vague area of

Fig. 4. pCR. Post-treatment mastectomy demonstrating an irregular area of whitish fibrous tissue that on microscopic examination revealed complete pathologic response.

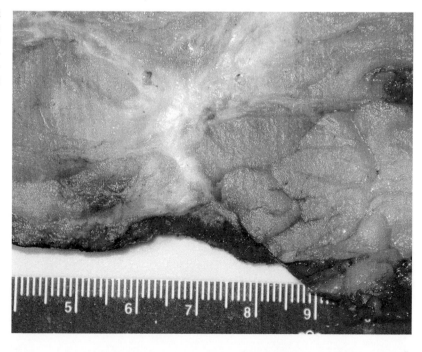

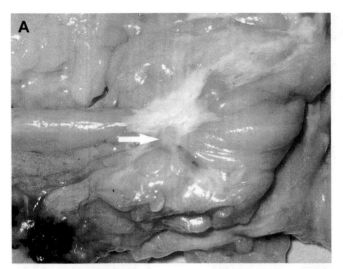

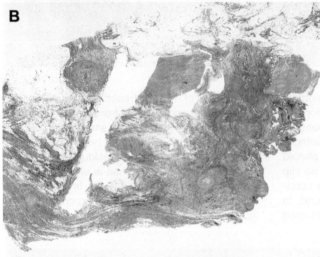

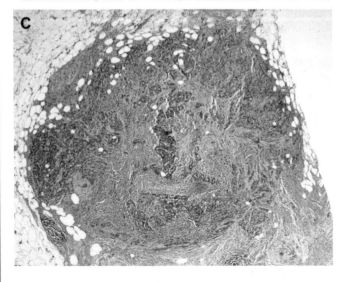

Fig. 5. Pathologic PR. (*A*) Post-treatment lumpectomy specimen with a grossly visible irregular area of fibrotic tumor bed with a small, tan nodule of residual invasive carcinoma (*arrow*). (*B*) On pathologic examination, this patient had small foci of residual tumor in a large fibrotic tumor bed (low-power view). (*C*) High-power view of the residual focus of carcinoma shows little change of cellularity after treatment.

irregular rubbery fibrous tissue that is difficult to distinguish from normal breast (**Fig. 4**). Residual invasive carcinoma is sometimes visible as tan nodules within the tumor bed (**Fig. 5**). In many cases, however, the residual carcinoma is scattered throughout the bed as small foci and may not be grossly evident. The size of the tumor bed and recognizable residual tumor should be documented and the relationship to the margins noted,

when possible. Specimens should be differentially inked to assess margins.

At least one section per centimeter of the pretreatment carcinoma size is suggested if the tumor bed is large (≥5 cm). Sampling a complete cross-section of the tumor bed is helpful to estimate the overall cellularity. If residual invasive carcinoma is documented microscopically on the initial sections, additional sampling is not

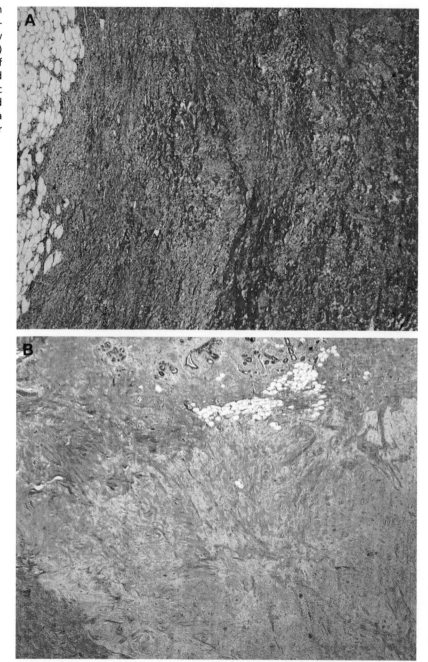

Fig. 6. Tumor bed with complete pathologic response (low-power view of 2 different cases). (*A*) Tumor bed with sheets of microphages distibuted throughout the fibrotic stroma. (*B*) Hyalinized loose collagenous stroma that is lacking glandular breast elements.

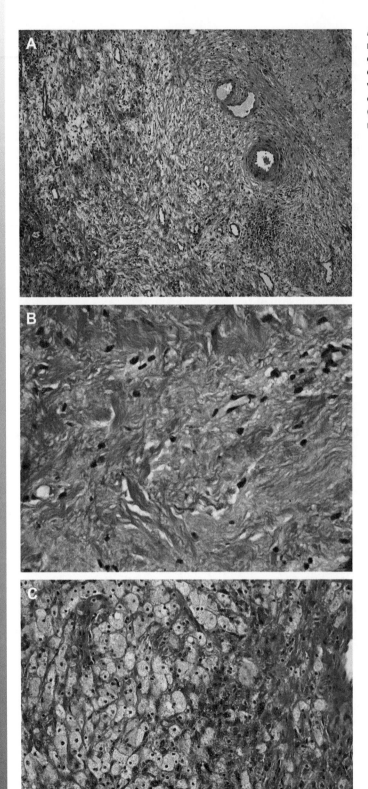

Fig. 7. Tumor bed, complete pathologic response. (*A*) Loose vascular stroma demonstrating edema, elastosis and chronic inflammatory cells (low-power view). (*B*) Tumor bed with prominent edema and elastosis (high-power view). (*C*) Tumor bed with large sheets of macrophages and hemosiderinpigment.

necessary. If no residual invasive carcinoma is found, additional sampling may be considered to document pCR. If the residual tumor bed is small (≤3 cm), the entire area should be sampled for pathologic examination.

Lymph Nodes

Lymph nodes may be difficult to recognize after chemotherapy because of atrophy and fibrosis.[37] Although one study reported low axillary lymph node counts after chemotherapy,[38] other studies have found little or no difference.[39,40] All nodes should be thinly sectioned along the long axis and completely submitted for microscopic examination.

MICROSCOPIC EVALUATION

All prognostic and predictive factors that are important in untreated tumors are also important in tumors treated with NAT. The interpretation of

Fig. 8. Loss of tumor cellularity after therapy. (*A*) Pretreatment core biopsy of a high-grade invasive ductal carcinoma. (*B*) Foci of residual tumor nodules separated by fibrous stroma.

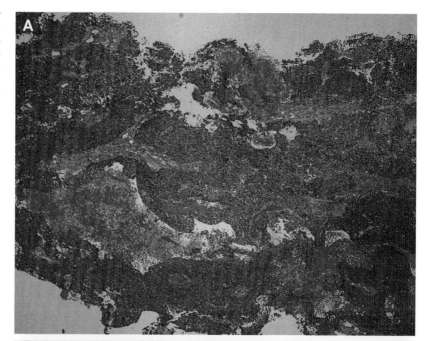

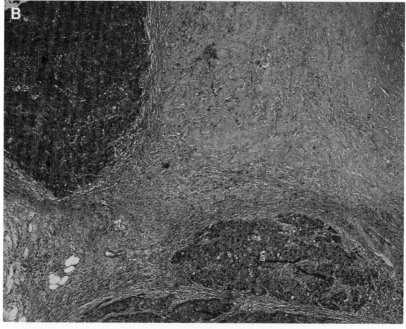

these factors, however, is often more difficult in the post-treatment specimen. Evaluation of the extent of response and quantification of any residual carcinoma are additional but important prognostic factors.

Tumor Bed

The presence of residual carcinoma or a tumor bed must be confirmed microscopically. The tumor bed is characterized by loose collagenous stroma without the presence of normal glandular structures (**Fig. 6**). The stroma is often associated with edema and myxoid change (**Fig. 6**). A sprinkling of lymphocytes, plasma cells, and macrophages, sometimes in large sheets, and hemosiderin pigment in the stroma are common findings (**Fig. 7**). If histologic features of a tumor bed and/or residual carcinoma are not seen in the region of a clip, additional sampling is

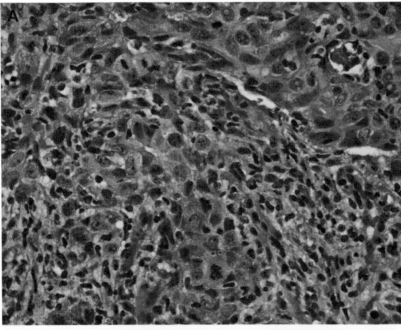

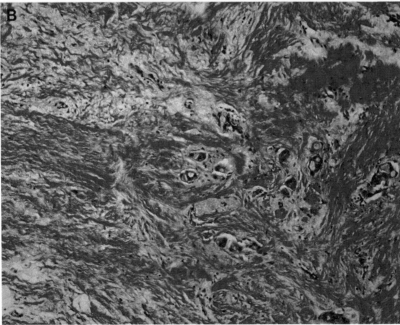

Fig. 9. Post-treatment tumor with marked loss of cellularity. (*A*) Pretreatment core biopsy of a high-grade invasive ductal carcinoma. (*B*) Scattered residual tumor cells within the tumor bed.

warranted. It is possible the clip did not deploy in the location of the carcinoma or was dislodged during surgery or gross examination.

Tumor Size

If there has been a minimal response, the carcinoma may appear slightly smaller than the pretreatment size with a peripheral rim of fibrous tissue. When there has been a marked response, multiple small nodules of invasive carcinoma or scattered single tumor cells are typically interspersed within a large, difficult-to-delineate tumor bed, making a determination of tumor size difficult (**Fig. 8**B, **9**B). Nonetheless, tumor size remains a good prognostic factor after NAT.[9,41,42] In one study, patients who underwent breast-conserving surgery and radiation therapy after NAT and had residual tumors larger than 2 cm had higher rates of locoregional recurrence.[43] The size of the largest

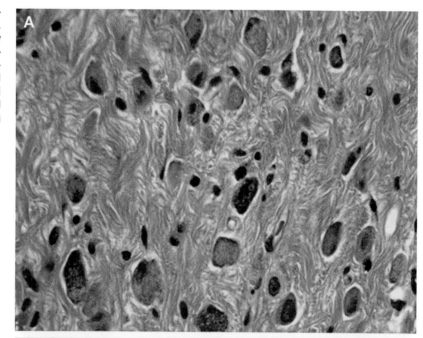

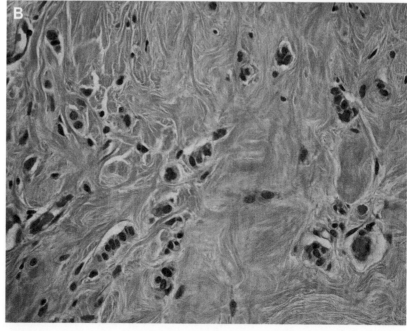

Fig. 10. Post-treatment tumor with treatment effect. (*A*) Post-treatment biopsy of an invasive lobular carcinoma resembling macrophages. (*B*) Single residual tumor cells of a ductal carcinoma with marked therapy effect, mimicking lobular carcinoma.

contiguous focus of invasive carcinoma and the number of foci are useful information for assessing the extent of residual carcinoma.

Tumor Cellularity

Carcinomas often become less cellular after treatment (**Fig. 9**B, **10**). An estimation of cellularity averaged over the tumor bed is used in some classifications of PR. The degree of change in cellularity from pretreatment to post-treatment can only be determined with certainty if the pretreatment carcinoma is available for comparison.

In cases of near-complete response, scattered single tumor cells may be difficult to detect on routine stains. Immunohistochemistry (IHC) in such cases is helpful to distinguish between epithelial cells (positive for cytokeratins AE1/AE3 or cytokeratin 7) and macrophages (CD68 positive).

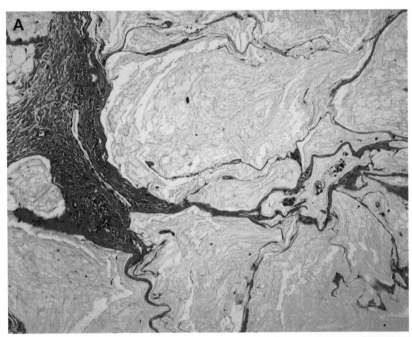

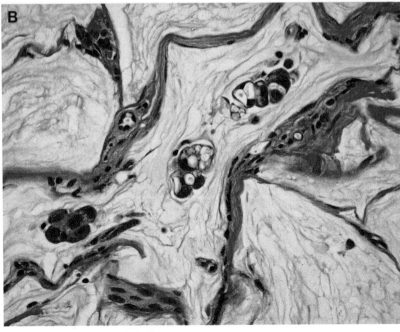

Fig. 11. Post-treatment mucinous carcinoma with pools of extracellular mucin and rare scattered tumor cells. (*A*) Low power view. (*B*) High power view of the same case demonstrating treatment effect in the form of cytoplasmic vacuoles.

Decreased cellularity is seen with both chemotherapy and hormonal therapy and has been shown to correlate with better outcome.[16,44] Additionally, a central fibrotic zone has been described in cancers treated with aromatase inhibitors.[45] A strong correlation between the reduction in tumor volume and 5-year OS has been shown in a study using a formula that requires pretreatment and post-treatment tumor size and tumor cellularity.[31]

Histologic Type

The histologic type of carcinoma does not change after NAT. Lobular carcinomas can be particularly difficult to detect because these cancers can be paucicellular and associated with minimal to no stromal response before treatment. After treatment, the tumor cells may be sparse and may have abundant foamy cytoplasm, closely resembling histiocytes (**Fig. 10**A). After a marked

Fig. 12. Ductal carcinoma in situ with treatment effect. (*A*) The residual neoplastic cells with enlarged nuclei. (*B*) Residual DCIS duct replaced by histiocytes with rare neoplastic cells.

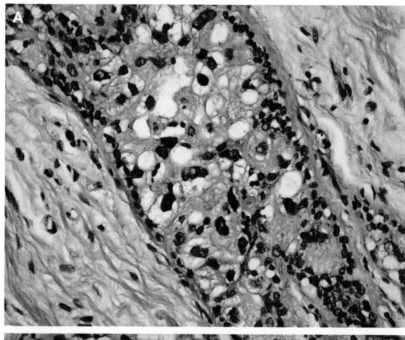

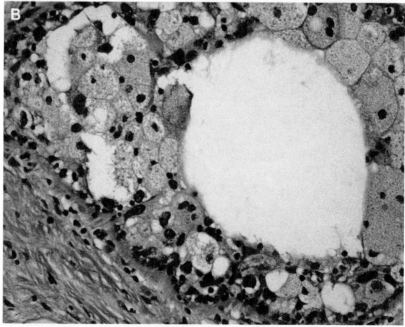

response, residual invasive ductal carcinoma cells may be distributed singly in tumor bed mimicking lobular carcinoma (see **Fig. 10B**). After treatment, mucin pools may be all that remains of a mucinous carcinoma. If tumor cells are not present, this finding should not be classified as residual disease (**Fig. 11**).

DCIS is relatively resistant to chemotherapy compared with invasive carcinoma and may be the only residual disease present after NAT.[46] Residual DCIS may or may not show morphologic alterations after therapy. DCIS may show replacement of neoplastic cells by macrophages or marked nuclear atypia in the residual neoplastic cells (**Fig. 12**).[19] Residual DCIS foci in a fibrotic tumor bed may mimic invasive carcinoma. In difficult cases, IHC for myoepithelial cells (eg, p63 or muscle-specific actin) is helpful in classifying carcinomas as in situ or invasive. It is important to make this distinction because residual DCIS does not preclude a pCR.

Histologic Grade

In the majority of cases, the histologic grade does not change after treatment. Changes in the mitotic count (may be low) and in the appearance of nuclei, however, may occur after treatment, affecting the grade of the residual tumor.[2,11,46] Additional treatment-related changes include distortion of glandular architecture, cytomegaly, cytoplasmic vacuolization and eosinophilic change, and pleomorphic and bizarre nuclei.

Occasionally, untreated tumors can show marked cytologic atypia that resembles therapy effect (**Fig. 13**). Therefore, cytologic changes cannot be attributed to the treatment unless the pretreatment cancer is available for comparison (**Fig. 14**). A change in overall grade has not been correlated with clinical outcome.

Lymphovascular Invasion

In some cases, the only residual carcinoma may be in the lymphatic channels. This finding confers a poorer prognosis (**Fig. 15**).[47,48] After chemotherapy, nests of tumor cells tend to shrink away from the stroma. This feature should not be misinterpreted as lymphatic or vascular invasion.

Tumor Markers

Changes in ER, PgR, and HER2 occur in a subset of cancers with residual disease after NAT. Confounding technical factors, such as variability in tissue processing and fixation, laboratory error in testing, and criteria for interpretation, should be considered before attributing the results as treatment related. In untreated tumors, minimal discordance between core needle biopsy and excisional biopsy for ER (discordance 1.8%), PgR (discordance 15%), and HER2 (discordance 1.2%) has been reported.[49] With NAT, however, the discordance rate between pretreatment and posttreatment specimens is higher and more frequent in tumors treated with targeted agents. Many cases of discordance are likely due to undetected

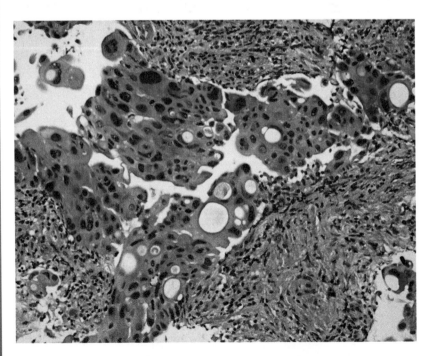

Fig. 13. Pretreatment diagnostic core biopsy of an invasive ductal carcinoma exhibiting marked cytologic atypia before any treatment.

Fig. 14. Post-treatment tumor with treatment effect. (*A*) Pretreatment core biopsy of a high-grade invasive ductal carcinoma. (*B*) Same tumor as in (*A*) showing marked cytomegaly and nucleomegaly and cyto-plasmic vacuoles related to therapy.

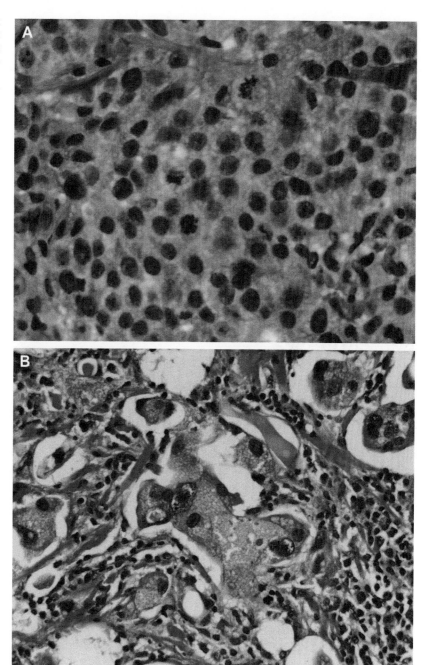

heterogeneity in the pretreatment cancer with selection of subclones by the treatment (Fig. 16A, B). In other cases, there may be a true change in marker expression (see Fig. 16C). Little is known about whether the pretreatment or post-treatment expression profile will be more predictive of the pattern in future recurrences or distant metastases. A change from a positive result to a negative result

is of uncertain significance because the change may be transient or may not occur in all residual carcinoma (eg, carcinoma at metastatic sites). A change from negative to positive may have greater clinical significance, because this finding identifies an additional means of treatment.

A change in HR status has been reported as high as 8% to 33%, particularly in studies where

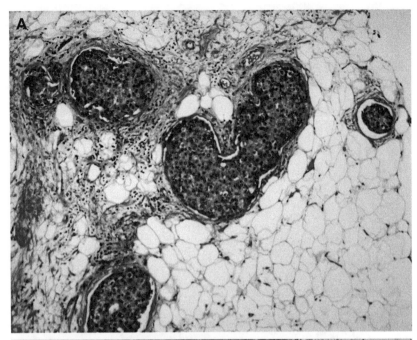

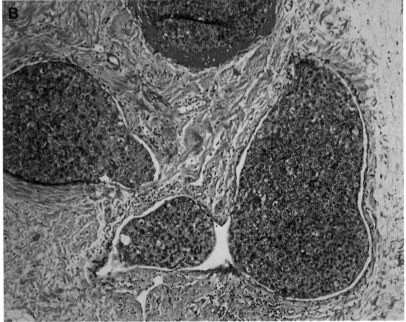

Fig. 15. Post-treatment tumor bed with residual tumor mostly in the lymphatics. (*A*) and (*B*) are from two different cases.

endocrine agents were used.[50] For ER, approximately half of discordances after chemotherapy are from a negative to a positive result. In two studies, patients whose cancers became ER positive benefited from hormonal therapy compared with similar patients who were not treated.[51,52] For PgR, changes from a positive to a negative result occur more commonly than seen for ER.

This is particularly marked after aromatase inhibitor treatment, as reported in 2 studies in which 70% and 94% of cancers lost PgR expression.[53,54] In contrast, fewer than 10% of tamoxifen treated cancers lost PgR expression and some cancers had an increase in the degree of positivity. These changes have not been linked to tumor response or survival.

Fig. 16. Possible reasons for change in tumor markers after NAT. The white circles represent one value (such as positive or negative) for a biologic marker (eg, ER, PR, or HER2) and the black circles represent the opposite result. (*A*) Some carcinomas are heterogeneous for markers and this heterogeneity may not be detected by core needle biopsy. The residual tumor may appear to have changed status for the marker, particularly if the treatment may be selective for expression. (*B*) Some patients have multiple carcinomas with variable expression. As in (*A*), an apparent change in expression can be due to selective response and sampling. (*C*) In some cases, there may be a true change in marker expression in tumor cells after treatment.

Pre-treatment   **Post-treatment**

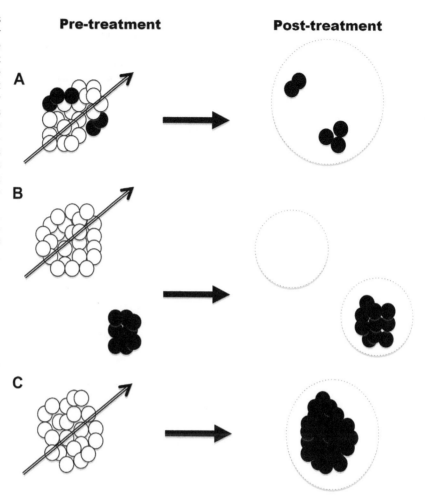

Changes in HER2 status after nontargeted chemotherapy are uncommon, particularly when evaluated by fluorescence in situ hybridization (FISH).[55–57] Loss of expression occurs in 0% to 17% (on average 13%) and gain of expression in 0% to 12% (on average 5%). In one study, loss of overexpression by both IHC and FISH was reported in 41% of HER2+ tumors treated with only an aromatase inhibitor.[58]

When NAT includes HER2-targeted therapy, trastuzumab, loss of HER2 expression is reported as high as 32% and 43% of the carcinomas, respectively.[59,60] The carcinomas no longer show gene amplification, supporting that the treatment is effective for a subclone of tumor cells and that loss is not a transient change in expression. Loss of HER2 in the post-treatment tumor is associated with poor recurrence-free survival.[59]

Change in proliferation index as determined by IHC for Ki-67 (MIB-1) have been suggested as a means to measure response to therapy, particularly in patients with HR+ tumors receiving hormonal agents.[61] A significant change in proliferation index after treatment has been linked to survival benefit.[62–65] A low post-treatment Ki-67 has been shown an independent predictor of recurrence-free survival and OS in both HR+ and HR− tumors.[22,64]

Margins

It is uncommon to have a single focus of residual carcinoma after a significant response to NAT. The more common pattern is to find multiple small foci scattered over the tumor bed. The significance of tumor bed at a margin is unclear in cases where no residual carcinoma is identified. If invasive carcinoma or DCIS is present throughout the tumor bed, however, tumor bed transected at a margin is more likely to be associated with residual carcinoma in the breast (**Fig. 17**).

Changes in Non-Neoplastic Breast Parenchyma

The cytotoxic effects of therapy in the normal breast parenchyma are more pronounced with radiation therapy than with chemotherapy. Scattered epithelial cells of the terminal duct–lobular unit can exhibit cellular atypia and sclerosis of basement membranes (Fig. 18). These changes should not be misinterpreted as residual in situ carcinoma, particularly when present near a margin. In some cases, however, it may be impossible to distinguish residual DCIS with treatment-related changes from alterations in normal glandular cells or benign lesions.

Lymph Nodes

Some nodes may show pronounced lymphoid depletion, fibrous scarring with little or no residual

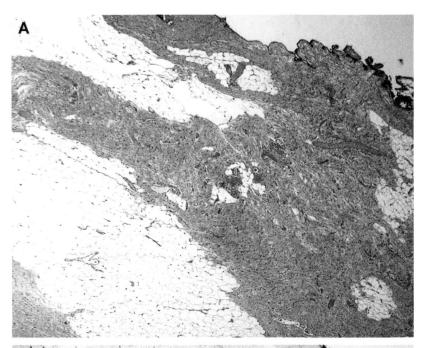

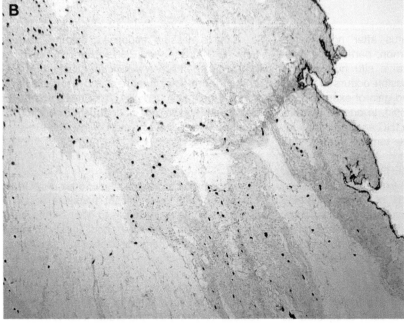

Fig. 17. Tumor bed at margin. (A) Scattered residual single tumor cells with marked loss of cellularity extending to an inked margin. (B) IHC stain for cytokeratin highlights the tumor cells.

Fig. 18. Normal terminal duct lobular unit with therapy effect manifested as scattered atypical ductal cells (inset showing high-power view of the atypical cell).

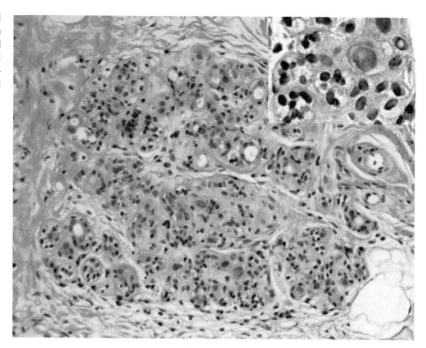

carcinoma, whereas other nodes may have metastases with little evidence of treatment effect. Lymph node metastases that show complete response to therapy are often replaced by fibrosis, aggregates of macrophages, or mucin pools without viable tumor cells (**Fig. 19**).[37] Metastases in nodes with a PR to therapy usually have single or small clusters of tumor cells, sometimes surrounded by thin or thick hyaline fibrosis (**Fig. 20**). IHC stains for cytokeratin are helpful to identify atypical cells that are difficult to classify on routine hematoxylin-eosin (H&E) stains (see **Fig. 20**).

Post-treatment lymph node status is the most important prognostic factor in patients who receive NAT.[14,66,67] Patients who have no residual tumor in the breast but residual tumor in the lymph nodes fare worse compared with patients who have negative nodes but residual tumor in breast.[7,14,67] Patients with an increasing number of residual positive nodes had progressively worse distant DFS and OS compared with patients with negative nodes.[68,69]

The significance of the size of a metastatic deposit in a lymph node depends on whether or not the patient has been treated with chemotherapy before surgery. In the National Surgical Adjuvant Breast and Bowel Project protocol B-18, at 9 years of follow-up, patients in the adjuvant arm with negative nodes or micrometastases had identical survival, whereas patients with macrometastases had a worse prognosis. In contrast, survival of patients in the NAT arm with minimetastases (<1.0 mm) and micrometastases (<2.0 mm) in nodes were similar to patients with macrometastases but significantly worse than those with no nodal disease.[2] Similar results have been reported by other studies.[68] This may be attributed to the fact that micrometastases in lymph nodes probably represent macrometastasis that have responded to therapy. No significant difference in DFS or OS is found between patients with and without isolated tumor cells found on keratin stain after a median follow-up of at least 62 months.[69,70] Routine IHC on negative nodes is not recommended unless part of a research study to determine their prognostic significance.

Metastatic tumor may completely respond without scarring or may leave a small fibrous scar, making it difficult to ascertain prior metastatic involvement. In one study, 35% of fine-needle aspiration proved metastases resolved without histologic evidence of prior involvement.[71] Therefore, it is important to document the presence of metastatic carcinoma before treatment.

SYSTEMS FOR EVALUATING DEGREE OF RESPONSE TO NAT

The prognosis of breast cancer patients treated with NAT is influenced by the pretreatment clinical stage, the post-treatment pathologic stage, and

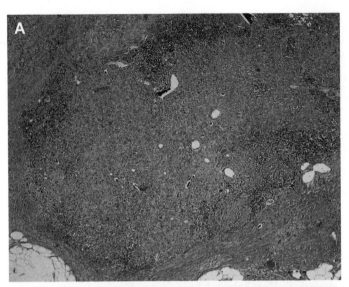

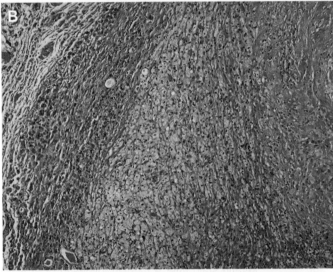

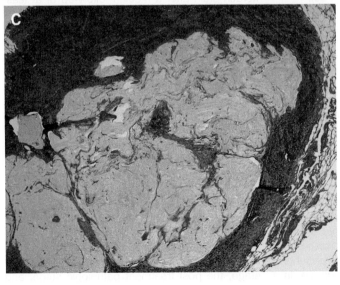

Fig. 19. Lymph node with complete response to therapy. (*A*) Lymph node with extensive fibrous scarring and marked depletion of lymphocytes. (*B*) Lymph node with sheets of foamy macrophages without viable tumor cells. (*C*) Metastatic mucinous carcinoma after therapy has only extracellular mucin without visible tumor cells.

Fig. 20. Lymph node with PR to therapy. (*A*) Post-therapy lymph node with isolated enlarged single tumor cells surrounded by thin fibrous bands. (*B*) Cytokeratin AE1/3 stain highlights single tumor cells.

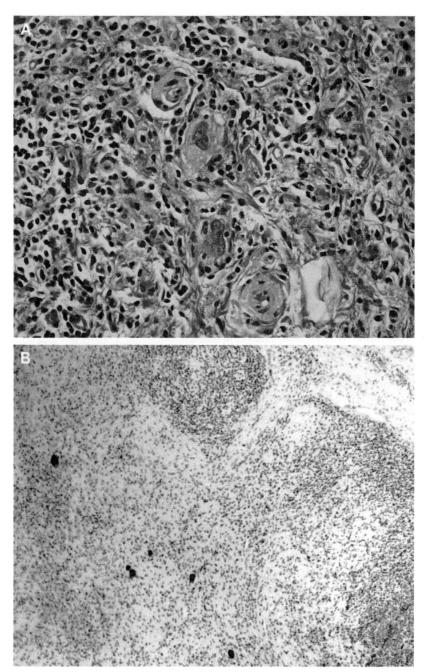

many other features (described previously).[72] The patients with the most favorable prognosis are those who experience complete resolution of their carcinoma in the breast and nodes (pCR), but this accounts for a minority of the patients.[8,9,16,27,73] Many pathologic classification systems have been developed to subclassify the larger group of patients with PR. The number of categories of PR varies from study to study and some systems quantify response as a continuous variable. No single method of assessing response has been shown superior in predicting clinical outcome. Some of the systems are discussed, with a brief description of the classification and category of responses.

THE AMERICAN JOINT COMMITTEE ON CANCER SYSTEM (SEVENTH EDITION)

The American Joint Committee on Cancer[74] (AJCC) pretreatment stage is based on imaging findings confirmed by biopsy. If a patient has a pretreatment stage IV (distant metastasis, M1) disease, the post-treatment classification does not change regardless of the response to therapy. Post-treatment carcinomas are assigned T and N categories indicated by the prefix "y"; "p" refers to pathologic classification. The post-treatment pathologic tumor size (ypT) is based on the largest contiguous focus of invasive carcinoma. If there are multiple scattered foci of carcinoma, this is designated with a modifier "m." Measurement of the largest tumor focus should not include areas of fibrosis within the tumor bed. Although this system does not include change in cellularity in the classification, it is recommended that additional information regarding extent of residual disease and overall tumor cellularity is included in the report to assist clinicians in the assessment of treatment response.

The post-treatment ypN categories are the same as those used for untreated tumors (pN). For example, isolated tumor cells (metastases no greater than 0.2 mm or fewer than 200 cells) are classified as ypN0 (i+). Patients with this finding, however, are excluded from being classified as pCR at this time and should be identified as a separate group.

The clinical-pathologic stage (CPS) based on the AJCC pretreatment clinical stage (CS) and post-treatment pathologic stage (PS) can be combined with estrogen receptor status (E) and grade (G) into a scoring system (CPS + EG staging system) that categorizes patients into a more refined subgroups by outcome than CS or final PS defined by the AJCC staging system.[75] A Web site (http://www.mdanderson.org/postchemotherapystaging) allows free access to use this system through a prognostic calculator.

THE MILLER-PAYNE SYSTEM FOR GRADING TUMOR CELLULARITY

The Miller-Payne system for grading tumor cellularity is based solely on changes in cellularity after NAT and, therefore, requires knowledge about the pretreatment core needle biopsy. Response is divided into 5 grades based on the percentage of change.[16] In this study, a grade 4 response (almost complete response) had a worse prognosis than a pCR (grade 5), providing evidence that pCR should be kept as a separate group. This system did not include, however, the response in lymph nodes for classification of pCR. Thus, it is possible that the patients with a grade 4 response who did poorly could have had residual tumor in the lymph nodes.

RESIDUAL CANCER BURDEN SYSTEM

This system was developed to calculate residual cancer burden (RCB) in 382 patients in 2 different treatment cohorts for prediction of distant relapse-free survival.[9] The system used residual invasive carcinoma cellularity, the number of lymph nodes with metastases, and the size of the largest metastasis. The extent to which DCIS contributes to residual carcinoma is excluded. These factors are combined mathematically to provide a continuous parameter of response (RCB index) and 4 classes of RCB (RCB-0 through RCB-III). Based on the RCB classes, patients with minimal residual disease (RCB-I) had the same 5-year survival as those with pCR (RCB-0). Patients who had moderate or extensive residual disease (RCB-II and RCB-III) and received adjuvant hormonal therapy, however, had greater survival benefit than those who did not.

Although this system requires the use of a complicated formula, a Web-based calculation script (http://www.mdanderson.org/breastcancer_RCB) is freely available to calculate the scores and the RCB class. The Web site also provides a stepwise guide for the pathologic evaluation of post-treatment breast specimens along with links to illustrative examples.

REPORTING POST-TREATMENT SPECIMENS

The following information in the surgical pathology report helps management and prognostication.

BREAST SPECIMEN

1. Documentation of tumor bed: essential in cases with pCR—report size in 2-D, if possible
2. Size and extent of residual invasive carcinoma
   a. Linear dimension of the largest contiguous area of invasive carcinoma
   b. Number of invasive foci or number of blocks with invasive carcinoma
3. Histologic grade—in addition to mitotic count, proliferation as determined by Ki-67 may be requested
4. Histologic type
5. Average tumor cellularity over the entire tumor bed (compare with pretreatment carcinoma if available)
6. Presence of lymphovascular invasion

7. Presence and extent of ductal carcinoma in situ (percentage of in situ carcinoma when using the RCB system)
8. Margins with respect to tumor bed, invasive carcinoma, and DCIS
9. A comment on the overall response to treatment—use of a classification system, when appropriate
10. Tumor markers (ER, PgR, and HER2) if sufficient residual invasive carcinoma is present

LYMPH NODES

1. Total number of lymph nodes examined
2. Number of lymph nodes with metastases
3. Size of the largest metastasis: it is helpful to include number of nodes with macrometastases, micrometastases, and isolated tumor cells

Pitfalls
GUIDE FOR EVALUATION OF POST-TREATMENT BREAST CARCINOMA

! Pathologists must be aware that patients have been treated to avoid misinterpretation of treatment-related changes—a long time interval between a diagnostic core needle biopsy and the definitive excision can be an important clue.

! To guide tissue sampling and to fully evaluate therapy response, pathologists should have knowledge of pretreatment size, number, and location of the tumor; relationship of the tumor to skin and chest wall, results of the prior biopsy and tumor markers, information regarding pretreatment lymph node evaluation and result of clinical/radiologic response to therapy.

! A specimen radiograph to confirm the presence of clips marking the tumor site may be essential if there has been a complete or near-complete clinical response.

! Failure to find the tumor bed can result in an erroneous conclusion that there has been a complete response.

! Residual tumor that has undergone a marked response is difficult to measure, because multiple small foci of invasive carcinoma or single tumor cells are often scattered throughout the tumor bed.

! In some cases, distinguishing residual in situ and invasive carcinoma can be difficult—IHC for myoepithelial markers should be used, if necessary, because residual DCIS does not preclude a pCR.

4. Presence of extranodal extension
5. Number of lymph nodes with evidence of prior metastatic involvement but without tumor cells (ie, fibrosis, necrosis, mucin pools, macrophages, and so forth)

REFERENCES

1. van der Hage JA, van de Velde CJ, Julien JP, et al. Preoperative chemotherapy in primary operable breast cancer: results from the European Organization for Research and Treatment of Cancer trial 10902. J Clin Oncol 2001;19:4224–37.
2. Fisher ER, Wang J, Bryant J, et al. Pathobiology of preoperative chemotherapy: findings from the National Surgical Adjuvant Breast and Bowel (NSABP) protocol B-18. Cancer 2002;95:681–95.
3. Mauri D, Pavlidis N, Ioannidis JP. Neoadjuvant versus adjuvant systemic treatment in breast cancer: a meta-analysis. J Natl Cancer Inst 2005;97:188–94.
4. Makris A, Powles TJ, Ashley SE, et al. A reduction in the requirements for mastectomy in a randomized trial of neoadjuvant chemoendocrine therapy in primary breast cancer. Ann Oncol 1998;9:1179–84.
5. Mieog JS, van der Hage JA, van de Velde CJ. Preoperative chemotherapy for women with operable breast cancer. Cochrane Database Syst Rev 2007;(2):CD005002.
6. Chen AM, Meric-Bernstam F, Hunt KK, et al. Breast conservation after neoadjuvant chemotherapy. Cancer 2005;103:689–95.
7. Hennessy BT, Hortobagyi GN, Rouzier R, et al. Outcome after pathologic complete eradication of cytologically proven breast cancer axillary node metastases following primary chemotherapy. J Clin Oncol 2005;23:9304–11.
8. Rouzier R, Pusztai L, Delaloge S, et al. Nomograms to predict pathologic complete response and metastasis-free survival after preoperative chemotherapy for breast cancer. J Clin Oncol 2005;23:8331–9.
9. Symmans WF, Peintinger F, Hatzis C, et al. Measurement of residual breast cancer burden to predict survival after neoadjuvant chemotherapy. J Clin Oncol 2007;25:4414–22.
10. Precht LM, Lowe KA, Atwood M, et al. Neoadjuvant chemotherapy of breast cancer: tumor markers as predictors of pathologic response, recurrence, and survival. Breast J 2010;16:362–8.
11. Sahoo S, Lester SC. Pathology of breast carcinomas after neoadjuvant chemotherapy: an overview with recommendations on specimen processing and reporting. Arch Pathol Lab Med 2009;133:633–42.
12. Chen JH, Feig B, Agrawal G, et al. MRI evaluation of pathologically complete response and residual tumors in breast cancer after neoadjuvant chemotherapy. Cancer 2008;112:17–26.

13. Partridge SC, Vanantwerp RK, Doot RK, et al. Association between serial dynamic contrast-enhanced MRI and dynamic 18F-FDG PET measures in patients undergoing neoadjuvant chemotherapy for locally advanced breast cancer. J Magn Reson Imaging 2010;32:1124–31.

14. Rouzier R, Extra JM, Klijanienko J, et al. Incidence and prognostic significance of complete axillary downstaging after primary chemotherapy in breast cancer patients with T1 to T3 tumors and cytologically proven axillary metastatic lymph nodes. J Clin Oncol 2002;20:1304–10.

15. von Minckwitz G, Untch M, Nuesch E, et al. Impact of treatment characteristics on response of different breast cancer phenotypes: pooled analysis of the German neo-adjuvant chemotherapy trials. Breast Cancer Res Treat 2011;125(1):145–56.

16. Ogston KN, Miller ID, Payne S, et al. A new histological grading system to assess response of breast cancers to primary chemotherapy: prognostic significance and survival. Breast 2003;12:320–7.

17. Jones RL, Lakhani SR, Ring AE, et al. Pathological complete response and residual DCIS following neoadjuvant chemotherapy for breast carcinoma. Br J Cancer 2006;94:358–62.

18. Mazouni C, Peintinger F, Wan-Kau S, et al. Residual ductal carcinoma in situ in patients with complete eradication of invasive breast cancer after neoadjuvant chemotherapy does not adversely affect patient outcome. J Clin Oncol 2007;25:2650–5.

19. Chen YY, DeVries S, Anderson J, et al. Pathologic and biologic response to preoperative endocrine therapy in patients with ER-positive ductal carcinoma in situ. BMC Cancer 2009;9:285.

20. Purushotham A, Pinder S, Cariati M, et al. Neoadjuvant chemotherapy: not the best option in estrogen receptor-positive, HER2-negative, invasive classical lobular carcinoma of the breast? J Clin Oncol 2010; 28:3552–4.

21. Schneeweiss A, Katretchko J, Sinn HP, et al. Only grading has independent impact on breast cancer survival after adjustment for pathological response to preoperative chemotherapy. Anticancer Drugs 2004;15:127–35.

22. Keam B, Im SA, Lee KH, et al. Ki-67 can be used for further classification of triple negative breast cancer into two subtypes with different response and prognosis. Breast Cancer Res 2011;13:R22.

23. Petit T, Wilt M, Velten M, et al. Comparative value of tumour grade, hormonal receptors, Ki-67, HER-2 and topoisomerase II alpha status as predictive markers in breast cancer patients treated with neoadjuvant anthracycline-based chemotherapy. Eur J Cancer 2004;40:205–11.

24. Pu RT, Schott AF, Sturtz DE, et al. Pathologic features of breast cancer associated with complete response to neoadjuvant chemotherapy: importance of tumor necrosis. Am J Surg Pathol 2005;29:354–8.

25. Denkert C, Loibl S, Noske A, et al. Tumor-associated lymphocytes as an independent predictor of response to neoadjuvant chemotherapy in breast cancer. J Clin Oncol 2010;28:105–13.

26. Carey LA, Dees EC, Sawyer L, et al. The triple negative paradox: primary tumor chemosensitivity of breast cancer subtypes. Clin Cancer Res 2007;13:2329–34.

27. Bhargava R, Beriwal S, Dabbs DJ, et al. Immunohistochemical surrogate markers of breast cancer molecular classes predicts response to neoadjuvant chemotherapy: a single institutional experience with 359 cases. Cancer 2010;116:1431–9.

28. Untch M, Rezai M, Loibl S, et al. Neoadjuvant treatment with trastuzumab in HER2-positive breast cancer: results from the GeparQuattro study. J Clin Oncol 2010;28:2024–31.

29. Gianni L, Eiermann W, Semiglazov V, et al. Neoadjuvant chemotherapy with trastuzumab followed by adjuvant trastuzumab versus neoadjuvant chemotherapy alone, in patients with HER2-positive locally advanced breast cancer (the NOAH trial): a randomised controlled superiority trial with a parallel HER2-negative cohort. Lancet 2010;375:377–84.

30. Buzdar AU, Valero V, Ibrahim NK, et al. Neoadjuvant therapy with paclitaxel followed by 5-fluorouracil, epirubicin, and cyclophosphamide chemotherapy and concurrent trastuzumab in human epidermal growth factor receptor 2-positive operable breast cancer: an update of the initial randomized study population and data of additional patients treated with the same regimen. Clin Cancer Res 2007;13:228–33.

31. Bhargava R, Dabbs DJ, Beriwal S, et al. Semiquantitative hormone receptor level influences response to trastuzumab-containing neoadjuvant chemotherapy in HER2-positive breast cancer. Mod Pathol 2011;24(3):367–74.

32. Rouzier R, Perou CM, Symmans WF, et al. Breast cancer molecular subtypes respond differently to preoperative chemotherapy. Clin Cancer Res 2005; 11:5678–85.

33. de Ronde JJ, Hannemann J, Halfwerk H, et al. Concordance of clinical and molecular breast cancer subtyping in the context of preoperative chemotherapy response. Breast Cancer Res Treat 2010;119:119–26.

34. Goldstein NS, Decker D, Severson D, et al. Molecular classification system identifies invasive breast carcinoma patients who are most likely and those who are least likely to achieve a complete pathologic response after neoadjuvant chemotherapy. Cancer 2007;110:1687–96.

35. Gianni L, Zambetti M, Clark K, et al. Gene expression profiles in paraffin-embedded core biopsy

tissue predict response to chemotherapy in women with locally advanced breast cancer. J Clin Oncol 2005;23:7265–77.

36. Rodriguez AA, Makris A, Wu MF, et al. DNA repair signature is associated with anthracycline response in triple negative breast cancer patients. Breast Cancer Res Treat 2010;123:189–96.

37. Donnelly J, Parham DM, Hickish T, et al. Axillary lymph node scarring and the association with tumour response following neoadjuvant chemoendocrine therapy for breast cancer. Breast 2001;10:61–6.

38. Neuman H, Carey LA, Ollila DW, et al. Axillary lymph node count is lower after neoadjuvant chemotherapy. Am J Surg 2006;191:827–9.

39. Sahoo S, Chagnar AB. Low lymph node count after neoadjuvant chemotherapy for breast cancer should not be assumed to represent complete axillary dissection. Mod Pathol 2008;21:1636.

40. Boughey JC, Donohue JH, Jakub JW, et al. Number of lymph nodes identified at axillary dissection: effect of neoadjuvant chemotherapy and other factors. Cancer 2010;116:3322–9.

41. Carey LA, Metzger R, Dees EC, et al. American Joint Committee on Cancer tumor-node-metastasis stage after neoadjuvant chemotherapy and breast cancer outcome. J Natl Cancer Inst 2005;97:1137–42.

42. Chollet P, Amat S, Belembaogo E, et al. Is Nottingham prognostic index useful after induction chemotherapy in operable breast cancer? Br J Cancer 2003;89:1185–91.

43. Chen AM, Meric-Bernstam F, Hunt KK, et al. Breast conservation after neoadjuvant chemotherapy: the MD Anderson cancer center experience. J Clin Oncol 2004;22:2303–12.

44. Rajan R, Poniecka A, Smith TL, et al. Change in tumor cellularity of breast carcinoma after neoadjuvant chemotherapy as a variable in the pathologic assessment of response. Cancer 2004;100:1365–73.

45. Thomas JS, Julian HS, Green RV, et al. Histopathology of breast carcinoma following neoadjuvant systemic therapy: a common association between letrozole therapy and central scarring. Histopathology 2007;51:219–26.

46. Sharkey FE, Addington SL, Fowler LJ, et al. Effects of preoperative chemotherapy on the morphology of resectable breast carcinoma. Mod Pathol 1996; 9:893–900.

47. Hasebe T, Tamura N, Iwasaki M, et al. Grading system for lymph vessel tumor emboli: significant outcome predictor for patients with invasive ductal carcinoma of the breast who received neoadjuvant therapy. Mod Pathol 2010;23:581–92.

48. Uematsu T, Kasami M, Watanabe J, et al. Is lymphovascular invasion degree one of the important factors to predict neoadjuvant chemotherapy efficacy in breast cancer? Breast Cancer 2011;18(4): 309–13.

49. Arnedos M, Nerurkar A, Osin P, et al. Discordance between core needle biopsy (CNB) and excisional biopsy (EB) for estrogen receptor (ER), progesterone receptor (PgR) and HER2 status in early breast cancer (EBC). Ann Oncol 2009;20:1948–52.

50. van de Ven S, Smit VT, Dekker TJ, et al. Discordances in ER, PR and HER2 receptors after neoadjuvant chemotherapy in breast cancer. Cancer Treat Rev 2011;37(6):422–30.

51. Hirata T, Shimizu C, Yonemori K, et al. Change in the hormone receptor status following administration of neoadjuvant chemotherapy and its impact on the long-term outcome in patients with primary breast cancer. Br J Cancer 2009;101:1529–36.

52. Tacca O, Penault-Llorca F, Abrial C, et al. Changes in and prognostic value of hormone receptor status in a series of operable breast cancer patients treated with neoadjuvant chemotherapy. Oncologist 2007;12:636–43.

53. Kurosumi M, Takatsuka Y, Watanabe T, et al. Histopathological assessment of anastrozole and tamoxifen as preoperative (neoadjuvant) treatment in postmenopausal Japanese women with hormone receptor-positive breast cancer in the PROACT trial. J Cancer Res Clin Oncol 2008;134:715–22.

54. Miller WR, Dixon JM, Cameron DA, et al. Biological and clinical effects of aromatase inhibitors in neoadjuvant therapy. J Steroid Biochem Mol Biol 2001;79: 103–7.

55. Taucher S, Rudas M, Mader RM, et al. Influence of neoadjuvant therapy with epirubicin and docetaxel on the expression of HER2/neu in patients with breast cancer. Breast Cancer Res Treat 2003;82: 207–13.

56. Varga Z, Caduff R, Pestalozzi B. Stability of the HER2 gene after primary chemotherapy in advanced breast cancer. Virchows Arch 2005;446: 136–41.

57. Vincent-Salomon A, Jouve M, Genin P, et al. HER2 status in patients with breast carcinoma is not modified selectively by preoperative chemotherapy and is stable during the metastatic process. Cancer 2002;94:2169–73.

58. Zhu L, Chow LW, Loo WT, et al. Her2/neu expression predicts the response to antiaromatase neoadjuvant therapy in primary breast cancer: subgroup analysis from celecoxib antiaromatase neoadjuvant trial. Clin Cancer Res 2004;10:4639–44.

59. Mittendorf EA, Wu Y, Scaltriti M, et al. Loss of HER2 amplification following trastuzumab-based neoadjuvant systemic therapy and survival outcomes. Clin Cancer Res 2009;15:7381–8.

60. Hurley J, Doliny P, Reis I, et al. Docetaxel, cisplatin, and trastuzumab as primary systemic therapy for human epidermal growth factor receptor 2-positive locally advanced breast cancer. J Clin Oncol 2006; 24:1831–8.

61. Dowsett M, Ebbs SR, Dixon JM, et al. Biomarker changes during neoadjuvant anastrozole, tamoxifen, or the combination: influence of hormonal status and HER-2 in breast cancer—a study from the IMPACT trialists. J Clin Oncol 2005;23:2477–92.

62. Lee J, Im YH, Lee SH, et al. Evaluation of ER and Ki-67 proliferation index as prognostic factors for survival following neoadjuvant chemotherapy with doxorubicin/docetaxel for locally advanced breast cancer. Cancer Chemother Pharmacol 2008;61: 569–77.

63. Jones RL, Salter J, A'Hern R, et al. The prognostic significance of Ki67 before and after neoadjuvant chemotherapy in breast cancer. Breast Cancer Res Treat 2009;116:53–68.

64. Decensi A, Guerrieri-Gonzaga A, Gandini S, et al. Prognostic significance of Ki-67 labeling index after short-term presurgical tamoxifen in women with ER-positive breast cancer. Ann Oncol 2011;22(3):582–7.

65. Toi M, Saji S, Masuda N, et al. Ki67 index changes, pathological response and clinical benefits in primary breast cancer patients treated with 24 weeks of aromatase inhibition. Cancer Sci 2011; 102:858–65.

66. Kuerer HM, Newman LA, Smith TL, et al. Clinical course of breast cancer patients with complete pathologic primary tumor and axillary lymph node response to doxorubicin-based neoadjuvant chemotherapy. J Clin Oncol 1999;17:460–9.

67. Escobar PF, Patrick RJ, Rybicki LA, et al. Prognostic significance of residual breast disease and axillary node involvement for patients who had primary induction chemotherapy for advanced breast cancer. Ann Surg Oncol 2006;13:783–7.

68. Klauber-DeMore N, Ollila DW, Moore DT, et al. Size of residual lymph node metastasis after neoadjuvant chemotherapy in locally advanced breast cancer patients is prognostic. Ann Surg Oncol 2006;13: 685–91.

69. Loya A, Guray M, Hennessy BT, et al. Prognostic significance of occult axillary lymph node metastases after chemotherapy-induced pathologic complete response of cytologically proven axillary lymph node metastases from breast cancer. Cancer 2009; 115:1605–12.

70. Sakakibara M, Nagashima T, Kadowaki M, et al. Clinical significance of axillary microresiduals after neoadjuvant chemotherapy in breast cancer patients with cytologically proven metastases. Ann Surg Oncol 2009;16:2470–8.

71. Brown AS, Hunt KK, Shen J, et al. Histologic changes associated with false-negative sentinel lymph nodes after preoperative chemotherapy in patients with confirmed lymph node-positive breast cancer before treatment. Cancer 2010;116:2878–83.

72. Gonzalez-Angulo AM, McGuire SE, Buchholz TA, et al. Factors predictive of distant metastases in patients with breast cancer who have a pathologic complete response after neoadjuvant chemotherapy. J Clin Oncol 2005;23:7098–104.

73. Rastogi P, Anderson SJ, Bear HD, et al. Preoperative chemotherapy: updates of National Surgical Adjuvant Breast and Bowel Project Protocols B-18 and B-27. J Clin Oncol 2008;26:778–85.

74. Edge SB, Byrd DR, Compton CC, editors. AJCC cancer staging mannual. 7th edition. New York: Springer; 2010.

75. Mittendorf EA, Jeruss JS, Tucker SL, et al. Validation of a novel staging system for disease-specific survival in patients with breast cancer treated with neoadjuvant chemotherapy. J Clin Oncol 2011;29: 1956–62.

PROGNOSTIC FACTORS FOR PATIENTS WITH BREAST CANCER: TRADITIONAL AND NEW

Amy Ly, MD*, Susan C. Lester, MD, PhD, Deborah Dillon, MD

KEYWORDS

• Breast cancer • Prognosis • Tumor classification

ABSTRACT

At the time of breast cancer diagnosis, multiple features of the tumor are routinely assessed to evaluate for prognostic and predictive factors. Prognostic factors provide information about the patient's likely clinical course, and include tumor stage (composed of lymph node status, tumor size, and presence of chest wall involvement), tumor histologic type and grade, estrogen and progesterone receptor expression, and HER2 status. These traditional prognostic factors are reviewed with particular attention to problematic areas in classification. Several newer prognostic tests may be able to provide information beyond the traditional prognostic factors and are presented.

OVERVIEW

Considerable progress has been made in recent years in elucidating the molecular alterations that contribute to the development of breast cancer; however, except for the evaluation of estrogen receptor (ER), progesterone receptor (PR), and human epidermal growth factor receptor 2 (HER2), very little of this information has had much impact on current clinical management of breast cancer. Aside from hormone receptor and HER2 status, most clinically relevant information is obtained through the careful histopathological examination of resected breast tissue.[1,2] Lymph node status and tumor size remain powerful prognostic indicators, yet there are still problematic areas in making these determinations in some cases. Standard prognostic factors in the histopathologic evaluation of breast cancer, including lymph node status, tumor size, histologic type and grade, presence of lymphovascular invasion, and skin/chest wall involvement are useful guides for clinical treatment (**Box 1**). Several new prognostic assays, including Oncotype DX, MammaPrint, and CellSearch, have the potential to provide additional information beyond the traditional prognostic factors in breast cancer; however, each of these new prognostic assays has its own strengths and limitations.

LYMPH NODE STATUS

The number of axillary lymph nodes involved by metastatic carcinoma has been repeatedly demonstrated to be the single most important prognostic indicator for patients with breast cancer.[3–5] Current American Joint Committee on Cancer (AJCC) staging for lymph nodes[6] places patients into the following 4 categories:

1. No positive nodes
2. 1 to 3 positive nodes
3. 4 to 9 positive nodes
4. 10 or more involved nodes

A node is considered positive in this scheme if the tumor deposit is greater than 0.02 cm in size. This approach stratifies patients according to clinical outcome. Patients without nodal involvement

The authors have nothing to disclose.
Department of Pathology, Brigham and Women's Hospital, Harvard Medical School, 75 Francis Street, Boston, MA 02115, USA
* Corresponding author.
E-mail address: aly1@partners.org

Box 1
Traditional prognostic factors in breast cancer

- Lymph node status
- Tumor size
- Tumor histology and grade
- Lymphovascular invasion
- Involvement of skin/chest wall
- Hormone receptor and HER2 expression

---

generally fare well, in one study showing a 4-year 90% overall survival after radical mastectomy[3] and an 8-year survival of 82% postmastectomy in another.[4] As the number of positive lymph nodes increases, disease-free survival and overall survival decrease.[7,8] Approximately 40% to 50% of patients with early-stage disease have at least 1 positive axillary lymph node.

Axillary dissection remains the gold standard for evaluating nodal status; however, sentinel lymph node sampling allows for evaluation of lymph nodes without performing a complete axillary dissection, which can lead to significant morbidity, such as lymphedema. Depending on the method used, a sentinel node may be successfully identified in up to 96% of breast cancer cases.[9] The sentinel lymph node is usually located in the axilla; however, sentinel lymph nodes can occasionally be found in internal mammary, intramammary, and clavicular sites.[10]

Given the importance of lymph node status in determining prognosis, methods for the evaluation of lymph nodes are beginning to be standardized. The detection of lymph node metastases is dependent on several factors, including the size of the metastasis, the size of the lymph node, and the number of sections examined.[11] The current recommendation from the College of American Pathologists (CAP) for evaluating lymph nodes is to slice the lymph node tissue into 2-mm sections, embed all tissue sections, and review 1 hematoxylin and eosin–stained (H&E) slide from each block (**Box 2**). Importantly, sectioning at 2-mm intervals

ensures that macrometastases will not be missed. Multilevel sectioning and immunohistochemistry are not required; however, some institutions choose to perform multiple serial H&E-stained sections and may routinely perform cytokeratin immunohistochemical staining on nodes that are not grossly involved by tumor. These practices increase the likelihood of detecting micrometastases and isolated tumor cells (ITCs).

The clinical significance of detecting micrometastases and ITCs has been a subject of some controversy. Several large studies have shown that the presence of micrometastases and ITCs detected by serial sectioning and/or immunohistochemistry is associated with a small but significant decrease in disease-free and/or overall survival.[12,13] Such studies have been difficult to evaluate because they are rarely controlled for factors involved in lymph node processing. A recent large prospective randomized study with carefully controlled lymph node processing and examination found that women with occult metastases on subsequent deeper levels and keratin immunohistochemistry had a very small but significantly worse overall survival at 5 years compared with women without occult metastases (94.6% versus 95.8%). In this study, micrometastases conferred slightly worse survival compared with ITCs.[14] Although this study did confirm poorer survival in patients with micrometastases, based on the very small size of the difference, the investigators concluded that clinical decisions should not be based on the presence of these very small metastases and, therefore, additional studies to find them are not warranted.[14] The lack of clinical significance of small metastases is further supported by the findings of the American College of Surgeons Z0011 Trial. This study was designed to examine the value of completion axillary dissection in a selected group of patients with sentinel lymph node metastases. The results of this trial demonstrated no local disease control or survival advantage of patients undergoing complete axillary dissection versus those with only sentinel lymph node examination.[15]

Current AJCC lymph node classification categories have refined the definitions and classification of ITCs and micrometastases. According to AJCC,[6] tumor deposits larger than 0.02 cm up to 0.2 cm (or more than 200 cells) are classified as micrometastases and deposits not more than 0.02 cm (or up to 200 cells) are classified as ITCs (**Box 3**). Lymph nodes with ITCs are not considered positive for staging purposes. For pT1 tumors, patients with only micrometastases (pN1mi), previously classified as Stage II, are now classified as Stage IB. Categorizing a nodal

---

Box 2
CAP guidelines for lymph node examination

1. Section all lymph node tissue into 2-mm slices
2. Embed all tissue sections
3. Review 1 H&E slide from each block

deposit as an ITC or a micrometastasis may be challenging in cases in which the tumor cells are scattered singly throughout the node, or if tumor cells form multiple, closely arranged, small clusters that do not touch (**Fig. 1**). The most recent CAP protocol for invasive breast cancer (www. cap.org) includes detailed suggestions for reporting challenging cases.

TUMOR SIZE

Tumor size is closely correlated with the probability of lymph node metastasis and is also a strong independent prognostic factor. Although reporting of pathologic size has not been standardized, numerous studies have demonstrated that it is the size of the invasive component that correlates with outcome. For this reason, the seventh edition of the *AJCC Cancer Staging Manual*[6] specifies that the pathologic tumor size for the T classification is based on measurement of only the invasive component. A number of problematic areas remain in the reporting of tumor size, particularly when the size is at or close to staging and treatment cutoff points, including determination of microinvasion, very small tumors, multifocal tumors, and tumors removed in more than one specimen.

Microinvasion

The current *AJCC Cancer Staging Manual*[6] definition of microinvasion is the extension of tumor cells beyond the basement membrane into the adjacent tissues with no focus more than 0.1 cm in greatest dimension. The microinvasive tumor cells are not connected to any adjacent ductal carcinoma in situ (DCIS) and may be associated with a marked lymphocytic infiltrate or reactive stromal changes. When multiple foci of microinvasion are present, it is the size of only the largest focus that is used to assign the T classification and not the sum of the microinvasive foci or including the space between foci of microinvasion (**Fig. 2**). Microinvasion is more likely to be found in cases of high-grade DCIS with adjacent stromal reaction. Histologic mimics of microinvasion include distortion of DCIS by biopsy-related changes or other sclerosing process, crush artifact in DCIS, and DCIS involvement of small acini in a lobule. Immunohistochemical staining for myoepithelial markers can be

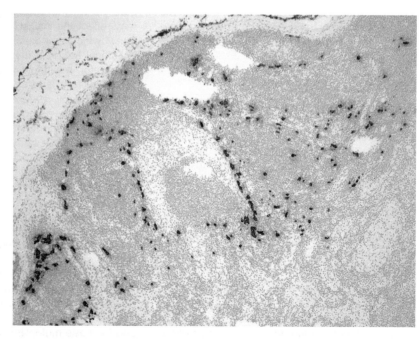

Fig. 1. Lymph node classification. On immunohistochemistry for pankeratin, the tumor cells in this lymph node are difficult to classify because of the pattern of multiple clusters with intervening spaces. Although the size of the metastatic deposit is generally based on the size of the largest contiguous cluster of tumor cells, in this case the total volume of metastatic tumor appears to be greater than the size of the largest contiguous cluster. In such cases, the pathologist should use his or her judgment in assigning the N category. Given the presence of more than 200 cells, this case was classified as a micrometastasis rather than ITCs (H&E stain, 40×).

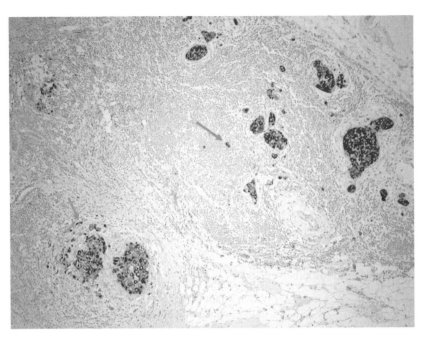

Fig. 2. Diagnosis of micro-invasion. When multiple foci of microinvasion are present, the size of only the largest focus is used to assign the T classification and not the sum of the microinvasive foci or including the space between foci of microinvasion. In this case, the most conservative interpretation is to consider that there are at least 2 foci of microinvasion (*arrows*) (each less than 0.1 cm and associated with a focus of DCIS) rather than including the size of the intervening tissue (Combined p63/AE1/AE3 immunohistochemical stain, 40×).

helpful in evaluating such foci. If microinvasion is present, the tissue should be well sampled to exclude a larger invasive carcinoma. Most studies have shown that the prognosis of DCIS with microinvasion (up to 0.1 cm) is similar to the prognosis of DCIS alone.[16] The clinical significance of multiple foci of microinvasion is unknown; however, in rare cases, women with numerous foci of microinvasion have developed distant metastases.[16] It seems advisable for the pathologist to report an estimate of the number of foci if multifocal microinvasion is present.

Small Tumors (T1a and T1b)

As the use of radiologic screening increases, more tumors are discovered at earlier stages. The size of small carcinomas is often difficult to determine accurately because of poor gross visualization, suboptimal sectioning, tissue shrinkage following fixation, and distortion from prior core-needle biopsies; however, determination of tumor size around staging cutoff points can be of critical importance. Careful gross and microscopic measurement of these small lesions, along with radiologic correlation, will provide the best determination of tumor size.

Multiple Carcinomas

It can be difficult to determine the size of multifocal carcinomas. For staging purposes, the size of the largest focus of invasive carcinoma is used to determine the T classification. In difficult cases, radiologic correlation can be very helpful in determining the best T classification.[17] There is some evidence to suggest that invasive carcinomas with multiple foci of invasion have higher rates of lymph node metastasis with worse survival than unifocal tumors, and that the number of lymph node metastases is predicted best by the aggregate size of the invasive foci[18–20]; however, this may reflect the inclusion of cases that are multifocal owing to intramammary spread. In cases of multifocal tumor, it may be possible to note the reason for multifocality; for example, separate foci of invasion arising in association with extensive intraductal carcinoma, separate foci of invasion arising in association with lymphovascular invasion, or completely independent foci.[21] Although current staging is determined by the size of the largest focus only, it has been suggested that this practice may underestimate the stage of some patients with multifocal/multicentric disease. For multifocal tumors, grossly distinct tumor masses found in separate quadrants should be staged as separate tumors. Multiple tumors should also be staged separately if the immunophenotype is distinct; however, if imaging studies show a single lesion, then multiple foci may be measured in aggregate and an overall size given. Rare cases of invasive carcinoma can be particularly difficult to measure if no mass is seen grossly and the pattern of infiltration is discontinuous (eg, some cases of invasive lobular carcinoma). In these cases, the pathology report can provide an indication of the total disease burden (eg, the total number of blocks involved), as well as the largest focus seen in a single block and suggest radiologic correlation for best estimate of tumor size.

Carcinomas Removed in More Than One Specimen

Carcinomas removed in more than one specimen can be difficult to measure because of obscuring biopsy site changes and difficulties in orienting the specimens and reexcisions. Care should be taken, particularly with small tumors, to correlate with imaging studies and not simply to add the size from the biopsy to the size in the excision. Biopsy site changes may contribute to the gross size measurement in the excision of a small tumor; thus, correlation with prebiopsy imaging studies, as well as the size of the tumor in the prior core-needle biopsy, is suggested. Adding all tumor measurements in excisions with positive margins and subsequent reexcisions can also result in overestimating tumor size. Again, imaging studies may provide the most accurate estimation of tumor size in such cases. Additional discussion of these and other problematic areas in tumor size determination can be found in the CAP protocol for reporting of invasive carcinomas (www.cap.org).

HISTOLOGIC TYPE AND GRADE

Histologic grade correlates with disease-free and overall survival independently of lymph node status and tumor size.[22,23] It is not included in the TNM staging system but is routinely reported. The most commonly used histologic grading system is the Elston-Ellis modification of the Scarff-Bloom-Richardson grading system[22,24] (Box 4). This semiquantitative system uses a 1-point to 3-point scale to score tubule formation, nuclear pleomorphism, and mitotic rate. The reproducibility of tumor grading with this method is moderate to good.[25–28] In this grading system, tubular carcinoma is by definition well differentiated, and medullary carcinoma is by definition poorly differentiated, but otherwise, all histologic tumor types are graded, including lobular carcinomas. When invasive lobular carcinomas are graded according to this grading system, the survival curves by histologic grade are almost identical to the survival curves of invasive ductal carcinomas of no special type.[22]

Certain histologic types, most notably tubular, mucinous, invasive cribriform, and adenoid cystic carcinoma, are associated with a particularly favorable outcome in most studies. If strict

Box 4 Modified Scarff-Bloom-Richardson grading	
Tubule formation	
Majority of tumor: >75%	1
Moderate: 10%–75%	2
Minimal: <10%	3
Nuclear pleomorphism	
Small regular nuclei	1
Moderate increase in size/nucleoli	2
Marked variation in size, chromatin clumping	3
Mitotic count (per 10 high-power fields)	
0–5	1
6–10	2
>11	3

diagnostic criteria are used, the prognosis (20-year disease-free survival) of these favorable histologic types 1.1 cm to 3.0 cm in size is similar to that of invasive ductal carcinomas 1.0 cm and smaller.[29] CAP recommends using the World Health Organization classification for the determination of histologic type. There are data to suggest that the presence of micropapillary features anywhere in the invasive carcinoma is associated with a slightly worse prognosis than invasive ductal carcinoma not otherwise specified (NOS) because of higher rates of lymph node involvement.[30] Metaplastic carcinoma in some studies is also associated with slightly worse prognosis despite having a lower frequency of axillary lymph node involvement at the time of diagnosis compared with invasive carcinoma NOS.[31,32]

SKIN/CHEST WALL INVOLVEMENT

Several specific forms of skin and chest wall involvement are adverse prognostic indicators in breast cancer, associated with shorter time to recurrence and lower overall survival rates. These features of locally advanced stages warrant a pT4 classification in the AJCC staging system.[6] pT4a refers to tumor of any size with extension to the chest wall, defined as invasion of the ribs, intercostal muscles, or serratus anterior. This designation does not include invasion of the pectoralis muscle. pT4b refers to tumor of any size with skin involvement, defined as clinically evident edema, ulceration of the skin, or satellite skin nodules confined to the same breast. Tumors with other skin changes, including dimpling, nipple retraction, and histologic skin involvement (confined to the dermis) have a much better prognosis; these changes alone are not sufficient for classification as pT4b.[33] The diagnosis of inflammatory breast carcinoma also deserves clarification. Although the clinical presentation of inflammatory breast cancer (breast erythema and edema) is attributable to tumor present in the dermal lymphatics, the diagnosis of inflammatory breast carcinoma (classified as T4d) requires both the clinical findings and the histologic documentation of carcinoma in the breast (either in lymphatics or within the breast parenchyma itself). Histologic evidence of dermal lymphatic invasion without clinical signs of inflammatory breast cancer has a better prognosis and is not classified as T4d.[34] The histologic finding of dermal lymphatic invasion alone is neither required nor sufficient for a diagnosis of inflammatory breast cancer. These distinctions are important because inflammatory breast cancer is an aggressive disease that carries the worst prognosis of all breast malignancies, with an overall survival of less than 30% at 10 years.[35,36]

LYMPHOVASCULAR INVASION

When tumor emboli are seen, they are usually within thin-walled vascular channels. Whether these represent lymphatics, capillaries, or venules cannot be determined with certainty and does not appear to have prognostic importance. We have chosen to use the broad term "lymphovascular" to encompass all of these. Most studies show that the presence of extratumoral lymphovascular invasion (LVI) is significantly associated with lymph node metastasis and indicates poor prognosis in lymph node–negative patients.[37–45] Considerable variation in the reported frequency of LVI (20%–54%) likely reflects differences both in study populations and in criteria for diagnosis (Box 5).

Distinguishing LVI from retraction artifact (tissue shrinkage during processing) around foci of invasive carcinoma can be difficult. For this reason, and because the prognostic significance of intratumoral LVI is not known, it is suggested that LVI

be diagnosed only outside areas of invasive carcinoma.

Reporting of LVI is recommended, but not required, by CAP. This is the least reproducible prognostic factor among pathologists, with many possibilities for both overdiagnosis and underdiagnosis. We currently use the criteria proposed by Rosen for the diagnosis of LVI.[46] These include (1) that LVI should be diagnosed outside the border of the invasive carcinoma; (2) that tumor emboli usually do not conform exactly to the contours of the spaces in which they are found; and (3) that endothelial cell nuclei should be seen in the cells lining the space (Fig. 3). Red blood cells within the space can also be a helpful feature. The most common site for detection of LVI is 0.1 to 0.2 cm from the advancing edge of the carcinoma. Immunohistochemical studies for endothelial cell markers (eg, CD31, CD34, D2–40) can result in both false-positive and false-negative results and should be interpreted with caution.

HORMONE RECEPTOR STATUS

Patients with ER-positive and PR-positive tumors have longer disease-free and overall survival than those whose tumors are negative for one or both of these receptors.[47–49] However, to some degree, hormone receptor expression correlates with tumor grade, and its value as an independent prognostic factor is only weak to moderate.[50,51] The greatest utility of hormone receptor status is as a strong predictor of response to endocrine therapy.

Hormone receptor expression is typically determined by immunohistochemistry and a number of antibodies are available commercially for this purpose. Attention has been focused recently on the need for standardization of methodology and scoring to improve concordance among laboratories. CAP and the American Society of Clinical Oncology have recently published guidelines for the performance and reporting of hormone receptor expression studies.[52] Significant survival benefit is derived from hormonal therapy (tamoxifen, aromatase inhibitors) by patients with at least 1% of tumor cells expressing hormone receptors. Therefore, 1% expression is now considered to be the cutoff for hormone receptor positivity.

HER2

HER2 is a cell membrane–bound tyrosine kinase receptor that normally promotes cell growth and proliferation. The HER2 gene is amplified in 15% to 20% of breast cancers and overexpression of the HER2 protein is associated with poor

---

Box 5
Criteria for lymphovascular invasion

- Outside the area of the invasive carcinoma
- Tumor cells are nonconforming
- Endothelial cells should be present
- Presence of an associated vessel lends weight to interpretation as lymphatic space
- Beware of retraction artifact!

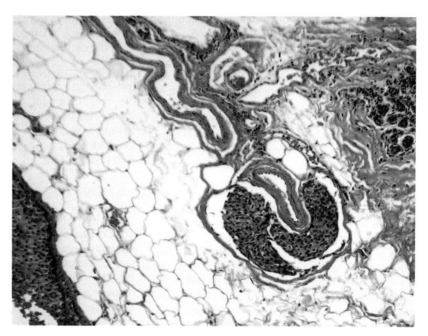

Fig. 3. Diagnosis of LVI. A tumor cell embolus is seen within a lymphatic channel circling a vessel. Although the tumor cells conform somewhat to the space, the location of the focus outside of the area of the invasive carcinoma, presence of endothelial cells, and association with a vessel all support interpretation as LVI (H&E stain, 200×).

prognosis. HER2 overexpression in invasive breast carcinoma correlates with high-grade histology, high mitotic activity, and frequent lymph node metastasis. In addition, amplification and overexpression of HER2 predicts response to anthracycline-based chemotherapies and is used to select patients for treatment with HER2-targeted therapies.[53] HER2 expression is typically determined by immunohistochemistry and fluorescence in situ hybridization (FISH). Care should be taken in cases in which there is a discrepancy between morphologically guided analysis, such as immunohistochemistry and FISH and HER2 status as reported by Oncotype DX, as the Oncotype DX methodology may be more susceptible to false-negative results.[54] Guidelines for the performance and reporting of HER2 assays have also recently been published in an effort to improve concordance among laboratories.[55]

PROGNOSIS FOLLOWING NEOADJUVANT THERAPY

In the setting of neoadjuvant chemotherapy, prognostic variables are the same as in the absence of preoperative treatment; however, the degree of response to chemotherapy constitutes an additional prognostic variable. The response to neoadjuvant therapy is best evaluated pathologically. The absence of residual carcinoma in the breast and lymph nodes indicates a complete pathologic response and portends the best possible

outcome. Several systems have been described for the evaluation of breast cancer following neoadjuvant therapy. For a detailed discussion of the evaluation and reporting of breast cancer following neoadjuvant chemotherapy, see the recent review by Sahoo and Lester[56] and the M.D. Anderson Cancer Center Web site (www.mdanderson.org/breastcancer_RCB).

NEW PROGNOSTIC TESTS

Recent methods for determining prognosis, including the St. Gallen criteria, the Nottingham Prognostic Index, and Adjuvant!Online (www.adjuvantonline.com), combine the traditional clinicopathologic features described into various combinations.[57–59] Although these risk categories are useful in assessing prognosis for groups of patients, they are less useful for determining prognosis in individual patients. Several novel molecular assays have been developed in an effort to address the need for better risk assessment for individual patients.

ONCOTYPE DX

The observation that women with lymph node–negative, ER-positive cancers have only a 15% chance of distant recurrence at 10 years (National Surgical Adjuvant Breast and Bowel Project B14 and B20) has led to interest in the identification of the subset of tumors likely to recur, with the rationale that the remaining 85% of women might be spared the effects of chemotherapy. Genomic Health, Inc. (Redwood City, CA) developed a 21-gene reverse transcriptase-polymerase chain reaction assay that can be performed on formalin-fixed paraffin-embedded tumor tissue to predict the likelihood of tumor recurrence in lymph node–negative ER-positive cancers. The assay is based on published data showing that the expression profile of this panel of genes correlated with the likelihood of distant recurrence in 668 patients in a retrospective study.[60] Recent data have shown the results of this assay to be prognostic for locoregional recurrence[61] and predictive of chemotherapy benefit in ER-positive lymph node–negative and lymph node–positive disease.[62,63] A prospective clinical trial to evaluate the added value of Oncotype DX, the TAILORx Trial (Trial Assigning Individualized Options for treatment), is currently under way.[64] Care should be taken in the interpretation of an intermediate to high Oncotype DX score in an otherwise low-grade histology tumor, as an associated inflammatory infiltrate may contribute to an apparently increased risk of recurrence by Oncotype DX.[65] Another recent study has determined that the Oncotype DX recurrence score adds little prognostic information beyond what is contained within standard histopathologic variables plus 4 immunohistochemical studies (IHC4; ER, PR, HER2, and Ki67).[66] Because most of these variables are included in standard reporting for invasive breast cancer, these data suggest that the IHC4 score may have general applicability in the future.

MAMMAPRINT

The US Food and Drug Administration (FDA)-cleared MammaPrint assay, marketed by Agendia (Amsterdam, the Netherlands), is based on the 70-gene Amsterdam breast cancer signature associated with high risk of distant recurrence. This signature was derived from gene expression array analysis of 117 invasive breast cancers of young patients with negative lymph nodes and any ER status.[67,68] Most of the genes in the signature have known biologic functions in growth, proliferation, transformation, cell death, DNA replication, and cell cycle control. In early validation studies, 90% of patients with a low-risk signature in this assay were free of distant metastasis at 10 years compared with 71% of patients with a high-risk signature.[68] The clinical utility of this assay is being assessed in 2 prospective multi-institutional clinical trials[69,70]:

1. MINDACT: Microarray In Node negative and 1 to 3 lymph node positive Disease may Avoid Chemotherapy Trial

2. I-SPY 2: Investigation of Serial studies to Predict your therapeutic response with imaging and molecular analysis 2 trial

Unlike Oncotype DX, MammaPrint can be used for patients with hormone receptor–negative disease. In the past, a disadvantage of this assay format has been the requirement for fresh tumor tissue; however, the test will be offered for formalin-fixed paraffin-embedded tissue beginning in early 2012.

CELLSEARCH FOR CIRCULATING TUMOR CELLS

The CellSearch system (Veridex LLC, Raritan, NJ) is currently the only FDA-approved in vitro diagnostic test for evaluating circulating tumor cells (CTCs) in the setting of clinically or radiologically measurable metastatic breast cancer. CTCs in the CellSearch system are defined as epCAM-positive, cytokeratin-positive, and CD45-negative, intact nucleated cells. Typically, a baseline CTC is drawn before the start of a new therapy regimen and CTC measurements may be repeated during the course of therapy. The presence of 5 or more CTCs in 7.5 mL of whole blood ("positive CTC test") at any time point is associated with a worse prognosis, manifesting as shorter time to recurrence and decreased survival. In addition, changes in CTC test results during or after the course of therapy likewise modify the patient's prognosis and suggest a measurable response to therapy.[71–73] CTC testing is intended for use in conjunction with all other clinical and radiologic findings, and can be used serially to follow patients clinically. CTC testing is not currently part of National Comprehensive Cancer Network and American Society of Clinical Oncology guidelines; however, some data show it is a prognostic marker independent of other established traditional factors and type of chemotherapy regimen, and is as accurate as radiology in monitoring response to therapy.[74]

SUMMARY

The traditional prognostic factors (tumor size, lymph node status, histologic type and grade, skin/chest wall involvement, and LVI) require careful gross and histopathologic examination of the resected breast tissue. These traditional prognostic factors have provided the foundation for accurate tumor staging, guiding the clinical treatment of breast cancer. Tremendous advances have resulted from the characterization of ER, PR, and HER2 and development of targeted therapies. It is reasonable to expect that in coming years the combined power of new high-throughput technologies and bioinformatics will result in the identification of molecular markers capable of even greater refinements in prognosis and better prediction of response to specific therapies. The close cooperation of basic scientists and clinicians and their patients is required for the evaluation of novel assays to determine if and when they might best be incorporated into routine clinical use.

REFERENCES

1. Goldhirsch A, Glick JH, Gelber RD, et al. Meeting highlights: international consensus panel on the treatment of primary breast cancer. J Natl Cancer Inst 1998;90(21):1601–8.

2. Fitzgibbons PL, Page DL, Weaver D, et al. Prognostic factors in breast cancer. College of American Pathologists Consensus Statement 1999. Arch Pathol Lab Med 2000;124(7):966–78.

3. Fisher ER, Palekar A, Rockette H, et al. Pathologic findings from the National Surgical Adjuvant Breast Project (Protocol No. 4) V. Significance of axillary nodal micro- and macrometastases. Cancer 1978; 42(4):2032–8.

4. Huvos AG, Hutter RV, Berg JW. Significance of axillary macrometastases and micrometastases in mammary cancer. Ann Surg 1971;173(1):44–6.

5. Fisher B, Ravdin RG, Ausman RK, et al. Surgical adjuvant chemotherapy in cancer of the breast: results of a decade of cooperative investigation. Ann Surg 1968;168(3):337–56.

6. Edge SB, Byrd DR, Compton CC, et al, editors. AJCC cancer staging manual. 7th edition. New York: Springer; 2010.

7. Smith JA, Gamez-Araujo JJ, Gallager HS, et al. Carcinoma of the breast. Analysis of total lymph node involvement versus level of metastasis. Cancer 1977;39(2):527–32.

8. Fisher B, Bauer M, Wickerham DL, et al. Relation of number of positive axillary nodes to the prognosis of patients with primary breast cancer. An NSABP update. Cancer 1983;52(9):1551–7.

9. Kim T, Giuliano AE, Lyman GH. Lymphatic mapping and sentinel lymph node biopsy in early-stage breast carcinoma: a metaanalysis. Cancer 2006; 106(1):4–16.

10. Estourgie SH, Nieweg OE, Olmos RA, et al. Lymphatic drainage patterns from the breast. Ann Surg 2004;239(2):232–7.

11. Wilkinson EJ, Hause L. Probability in lymph node sectioning. Cancer 1974;33(5):1269–74.

12. Dowlatshahi K, Fan M, Snider HC, et al. Lymph node micrometastases from breast carcinoma: reviewing the dilemma. Cancer 1997;80(7):1188–97.

13. Liberman L. Pathologic analysis of sentinel lymph nodes in breast carcinoma. Cancer 2000;88(5):971–7.

14. Weaver DL, Ashikaga T, Krag DN, et al. Effect of occult metastases on survival in node-negative breast cancer. N Engl J Med 2011;364(5):412–21.

15. Giuliano AE, Hunt KK, Ballman KV. Axillary dissection vs no axillary dissection in women with invasive breast cancer and sentinel node metastasis: a randomized clinical trial. JAMA 2011;305:569–75.

16. Padmore RF, Fowble B, Hoffman J, et al. Microinvasive breast carcinoma: clinicopathologic analysis of a single institution experience. Cancer 2000;88(6): 1403–9.

17. Connolly JL. Changes and problematic areas in interpretation of the AJCC Cancer Staging Manual, 6th edition, for breast cancer. Arch Pathol Lab Med 2006;130(3):287–91.

18. Andea AA, Bouwman D, Wallis T, et al. Correlation of tumor volume and surface area with lymph node status in patients with multifocal/multicentric breast carcinoma. Cancer 2004;100(1):20–7.

19. Coombs NJ, Boyages J. Multifocal and multicentric breast cancer: does each focus matter? J Clin Oncol 2005;23(30):7497–502.

20. Andea AA, Wallis T, Newman LA, et al. Pathologic analysis of tumor size and lymph node status in multifocal/multicentric breast carcinoma. Cancer 2002;94(5):1383–90.

21. Lester SC. Multiple breast cancers raise multiple questions. Am J Onc Rev 2004;31–5.

22. Elston CW, Ellis IO. Pathological prognostic factors in breast cancer. I. The value of histological grade in breast cancer: experience from a large study with long-term follow-up. Histopathology 1991; 19(5):403–10.

23. Rakha EA, El-Sayed ME, Lee AH, et al. Prognostic significance of Nottingham histologic grade in invasive breast carcinoma. J Clin Oncol 2008;26(19): 3153–8.

24. Bloom HJ, Richardson WW. Histological grading and prognosis in breast cancer; a study of 1409 cases of which 359 have been followed for 15 years. Br J Cancer 1957;11(3):359–77.

25. Dalton LW, Page DL, Dupont WD. Histologic grading of breast carcinoma. A reproducibility study. Cancer 1994;73(11):2765–70.

26. Frierson HF Jr, Wolber RA, Berean KW, et al. Interobserver reproducibility of the Nottingham modification of the Bloom and Richardson histologic grading scheme for infiltrating ductal carcinoma. Am J Clin Pathol 1995;103(2):195–8.

27. Meyer JS, Alvarez C, Milikowski C, et al. Breast carcinoma malignancy grading by Bloom-Richardson system vs proliferation index: reproducibility of grade and advantages of proliferation index. Mod Pathol 2005;18(8):1067–78.

28. Longacre TA, Ennis M, Quenneville LA, et al. Interobserver agreement and reproducibility in classification of invasive breast carcinoma: an NCI breast

cancer family registry study. Mod Pathol 2006;19(2): 195–207.

29. Rosen PP, Groshen S, Kinne DW, et al. Factors influencing prognosis in node-negative breast carcinoma: analysis of 767 T1N0M0/T2N0M0 patients with long-term follow-up. J Clin Oncol 1993;11(11): 2090–100.

30. Paterakos M, Watkin WG, Edgerton SM, et al. Invasive micropapillary carcinoma of the breast: a prognostic study. Hum Pathol 1999;30(12):1459–63.

31. Carter MR, Hornick JL, Lester S, et al. Spindle cell (sarcomatoid) carcinoma of the breast: a clinicopathologic and immunohistochemical analysis of 29 cases. Am J Surg Pathol 2006;30(3):300–9.

32. Yamaguchi R, Horii R, Maeda I, et al. Clinicopathologic study of 53 metaplastic breast carcinomas: their elements and prognostic implications. Hum Pathol 2010;41(5):679–85.

33. Guth U, Moch H, Herberich L, et al. Noninflammatory breast carcinoma with skin involvement. Cancer 2004;100(3):470–8.

34. Gruber G, Ciriolo M, Altermatt HJ, et al. Prognosis of dermal lymphatic invasion with or without clinical signs of inflammatory breast cancer. Int J Cancer 2004;109(1):144–8.

35. Chang S, Parker SL, Pham T, et al. Inflammatory breast carcinoma incidence and survival: the surveillance, epidemiology, and end results program of the National Cancer Institute, 1975–1992. Cancer 1998;82(12):2366–72.

36. Yang R, Cheung MC, Hurley J, et al. A comprehensive evaluation of outcomes for inflammatory breast cancer. Breast Cancer Res Treat 2009;117(3): 631–41.

37. Bettelheim R, Penman HG, Thornton-Jones H, et al. Prognostic significance of peritumoral vascular invasion in breast cancer. Br J Cancer 1984;50(6): 771–7.

38. Rosen PP, Saigo PE, Braun DW, et al. Occult axillary lymph node metastases from breast cancers with intramammary lymphatic tumor emboli. Am J Surg Pathol 1982;6(7):639–41.

39. Lauria R, Perrone F, Carlomagno C, et al. The prognostic value of lymphatic and blood vessel invasion in operable breast cancer. Cancer 1995;76(10): 1772–8.

40. Davis BW, Gelber R, Goldhirsch A, et al. Prognostic significance of peritumoral vessel invasion in clinical trials of adjuvant therapy for breast cancer with axillary lymph node metastasis. Hum Pathol 1985; 16(12):1212–8.

41. Orbo A, Stalsberg H, Kunde D. Topographic criteria in the diagnosis of tumor emboli in intramammary lymphatics. Cancer 1990;66(5):972–7.

42. Pinder SE, Ellis IO, Galea M, et al. Pathological prognostic factors in breast cancer. III. Vascular invasion: relationship with recurrence and survival in a large study with long-term follow-up. Histopathology 1994;24(1):41–7.

43. Locker AP, Ellis IO, Morgan DA, et al. Factors influencing local recurrence after excision and radiotherapy for primary breast cancer. Br J Surg 1989; 76(9):890–4.

44. O'Rourke S, Galea MH, Morgan D, et al. Local recurrence after simple mastectomy. Br J Surg 1994; 81(3):386–9.

45. Kuru B, Camlibel M, Gulcelik MA, et al. Prognostic factors affecting survival and disease-free survival in lymph node-negative breast carcinomas. J Surg Oncol 2003;83(3):167–72.

46. Rosen PP. Tumor emboli in intramammary lymphatics in breast carcinoma: pathologic criteria for diagnosis and clinical significance. Pathol Annu 1983;18:215–32.

47. Dunnwald LK, Rossing MA, Li CI. Hormone receptor status, tumor characteristics, and prognosis: a prospective cohort of breast cancer patients. Breast Cancer Res 2007;9(1):R6.

48. Knight WA, Livingston RB, Gregory EJ, et al. Estrogen receptor as an independent prognostic factor for early recurrence in breast cancer. Cancer Res 1977;37(12):4669–71.

49. Clark GM, McGuire WL, Hubay CA, et al. Progesterone receptors as a prognostic factor in Stage II breast cancer. N Engl J Med 1983;309(22):1343–7.

50. Tinnemans JG, Beex LV, Wobbes T, et al. Steroid-hormone receptors in nonpalpable and more advanced stages of breast cancer. A contribution to the biology and natural history of carcinoma of the female breast. Cancer 1990;66(6):1165–7.

51. Fisher B, Redmond C, Fisher ER, et al. Relative worth of estrogen or progesterone receptor and pathologic characteristics of differentiation as indicators of prognosis in node negative breast cancer patients: findings from National Surgical Adjuvant Breast and Bowel Project Protocol B-06. J Clin Oncol 1988;6(7):1076–87.

52. Hammond ME, Hayes DF, Dowsett M, et al. American Society of Clinical Oncology/College of American Pathologists guideline recommendations for immunohistochemical testing of estrogen and progesterone receptors in breast cancer. Arch Pathol Lab Med 2010;134(6):907–22.

53. Slamon DJ, Clark GM, Wong SG, et al. Human breast cancer: correlation of relapse and survival with amplification of the HER-2/neu oncogene. Science 1987;235(4785):177–82.

54. Dabbs DJ, Klein ME, Mohsin SK, et al. High false-negative rate of HER2 quantitative reverse transcription polymerase chain reaction of the Oncotype DX test: an independent quality assurance study. J Clin Oncol 2011;29(32):4279–85.

55. Wolff AC, Hammond ME, Schwartz JN, et al. American Society of Clinical Oncology/College of

American Pathologists guideline recommendations for human epidermal growth factor receptor 2 testing in breast cancer. Arch Pathol Lab Med 2007;131(1):18–43.

56. Sahoo S, Lester SC. Pathology of breast carcinomas after neoadjuvant chemotherapy: an overview with recommendations on specimen processing and reporting. Arch Pathol Lab Med 2009;133(4):633–42.

57. Goldhirsch A, Wood WC, Gelber RD, et al. Progress and promise: highlights of the international expert consensus on the primary therapy of early breast cancer 2007. Ann Oncol 2007;18(7):1133–44.

58. Goldhirsch A, Ingle JN, Gelber RD, et al. Thresholds for therapies: highlights of the St Gallen International Expert Consensus on the primary therapy of early breast cancer 2009. Ann Oncol 2009;20(8):1319–29.

59. Galea MH, Blamey RW, Elston CE, et al. The Nottingham Prognostic Index in primary breast cancer. Breast Cancer Res Treat 1992;22(3):207–19.

60. Paik S, Shak S, Tang G, et al. A multigene assay to predict recurrence of tamoxifen-treated, node-negative breast cancer. N Engl J Med 2004;351(27):2817–26.

61. Mamounas EP, Tang G, Fisher B, et al. Association between the 21-gene recurrence score assay and risk of locoregional recurrence in node-negative, estrogen receptor–positive breast cancer: results from NSABP B-14 and NSABP B-20. J Clin Oncol 2010;28:1677–83.

62. Tang G, Shak S, Paik S, et al. Comparison of the prognostic and predictive utilities of the 21-gene Recurrence Score assay and Adjuvant! for women with node-negative, ER-positive breast cancer: results from NSABP B-14 and NSABP B-20. Breast Cancer Res Treat 2011;127(1):133–42.

63. Albain KS, Barlow WE, Shak S, et al. Prognostic and predictive value of the 21-gene recurrence score assay in postmenopausal women with node-positive, oestrogen-receptor-positive breast cancer on chemotherapy: a retrospective analysis of a randomised trial. Lancet Oncol 2010;11(1):55–65.

64. Sparano JA, Paik S. Development of the 21-gene assay and its application in clinical practice and clinical trials. J Clin Oncol 2008;26(5):721–8.

65. Acs G, Esposito NN, Kiluk J, et al. A mitotically active, cellular tumor stroma and/or inflammatory cells associated with tumor cells may contribute to intermediate or high Oncotype DX Recurrence Scores in low-grade invasive breast carcinomas. Mod Pathol 2012;25(4):556–66.

66. Cuzick J, Dowsett M, Pineda S, et al. Prognostic value of a combined estrogen receptor, progesterone receptor, Ki-67, and human epidermal growth factor receptor 2 immunohistochemical score and comparison with the Genomic Health recurrence score in early breast cancer. J Clin Oncol 2011;29(32):4273–8.

67. van de Vijver MJ, He YD, van't Veer LJ, et al. A gene-expression signature as a predictor of survival in breast cancer. N Engl J Med 2002;347(25):1999–2009.

68. Buyse M, Loi S, van't Veer L, et al. Validation and clinical utility of a 70-gene prognostic signature for women with node-negative breast cancer. J Natl Cancer Inst 2006;98(17):1183–92.

69. Cardoso F, van't Veer L, Rutgers E, et al. Clinical application of the 70-gene profile: the MINDACT trial. J Clin Oncol 2008;26(5):729–35.

70. Barker AD, Sigman CC, Kelloff GJ, et al. I-SPY 2: an adaptive breast cancer trial design in the setting of neoadjuvant chemotherapy. Clin Pharmacol Ther 2009;86(1):97–100.

71. Cristofanilli M, Budd GT, Ellis MJ, et al. Circulating tumor cells, disease progression, and survival in metastatic breast cancer. N Engl J Med 2004;351(8):781–91.

72. Hayes DF, Cristofanilli M, Budd GT, et al. Circulating tumor cells at each follow-up time point during therapy of metastatic breast cancer patients predict progression-free and overall survival. Clin Cancer Res 2006;12(14):4218–24.

73. Dawood S, Broglio K, Valero V, et al. Circulating tumor cells in metastatic breast cancer: from prognostic stratification to modification of the staging system? Cancer 2008;113(9):2422–30.

74. Budd GT, Cristofanilli M, Ellis MJ, et al. Circulating tumor cells versus imaging—predicting overall survival in metastatic breast cancer. Clin Cancer Res 2006;12:6403–9.

Index

Note: Page numbers of article titles are in **boldface** type.

A

Adenoid cystic carcinoma (ACC), 686
  differential diagnosis of, adenomyoepithelial
    adenosis, 690
     basal-type carcinoma, 689
     collagenous spherulosis, 691–693
     cribiform DCIS, 689–693
     cylindroma, 690–691, 693
     invasive ductal carcinoma, 689–691
     pleomorphic adenomyoepithelioma, 690
  grading system for, 688
  immunoprofile of, 688–689
  immunostaining for, 690
    p63, 688
  key features of, 689
  microscopic features of, epithelial and
    myoepithelial cell types in, 687–688
    growth patterns in, 686–687
    infiltrative pattern, 688, 690
    prognosis for, 692–693
Adenomyoepithelioma, 668–669
  differential diagnosis of, benign conditions,
    673, 675
    clear cell hidradenoma, 674–675
    invasive ductal carcinoma, 675–676
    malignant tumors, 675
  immunohistochemical staining of, myoepithelial
    markers, 671–673
  microscopic features of, chondroid matrix
    resembling pleomorphic adenoma, 671
    cytologic, 669–670
    lobulated variant of, 671–672
    multilobulated and papillay patterns, 669
    with sebaceous metaplasia, 671
Adenomyoepithelipoma, differential diagnosis of,
  677, 679–680
  with malignant progression, 676–680
    microscopic features of, 677–678
Angiolipoma, microscopic features of, cellular,
  646–647
    fibrin microthrombi, 645–646
    mixture of adipose tissue and small vessels,
     645–646
  pathologic features of, 645
  vs. angiosarcoma, 647
  vs. atypical lipomatous tumor, 647
  vs. hemangioma, 647
Angiosarcoma. See also *Radiation-associated*
  cutaneous angiosarcoma.

  differential diagnosis of, 656–657
  microscopic features of, 656–657
  pathologic features of, 656
  primary, 655–658
  prognosis for, 657–658
  radiation-associated, 652–655
  vs. radiation-associated angiosarcoma, 655
Apcrine DCIS, 531, 533–534
Atypical vascular lesion(s) (AVLs), 651–652

B

Biopsy site marking devices, reactions to, 582–583
Breast cancer, differentiation from other
  malignancies, 719–720
  incidence of, 719
Breast carcinoma, diagnostic immunohistochemistry
  for, 730–741
    CK7/CK20, 730–731
    for site of origin, 741
    GCDFP-15, 731–732, 734, 738, 740
    in carcinomas of breast origin, 730–732
    mucin glycogen antigens, 738
    napsin a, 733–734
    PAX8, 734, 737–738
    thyroid transcription factor, 733
    WT-1, 734–735, 737
  differential diagnosis of, endometrium, 738–739
    lung, 732–734
    mammaglobin, 731–732, 734, 738
    melanoma, 738–739
    ovary, 734–738
    skin adnexa, 739–741
    stomach, 738, 740

C

Clear cell variants of DCIS, glycogen-rich, 530
  histiocytoid, 531–532
  lipid-rich, 530–531
  secretory, 531
  signet ring cell, 531–532
Clinging carcinoma, 531, 536–537
Collagenous spherulosis, immunostaining in, 665
  microscopic features of, 665–666
  vs. adenoid cystic carcinoma, 666–668
  vs. cribiform DCIS, 665–667
Cystic hypersecretory DCIS, 531, 534–535

Surgical Pathology 5 (2012) 787–791
http://dx.doi.org/10.1016/S1875-9181(12)00134-1
1875-9181/12/$ – see front matter © 2012 Elsevier Inc. All rights reserved

Moving?

Make sure your subscription moves with you!

To notify us of your new address, find your **Clinics Account Number** (located on your mailing label above your name), and contact customer service at:

Email: journalscustomerservice-usa@elsevier.com

800-654-2452 (subscribers in the U.S. & Canada)
314-447-8871 (subscribers outside of the U.S. & Canada)

Fax number: 314-447-8029

**Elsevier Health Sciences Division
Subscription Customer Service
3251 Riverport Lane
Maryland Heights, MO 63043**

ELSEVIER